INSTRUCTIONAL COURSES
Volume 4, 1991

Plastic Surgery Educational Foundation

INSTRUCTIONAL COURSES

Edited by
Robert C. Russell, M.D.   **Volume 4, 1991**

Professor of Surgery
Division of Plastic and Reconstructive Surgery
Southern Illinois University School of Medicine
Springfield, Illinois

with 404 illustrations

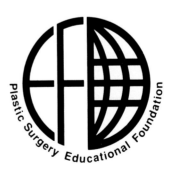

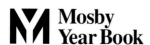 **Mosby**
Year Book

St. Louis   Baltimore   Boston   Chicago   London   Philadelphia   Sydney   Toronto

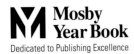
Mosby
Year Book
Dedicated to Publishing Excellence

Editor: Anne S. Patterson
Assistant Editor: Maura K. Leib
Project Manager: Carol Sullivan Wiseman
Production Editor: Lisa D. Cohen
Designer: Liz Fett

CL/MV 9 8 7 6 5 4 3 2 1

CONTRIBUTORS

Joseph R. Barnthouse, M.D.
Fellow, Reconstructive Surgery Foundation
Atlanta, Georgia

G. Kristine Bennett, M.D.
Atlanta Plastic Surgery, PA
Atlanta, Georgia

H. Hollis Caffee, M.D., F.A.C.S.
Professor of Surgery
University of Florida College of Medicine
Gainesville, Florida

Bruce F. Connell, M.D.
Clinical Professor of Surgery (Plastic)
University of California
Irvine, California

Elof Eriksson. M.D.
Professor of Plastic Surgery
Harvard University School of Medicine;
Chief, Division of Plastic Surgery
Brigham and Women's Hospital
Boston, Massachusetts

Jack Fisher, M.D., F.A.C.S.
Assistant Clinical Professor
Department of Plastic Surgery
Vanderbilt University;
The Institute for Aesthetic and Reconstructive Surgery
Baptist Hospital
Nashville, Tennessee

Lawrence J. Gottlieb, M.D.
Assistant Professor of Surgery
Department of Plastic and Reconstructive Surgery
University of Chicago School of Medicine
Chicago, Illinois

Jeffrey P. Groner, M.D.
Assistant Professor
Department of Plastic and Reconstructive Surgery
Washington University School of Medicine
St. Louis, Missouri

José Guerrerosantos, M.D., F.A.C.S.
Medical Director and Founder
Jalisco Institute for Reconstructive and Plastic Surgery;
Professor and Chairman
Division of Plastic and Reconstructive Surgery
Medical and Graduate Schools
University of Guadalajara
Guadalajara, Mexico

Carl R. Hartrampf, Jr., M.D.
Associate Professor
Department of Surgery
Division of Plastic Surgery
Emory University;
Atlanta Plastic Surgery, PA
Atlanta, Georgia

Neil Ford Jones, M.D.
Associate Professor of Plastic and Hand Surgery
University of Pittsburgh School of Medicine
Pittsburgh, Pennsylvania

Eric P. Kindwall, M.D.
Associate Professor
Department of Plastic and Reconstructive Surgery
Medical College of Wisconsin
Milwaukee, Wisconsin

Vasilios S. Lambros, M.D.
Clinical Instructor of Surgery
University of California
Irvine, California

Paul Y. Liu, M.D.
Clinical/Research Fellow in Surgery
Harvard University School of Medicine;
Division of Plastic Surgery
Brigham and Women's Hospital
Boston, Massachusetts

Timothy J. Marten, M.D.
Department of Plastic Surgery
St. Mary's Hospital and Medical Center;
Director In Chief, Sutter Street Plastic Surgery Center
San Francisco, California

Hani S. Matloub, M.D.
Associate Professor
Department of Plastic and Reconstructive Surgery
Medical College of Wisconsin
Milwaukee, Wisconsin

Thomas A. Mustoe, M.D.
Associate Professor
Department of Plastic and Reconstructive Surgery
Washington University School of Medicine
St. Louis, Missouri

David Netscher, M.D.
Assistant Professor
Division of Plastic Surgery
Baylor College of Medicine
Houston, Texas

Jeffrey C. Posnick, D.M.D., M.D., F.R.S.C.S.(C), F.A.C.S.
Medical Director, Craniofacial Program
Division of Plastic Surgery
The Hospital for Sick Children
Assistant Professor, Faculty of Medicine
Associate Professor, Faculty of Dentistry
University of Toronto
Toronto, Ontario, Canada

Kenneth E. Salyer, M.D., F.A.C.S., F.A.A.P., F.I.C.S.
Director, Founding Chairman
International Craniofacial Institute
Humana Advanced Surgical Institutes
Dallas, Texas

Melvin Spira, M.D.
Professor of Plastic Surgery
Division of Plastic Surgery
Baylor College of Medicine
Houston, Texas

Samuel Stal, M.D.
Associate Professor
Division of Plastic Surgery
Baylor College of Medicine
Houston, Texas

Linton A. Whitaker, M.D.
Professor of Surgery (Plastic)
University of Pennsylvania
School of Medicine;
Chief of Plastic Surgery
Hospital of the University of Pennsylvania
Philadelphia, Pennsylvania

Vernon Leroy Young, M.D.
Professor of Surgery (Plastic and Reconstructive)
Department of Surgery
Division of Plastic Surgery
Washington University School of Medicine;
Plastic Surgeon in Chief
Barnes West County Hospital;
Attending Surgeon
Barnes, St. Louis Children's, and St. Louis
Regional Hospitals
St. Louis, Missouri

M. John Yousif, M.D.
Assistant Professor
Department of Plastic and Reconstructive Surgery
Medical College of Wisconsin
Milwaukee, Wisconsin

PREFACE

For the past 3 years I have had the pleasure of serving as chairman of the Instructional Course Committee for the Plastic Surgery Educational Foundation (PSEF). The fourth volume of the Instructional Courses, published by Mosby—Year Book in conjunction with the PSEF, marks the end of my term as committee chairman and editor of this yearly publication. I have enjoyed a close association with the staff of ASPRS in the central office in Chicago and the challenge of planning the Instructional Course program for the annual meeting. I am sure the 1991 Instructional Course Committee headed by Riley Rees, M.D., will continue the tradition of selecting the most knowledgeable experts in our field as instructors for future Instructional Course programs. The Instructional Course format for the 1990 meeting, which included 1-, 2-, and 3-hour courses was well received by the membership and will be continued in the 1991 courses offered in Seattle. The Committee evaluated each of last year's couses, deleted some, and added new and exciting educational opportunities for us at the 1991 meeting. As our specialty expands and the areas of interest broaden, I am sure the Committee will continue to bring you the most up-to-date and thought-provoking courses, which should provide a wealth of information and material for future Instructional Course volumes. The courses selected for publication cover a wide spectrum of plastic surgery subspecialties and follow two broad categories: aesthetic and reconstructive plastic surgery.

It is an honor to be asked to give an Instructional Course at the annual meeting and even more so to be chosen to contribute to this text. The faculty members who voluntarily contribute their time and effort to each chapter are noted experts on the topics presented. This text is intended to be a concise summary of a given topic. Each Instructional Course volume offers the reader an in-depth look "in the mind's eye" of a noted expert and describes the specifics of how the experts get the best results from a certain procedure or technique. This text is not intended to take the place of conventional textbooks or the actual Instructional Courses themselves; however, the entire series offers the reader an excellent reference source for his or her personal library.

I would like to thank the authors who contributed to Instructional Courses volume 4 for their time and energy in producing their chapters and for sharing their expertise with us. I also wish to thank the Instructional Course Committee for 1991, who are listed below, for making the evaluation and selection process of the Instructional Courses for the 1991 annual meeting a success. I also wish to extend my thanks to Kim Restivo from the ASPRS-PSEF's central office in Chicago and the editorial staff of Mosby—Year Book for making this text possible.

Editing a textbook a year for the last 3 years has been arduous and, at times, both a learning and frustrating experience for me. I have enjoyed the opportunity to become more acquainted with many of the authors who have contributed chapters to the Instructional Course series over the last 3 years and have in the process of editing expanded my own knowledge. Our strength as a specialty is founded on research, education and training, and the highest standards of patient care. We must continue our pursuit of excellence in all of these areas if we are to maintain and extend our position as the world's premier organization of plastic and reconstructive surgeons. The Instructional Courses provided by our members at the annual meeting and the Instructional Course volume series is one part of the continuing medical educational experience that ultimately results in improved patient care. I hope you will join me in supporting our national organizations, continuing your own medical education with publications like this one, and attending our meetings.

Robert C. Russell, M.D.

CONTENTS

INSTRUCTIONAL COURSES
Volume 4, 1991

PART ONE

AESTHETIC SURGERY

CHAPTER 1

Capsule Contracture: Etiology, Prevention, and Treatment

H. Hollis Caffee

The use of breast implants for either reconstructive surgery or breast augmentation is in general a highly successful endeavor with good patient and surgeon satisfaction. However, every implant results in the formation of a scar capsule, and, if that capsule contracts, it will result in hardening and deformation of the breast.

The majority of implant patients are satisfied with the result of their surgery, including many who have some degree of contracture. However, of the few who are not entirely satisfied, there may be various reasons that may or may not include contracture. Very few patients will have contracture severe enough to cause pain or to produce enough visible deformity to create embarrassment. Seldom does a patient have enough symptoms from contracture to request that the implants be removed.

ASSESSMENT OF CONTRACTURE
Definition

Most clinical practitioners would agree that a firm breast after implant surgery sufficiently defines capsule contracture. However, to evaluate or conduct research on this problem requires a more precise definition. The capsule is a scar, and the problem is that scars tend to contract. In the case of a linear scar, contraction results in a decrease in length. Implant capsules are sheets of scar tissue and are therefore two dimensional. Contraction of an implant capsule results in a decrease in surface area. Capsule contracture is the most common cause of a firm breast, but other potential causes include infection, hematoma, fibrosis, tumor, or a hard implant.

Diagnosis

Ordinarily the diagnosis of contracture is easily made and only requires palpation to detect a lack of implant compressibility. It is not difficult to differentiate capsule contracture from other causes of a firm breast. The hand used to palpate should compress the implant, pinching its center until the two sides of the elastomer shell are within 1 centimeter of each other. The degree of compression achieved can be difficult to discern if there is a thick layer of tissue over the implant. Polyurethane-covered implants are less compressible than other types because of a more heavily cross-linked-silicone gel.

The problem in contracture diagnosis is not so much in detection as it is in the subjective nature of the examination through which it is usually determined. Because one surgeon might report a frequency of contracture vastly different from that of another surgeon who has examined the same group of patients, there is often confusion in reporting results. In 1981 Burkhardt et al reported a reduction in the incidence of contracture from 37% to 3% with the use of antibiotics.[7] This paper was criticized for its methodology, and to their credit, the authors repeated this study, using both objective criteria and "blind" examiners. In the second study, contracture was reduced from 41% to 19%.[6] This study demonstrated that for conclusions to be significant, it is essential to have some method of eliminating bias in reporting breast implant results.

There are two methods for eliminating bias in contracture studies. Either patients in clinical studies must be evaluated by a neutral examiner who is not aware of the method or variation that was used in a given study or objective measurement must be used.

Measurement

Objective measurements are important not only in the control of bias but also in the quantitation of contracture. Capsule contracture is not an all or none phenomenon, and therefore papers reporting a particular

3

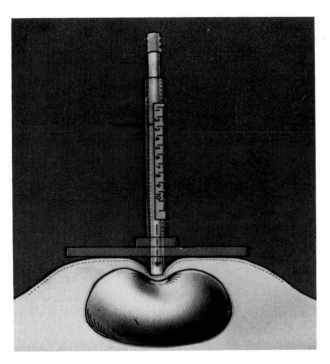

Fig. 1-1 One type of indentation tonometer uses a steel rod inside a plexiglass tube with a flange on the bottom. The weight of the rod pushes into the breast and then into the implant and capsule. The tube is lowered until the flange touches the surface of the breast on all sides. The depth of indentation is proportioned to the softness of the breast, capsule, and implant.

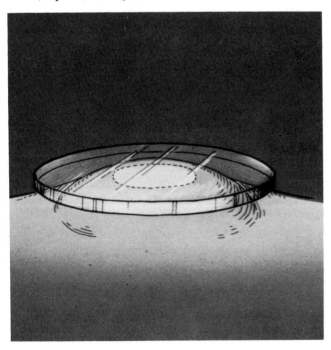

Fig. 1-2 Moore's applanation tonometer is a simple plexiglass disk. The weight of the disk will produce a flattened area. The size of the flattened area is proportional to the softness of the breast.

percentage of contracted implant capsules are not significant. Baker was the first to emphasize this point, and his grading system has become a classic.[3] However, actual measurements are much more useful than classifications, since they allow comparison of groups of implants by statistical analysis.

Standard method

Several methods for measuring capsule contracture have been proposed; most of which involve measurement of deformability, or softness. Usually a standard force is applied, and the degree of deformation is measured. There have been three basic types of devices for measuring softness. Indentation tonometers push straight into the implant and measure the depth of the dent[9,17,19] (Fig. 1-1). Applanation tonometers use a flat weight (normally a clear plastic disk) and measure the area of flattening[22] (Fig. 1-2). Calipers may be used to compress the implant between two tines, and the distance remaining is measured.[8]

All of the instruments for measuring deformability are subject to error. Minor differences in instrument positioning relative to the implant can influence the result. All of the instruments will produce more deformation of the overlying tissue than the implant. This is particularly true of applanation tonometers, which are reliable only in thin patients or animals. Deformation devices are much more reliable in laboratory studies where the implant capsule can be measured directly on a bench without overlying tissue.

Contracture methods
Capsule measurements

Another approach to diagnosis and measurement of contracture relates to the definition of contracture proposed earlier. As a capsule contracts, its surface area decreases. Theoretically, this could continue until the capsule becomes a sphere, since liquids are noncompressible, and a sphere has the smallest possible surface area for a given volume. In practice this never happens because implants tend to fold into fusiform shapes as they are compressed. Most implants are in the form of ellipsoids, although some high-profile implants might be classified somewhere between a cone and a hemisphere. Regardless of design, if the implant is viewed in profile, it has two readily measured dimensions: height and diameter. Typically diameter is about five times greater than height. As a capsule contracts, implant diameter decreases and height increases. In the laboratory the implant can be removed with its capsule intact and these quantities measured directly with the encapsulated implant on a flat surface. In the clinical setting the measurements can be obtained mammographically, using a cross table lateral view (Fig. 1-3).

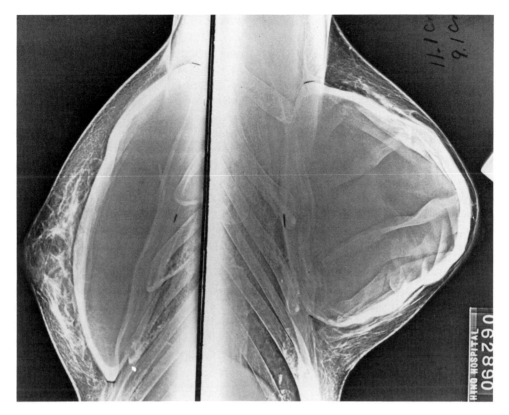

Fig. 1-3 A cross-table-lateral view of the breast is obtained with xeromammography. On the left is a soft (grade I) breast. The transverse diameter-to-height ratio is the same as that of the implant. A ruler is placed in the plane of the center of the implant to correct for projection magnification. On the right is a grade IV contracture, and the implant is identical to the one on the left. Note the decrease in transverse diameter and increase in height. The resulting decrease in the ratio is proportional to and therefore a good quantitative objective measurement of capsule contracture.

Ordinary mammograms are obtained with the patient upright and the breast compressed. For capsule measurement the patient must be in a supine-oblique position so that the breast points straight up. A ruler should be placed in the plane of the center of the breast to calculate projection error. The surgeon knows the dimensions of the implant before placement so that any decrease in diameter or increase in height would represent contracture. Even if implant dimensions are not known, the method can be used to compare one implant with another of the same design and to document changes in measurements over time or after treatment simply by calculating a ratio of diameter to height.[29]

The advantage of the mammographic measurement of capsules is that it measures deformation rather than deformability. It is not necessary to push through overlying tissue to deform the implant. However, there are some disadvantages. If an implant contracts asymmetrically, the diameter measurement will be greatly influenced by the viewing angle. This only becomes a factor in severe contractures. Submuscular implants, particularly in early stages, tend to be flattened by the tension of the muscle. This can result in a diameter-to-height ratio greater than before implantation.

Pressure measurements

Pressure measurement is an entirely different approach to contracture assessment. The relationship between contracture and intracapsular pressure is not linear and is influenced by the relationship of volume-to-surface area and, to a lesser extent, by compliance of the capsule and possibly the weight of overlying tissue or skin tension. Minor degrees of contracture will produce almost no change in pressure, making pressure measurements insensitive to the soft end of the spectrum. At the hard end of the spectrum, a very small increase in contracture will result in a huge increase in pressure, making the method too sensitive. This nonlinearity tends to exaggerate differences in capsules and make a trivial difference appear clinically significant. A variation of this technique is to inject additional volume into the implant and measure the resulting change in pressure. This tends to increase sensitivity, which can be helpful at the soft end but aggravates the excessive sensitivity at the hard end of the spectrum.

The biggest problem with pressure measurements is that normally they are invasive techniques. This is not much of a problem with expander-type implants, but it becomes a major problem for other types of implants. Currently, an internal pressure transducer, which can be interrogated by radio, is being developed but do not expect these to be available soon.

Measurements of capsule thickness have been used as a criterion of contracture in some reports. This method is not valid, since there is no direct relationship between capsule thickness and contracture.

These complex measurement systems should be of interest to clinical surgeons if they wish to understand the significance and reliability of reports of new techniques or implant designs. They are essential to any surgeon who wishes to report his results to others and be taken seriously.

CAUSES OF CAPSULE CONTRACTURE

The mechanism by which scar tissue contracts is believed to be through the interaction of actin and myosin. These proteins are normal components of muscle but are also found in myofibroblasts.[15] Myofibroblasts are known to be present in implant capsules and are believed to provide the force required for contraction.[16] However, identification of the responsible cell still does not explain why one capsule contracts and another does not. It is possible that contracture of scar capsules is purely a random event and merely represents part of the normal spectrum of healing. However, several potential stimulating influences have been proposed as contributing factors and include the following:

1. Irritants resulting in inflammatory or "foreign body reactions."
2. Silicone bleed.
3. Bacteria.
4. Hematoma.

The term *foreign body reaction* usually refers to histologic observations of white cell infiltrates, macrophages, and in the most severe cases, exudate and necrosis. The concept of foreign body reaction is difficult to relate to capsule contracture. As a foreign body itself, a smooth silicone elastomer produces minimal inflammatory reaction. The polyurethane-foam-covered implants produce the greatest degree of foreign body reaction and yet are believed to have the greatest resistance to contracture.

Implants are known to attract dust particles, and package inserts warn to avoid contact with paper or cloth and to remove all starch powder from gloves before handling implants. However, there is no evidence that particulate contamination has any effect on capsule contracture.

Sclerosing agents such as sodium tetradecyl can stimulate capsule contracture in experiments with laboratory animals. This observation is relevant only in experimental work where a contracture model is desired but has no relevance to clinical events.

The phenomenon of *silicone bleed* was recognized long ago but only recently has its significance been generally acknowledged. Many surgeons have suggested that saline-filled implants were less prone to contracture, however, it was not until Asplund's study[2] that reliable evidence was available. It would be difficult to account for the difference in contracture with gel-filled implants and saline-filled implants without invoking gel bleed. It has also been shown experimentally that low-bleed-gel implants have fewer contractures than high-bleed-gel implants, although they do not eliminate contracture.[10] The fact that contracture still occurs with saline-filled implants and low-bleed implants suggests that silicone bleed cannot be the only explanation for the contracture problem.

Whether the reduction in gel bleed provided by the newer implant designs is as effective as saline-filled implants in reducing contracture and in reducing the microscopic particles of silicone found in the capsule is unknown. Saline-filled implants are not entirely free of particles in their capsules, since the elastomer apparently sheds some of this material.

Manufacturers disagree as to how much reduction in gel bleed is required to qualify for the term *low bleed.* They also disagree as how to best measure gel bleed.

Contradicting reports have perpetuated the debate over the role of bacteria in capsule contraction. Dubin, who first suggested the theory, reported a high incidence of positive cultures at the time of open capsulotomy.[14] He suggested the use of an antibiotic irrigation to prevent contracture. Burkhardt et al produced a convincing randomized trial with blind evaluation and caliper measurements,[6] and concluded that antibiotic or antiseptic irrigations effectively reduced contractures occurring within the first 3 months. Regardless of whether the conclusions of this study are reliable, there is still no explanation for the large number of contractures that appear later than 3 months postoperatively.

An observation that challenges the bacterial theory is that systemic antibiotics can reduce the frequency of positive cultures yet do not appear to influence contracture. Although positive cultures are reported to occur frequently in breast wounds (usually growing staphylococcus epidermitis), it is well known from the surgical-infection literature that a minimum quantity of bacteria are required to produce an infection, but a single organism can produce a positive culture. Unpublished data on quantitative bacteriology of breast tissue suggests that bacteria are often present in breast tissue but only in minuscule quantities.

Currently, there is doubt as to whether bacteria have any role in the contracture phenomenon. However, the risk of systemic or local antibiotic therapy is small enough that either or both would reasonably be part of the routine.

Evidence that hematomas stimulate capsule contraction is quite weak. The hypothesis is attractive because it would be consistent with the random nature of the problem and the fact that relatively small collections of blood occur frequently. However, anecdotal reports have provided the only accounts suggesting that hematomas have a role in stimulating capsule contraction. In animal studies it was not possible to increase the contracture incidence or severity, even with large hematomas.[11]

PREVENTION OF CAPSULE CONTRACTURE

There are two logical approaches to prevent capsule contracture. The first and most obvious is to avoid known stimulants of contraction. The only acknowledged stimulant is gel bleed, and the use of saline or low-bleed gel-filled implants has been shown to reduce but not eliminate contracture. Even if bacteria are not a factor in producing contracture, it is hard to argue against the use of antibiotics and antiseptic irrigation. There can be no arguement against good hemostasis.

Another approach is perhaps more fatalistic because it implies that capsules naturally want to contract and that the clinical role is to actively try to stop them. The concept is therefore to take steps to influence wound healing. Several measures believed to influence healing at the implant-capsule interface include the following:

1. Drugs that modify healing.
2. Physical measures.
3. Implant surface design changes.
4. Implant tissue environment (submuscular vs. retromammary).

Drugs

Of the drugs that apparently modify wound healing, steroids are by far the most potent. Steroids were first applied to this problem by placing triamcinolone in the implant pocket at the time of augmentation.[28] Steroids used in this manner have never been shown to be effective because the drug is almost certainly gone before the contraction process begins. Intraprosthetic

methylprednisolone was later suggested to help overcome the short duration of action.[27] Intraprosthetic administration proved effective but also dangerous because many cases of atrophy, implant ptosis, and even extrusion were reported.[13,26] These difficulties can be greatly reduced by keeping the concentration of methylprednisolone below 20mg/100ml, using a gel-saline implant, and placing the implant submuscularly. Contractures can still occur when using steroids, and the necessity of using more complex (and expensive) implants and the dangers of the drug remaining in the implant too long have prevented universal acceptance of this approach. The ideal method of steroid use would be to administer the drug for 3 to 4 weeks after surgery in a form that would persist no longer than a few weeks. This method should be possible in the near future.

Other drugs believed to influence scarring include nonsteroidal-anti-inflammatory agents and vitamin E.[12] Each has some experimental evidence that suggests a beneficial effect, yet the degree of these effects are minor enough to render any clinical effect insignificant.

Physical measures

Physical measures intended to modify capsule contraction fall into two categories. The concept that the implant pocket be overly large and the implant moved about as the capsule forms to maintain this space seems superficially plausible but has never garnered any scientific support. Implant compression exercises to stretch the capsule as it forms is a related concept with the same principle involved in dynamic splinting of hands or in dilating strictures of hollow organs. The stretching of implant capsules has considerable theoretical merit based on what is known about other types of scars but has never been proved effective in implant patients. Patient compliance would be a major limiting factor.

Implant surface design changes

Implant surface modifications are available in two fundamentally different forms. The original breast implant was and still is a smooth silicone elastomer. Thin sheets of polyurethane foam have been added to the surface of implants using an adhesive.[1] Polyurethane-foam-covered implants are generally believed to be resistant to capsule contracture. It has been shown that the polyurethane foam alters the healing response with a much greater degree of inflammatory response, macrophages, and multinucleated giant cells. Exactly how these effects interfere with capsule contraction is not clear, but one hypothesis has been that the resulting collagen is distributed more randomly, and therefore the contracting forces tend to nullify each other rather than acting in concert.[5]

Despite numerous favorable reports supporting the suggestion that polyurethane foam interferes with capsule contraction, these implants have not gained overwhelming acceptance. The disadvantages of polyurethane include rashes, degradation, and aesthetic limitations. About one fourth of implant patients will experience an erythematous rash over the implants. The rash is self-limited, and its primary medical significance is that it might be confused with infection. Antihistamines have been recommended, based on the assumption that the rash is an allergic reaction. However, it is more likely that the rash is merely an inflammatory reaction and one component of a fairly dramatic foreign body response to the polyurethane material.

There have been some indications that the polyurethane foam may undergo hydrolysis. Reports have been inconsistent and largely based on the condition of implants removed for various problems such as contracture or infection.[18] Nevertheless, there have been reported cases in which polyurethane foam had apparently disappeared to some extent. If polyurethane is biodegradable, the longevity of the result and the metabolic fate and effects of the products of hydrolysis would be questioned.

The aesthetic problems with polyurethane-covered implants include firmness and wrinkles. Although the polyurethane-foam covering seems to resist capsule contracture, it does induce a significant fibrosis, causing some induration. In addition, the gel used in foam-covered implants is more heavily cross-linked, making the implant firmer than implants of other types. Therefore the best result obtained with polyurethane will never be as soft as a good result with a smooth-silicone gel or saline-filled implant. The problem of wrinkles results from adherence of the implant to the capsule. These wrinkles are typically vertically oriented in the upper half of the breast and most apparent when the patient leans forward. The wrinkle problem is more often seen in mature women with loose skin from postpartum atrophy or weight loss.

Concerns about some of the undesirable characteristics of polyurethane have led to the most recent development, the introduction of textured silicone. The new textured implants are based on the assumption that it is the physical structure of polyurethane rather than its chemical properties that explains the resistance to capsule contracture. However, it must be recognized that none of the several textured silicones currently available comes close to duplicating the physical properties of polyurethane. Polyurethane is used as an open-cell foam, whereas the textured silicones are provided with either projections or excavations that appear to merely roughen the surface in some types of implants or provide orderly rows of projections in others. Apparently, an open-cell foam of silicone would be too fragile to be practical. Open-cell foams of other polymers can be made (e.g., expanded polytetrafluroethylene (PTFE) but are too expensive to be of interest to the industry.

It is too early to know what effect these new textured implants will have in the clinical setting. The available data from experiments on laboratory animals are discouraging, but it is unlikely that the appropriate animal model has been found. Early clinical reports, although enthusiastic, are uncontrolled and without appropriate measures to control bias. There is a prospective, randomized, controlled study underway with one type of textured implant, but the results are not yet available. Early indications suggest that textured implants are not as bad as the laboratory animal experiments might have suggested, but neither do they appear to have any marked advantage.

Implant tissue environment

Placing implants behind the chest muscles is another measure believed to modify the host response to implants. Submuscular placement was originally beneath the pectoralis major but was later modified to include the serratus anterior.

The only situation in which the advantage of a muscle cover has been clearly established has been in mastectomy patients. For some reason, an implant under a skin flap is much more likely (some would say guaranteed) to develop capsule contracture than one behind a breast gland or behind muscle. The reasons for this are unclear, but one possibility is a difference in blood supply. Another possible explanation is that the muscle contraction compresses and therefore stretches the capsule. The advantage of a muscle cover over a glandular cover is not well established. The best controlled series advocating intraprosthetic steroids had submuscular implants as its control group. A substantial incidence of contracture was observed in the control group, suggesting minimal benefit from muscle coverage alone.[30] There are a number of disadvantages to submuscular implant placement in augmentation mammoplasty. It is difficult to dissect a submuscular pocket with local anesthesia. The early results are not as good with an undesirable convexity of the upper half of the breast and a relative lack of projection. The shape gradually improves as the muscle accommodates to the presence of the implant, but this takes several months. Vigorous contraction of the pectoralis muscles produces a gross distortion of the implants, but this does not occur with normal activities and is only occasionally a source of patient dissatisfaction. It is more difficult to get precise placement of the inframammary fold, but this can be overcome with experience.

The advantages of submuscular placement are a greater ease in concealing the implant in thin patients with very small breasts, and the fact that muscle coverage appears to enhance the safety of using intraprosthetic steroids.

TREATMENT OF ESTABLISHED CAPSULE CONTRACTURE

Presently, standard practice includes two possibilities for treating capsule contracture. These are open capsulotomy and closed capsulotomy. Closed capsulotomy was discovered accidently[4], and, when first reported, it was well received as an easy alternative to open capsulotomy. Closed capsulotomy, however, was quickly followed by disillusionment when reports of ruptured implants began to appear. Two large series on the complications of closed capsulotomy have been reported. Little and Baker reported 544 closed capsulotomies in 243 patients from a single practice.[20] They reported no implant ruptures and only three hematomas. However, their contractive recurrence rate was 30% in 1 year. Nelson reported a survey of 30,000 closed capsulotomies and 5,579 open capsulotomies by surgeons from all over North America.[24,25] The complication rate in these two groups was 9.97% and 6.24% respectively and included not only patient and implant injuries, but injuries to the surgeon's hands.

The other problem with closed capsulotomy has been recurrent contracture, which has been reported to exceed 50% and appears to increase with each successive closed release so that a fourth release is probably futile.[23]

If open capsulotomy is elected, it seems only logical to take some measure to reduce the risk of recurrence. Three possibilities will be discussed.

If a smooth implant was used in the first procedure, it can be replaced with a polyurethane-foam-covered implant.[21] If this choice is elected, the implant should be placed in contact with fresh tissue. In the case of retromammary implants, this is best accomplished with a capsulectomy. If the implant was submuscular, it can simply be moved to a retromammary position.

Another option is to use a double lumen implant with methylprednisolone in the outer lumen. Steroids are safer if the implant is moved to a submuscular position. A concentration that is both safe and effective has not been clearly established, but most of the problems reported with steroids have had methylprednisolone concentrations in excess of 20mg/100ml.

A third option would be to use temporary overexpansion, which is accomplished by replacing the implant with one of the permanent expanders. The expander is then left overinflated for a period of months and then deflated to the desired volume. The theory behind this method is that the capsule is splinted at a larger surface area until the contractile period ends. One problem is that no one knows when and if the contractile period ends. The other obvious problem is patient acceptance.

The problem of capsule contracture deserves our continued attention. None of the proposed explanations has been entirely satisfactory, and none of the preventive or therapeutic measures for this problem has been entirely effective. Capsule contraction is just one form of scar contraction and may provide us with a superb model for the study of this universal mamallian phenomenon. It is likely that the problem may be multifactorial and will be improved by advances in several of the areas mentioned.

REFERENCES

1. Ashley FL: A new type of breast prosthesis, Plast Reconstr Surg 45:421, 1970.
2. Asplund O: Capsule contracture in silicone gel and saline-filled breast implants after reconstruction, Plast Reconstr Surg 73:270, 1984.
3. Baker JL: Augmentation mammaplasty. In Owsley JQ and Peterson RA (eds): Symposium on aesthetic surgery of the breast, St. Louis, 1978, The CV Mosby Co.
4. Baker JL, Bartels RJ, and Douglas WM: Closed compression technique for rupturing a contracted capsule around a breast implant, Plast Reconstr Surg 58:137, 1976.
5. Brand KG: Polyurethane-coated silicone implants and the question of capsular contracture, Plast Reconstr Surg 73:498, 1984.
6. Burkhardt BR et al: A prospective study of the effect of local antibacterial agents, Plast Reconstr Surg 77:919, 1986.
7. Burkhardt BR et al: Capsules, infection, and intraluminal antibiotics, Plast Reconstr Surg 68:43, 1981.
8. Burkhardt BR et al: Objective clinical assessment of fibrous capsular contracture, Plast Reconstr Surg 69:794, 1982.
9. Caffee HH: External compression for the prevention of scar capsule contracture—a preliminary report, Ann Plast Surg 8:453, 1982.
10. Caffee HH: The influence of silicone bleed on capsule contracture. Ann Plast Surg 17:284, 1986.
11. Caffee HH: The effects of hematoma on implant capsules, Ann Plast Surg, 16:102, 1986.
12. Caffee HH: Vitamin E and capsule contracture, Ann Plast Surg 19:512, 1987.
13. Carrico TJ and Cohen IK: Capsular contracture and steroid-related complications after augmentation mammoplasty: a preliminary study, Plast Reconstr Surg 64:377, 1979.
14. Dubin DB: The etiology, pathophysiology, predictability, and early detection of spherical scar contracture of the breast: a detailed explanation and protocol for prevention of spherical scar contracture of the breast. Proceedings of 13th annual meeting of the American Society of Aesthetic Plastic Surgery, 1980.
15. Gabbiani G, Ryan GB, and Majno G: Presence of modified fibroblasts in granulation tissue and their possible role in wound contraction, Experimentation 27:549, 1971.
16. Guber S and Rudolph R: The myofibroblast, Surg Gynecol Obstet 146:641, 1978.
17. Hayes H and McLeod P: Indentation tonometry of breasts, Plast Reconstr Surg 63:13, 1979.

18. Jabaley ME: Late breast pain following reconstruction with polyurethane-covered implants, Plast Reconstr Surg 78:390, 1986.

19. Ksander GA, Vistnes LM, and Fogarty D: Experimental effects on surrounding fibrous capsule formation from placing steroid in a silicone bag-gel prosthesis before implantation, Plast Reconstr Surg 62:873, 1978.

20. Little G and Baker JL: Result of closed compression capsulotomy for treatment of contracted breast implant capsules, Plast Reconstr Surg 65:30, 1980.

21. Melmed EP: Treatment of breast contractures with open capsulotomy and replacement of gel prostheses with polyurethane-covered implants, Plast Reconstr Surg 86:270, 1990.

22. Moore JR: Applanation tonometry of breasts, Plast Reconstr Surg 63:9, 1979.

23. Moufarrege et al: Outcome of mammary capsulotomies, Ann Plast Surg 19:62, 1987.

24. Nelson GD: Complications of closed compression after augmentation mammaplasty, Plast Reconstr Surg 66:71, 1980.

25. Nelson GD: Complications from the treatment of fibrous capsular contracture of the breast, Plast Reconstr Surg 68:969, 1981.

26. O'Neal RM and Argenta LC: Late side effects related to inflatable breast prostheses containing soluble steroids, Plast Reconstr Surg 69:641, 1982.

27. Perrin ER: The use of soluble steroids within inflatable breast prostheses, Plast Reconstr Surg 57:163, 1976.

28. Peterson HD and Burt GB: The role of steroids in prevention of circumferential capsular scarring in augmentation mammaplasty, Plast Reconstr Surg 54:28, 1974.

29. Rotatori DS et al: Non-Invasive assessment of implant capsules, Plast and Reconstr Surg 87:703, 1991.

30. Spear SL et al: Methylprednisolone in double-lumen gel-saline submuscular mammary prostheses: a double-blind prospective clinical trait, Plast Reconstr Surg 87:483, 1991.

CHAPTER **2**

Face-Lift Surgery for the Active Man

Bruce F. Connell
Vasilios S. Lambros
Timothy J. Marten

In the past decade, increased numbers of men have sought facial rejuvenation as prevailing social attitudes have shifted. During this time, surgeons began to recognize the diminished margin for error imposed on these patients along with fewer options to disguise a mediocre result. This has led to a rethinking of techniques that had evolved mainly to treat facial aging in women. Today superior results can be achieved by surgeons who have artistic vision and a defined set of goals.

AESTHETIC CONSIDERATIONS

In most cultures, male facial aesthetics differ from those thought desirable in females. Attractive masculinity is not as closely equated with youth and beauty as is femininity. Certain aspects of facial aging in men may convey an element of strength, power, or wisdom, which are esteemed images that many men recognize. Men and women generally seek different results from facial rejuvenation surgery, with that of the man being arguably more complex. A sound surgical plan should recognize and address this fact.

SURGICAL AND ARTISTIC GOALS

A surgeon must recognize the components of facial aging and formulate a treatment plan for maximum improvement with safety and minimum detectability to obtain the best results. Committed study, careful planning, and good surgical technique should eliminate visible postoperative deformities that can preclude the intended good result.

PREOPERATIVE PLANNING

The preoperative evaluation must include an assessment and documentation of any natural, unrecognized facial asymmetry, both during animation and at rest. All attractive people have a bigger eye and a larger side of their face, and this fact should be made clear to each patient before their surgery. This helps in planning the procedure and eliminates postoperative misinterpretation by the patient, whose face will undoubtedly be subjected to closer and more critical scrutiny.

The entire face and neck should be evaluated with regard to skin redundancy, abnormal fat accumulations, platysma laxity, and salivary gland abnormalities. If the patient smiles and suddenly looks much older because of deep smile creases (crow's feet), this problem should be corrected as well.

Temporal incision

The difference between an excellent and an average result for all facial surgery lies in artistic vision, careful planning, and, to a lesser extent, technical proficiency. No better example exists than the planning and execution of the temporal portion of a face-lift incision. This portion of the incision has traditionally been placed well within the temporal hairline because of the belief that it would hide the resultant scar and minimize visibility. This was indeed true for small temporal skin shifts, but for many other patients, larger skin shifts resulted in an unnatural, unaesthetic, and obvious displacement of the temporal hair and sideburn (Fig. 2-1). Typically, women disfigured in this way were advised to restyle their hair to hide the deformity, a situation evident in many published postoperative photographs of face-lift patients. This recommendation is of little help to those patients who enjoy wearing their hair up or pulled back and who lead active lives outdoors where wind, water, and sport will displace camouflaging wisps of hair, creating a "slipped wig" appearance. Men, who in most cases wear short hairstyles, lack even this poor option. A traditional incision well within the temporal hairline may in some cases create additional problems for men by advancing small areas of "beard skip," sometimes present in Scandanavians and Northern Europeans, or red beard present in certain brown-haired men into darker temporal hair.

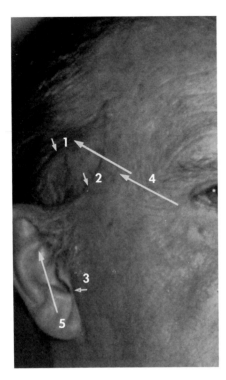

Fig. 2-1 Visible postsurgical deformities in the temple *1,* The hairline has been shifted posteriorly, creating an objectionable and aged appearance. *2,* The patient marked where he would like missing temporal hair. *3,* A change in color and texture around the preauricular scar makes this face-lift obvious. A better location would be to have the incision run along the edge of the tragus without an abrupt change in color anterior to the ear. *4,* The distance from the lateral canthus is much greater than 4 cm and makes this part of the face look old. *5,* The long axis of the earlobe is almost in alignment with the long axis of the ear. This suggests the patient has had a face-lift. A more natural-appearing result would have been obtained if the long axis of the earlobe had been rotated 12 to 15 degrees posterior to the long axis of the ear when the earlobe was reset.

Alternate incisions have been developed for a man's temple region to avoid these problems and prevent objectionable shift of the sideburn and temple hair. Incisions that should not be used include those that sweep below the sideburn to the corner of the eye, above the lateral brow, or along the entire temporal hairline (Fig. 2-2). These incisions may also lead to disruption of the delicate and aesthetically complex region just lateral to the eye by placing scars in an area subjected to considerable scrutiny. Incisions extending beneath the sideburn and above the lateral brow (Fig. 2-2) may also be visible and can create a disturbing diabolical or effeminate appearance by raising the lateral eyebrow. Incisions extending below the sideburn that parallel the temporal and frontotemporal hairline will

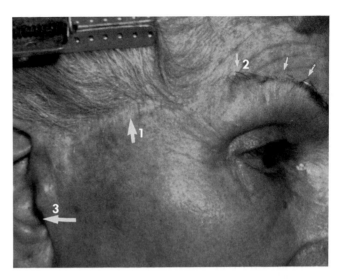

Fig. 2-2 Visible postsurgical deformities in the temporal and preauricular regions. *1,* The incision follows the hairline but raises it too high and then continues above the lateral portion of the eyebrow. *2,* The small arrows indicate the course of the surgical scar. Not only is the temporal hair too close to the eyebrows, but the lateral eyebrow is also raised, creating a diabolic look. *3,* The incisura intertragica has been obliterated, which spoils the beauty of this portion of the ear. This is prevented by designing the face-lift incision to form a distinct inferior border of the tragus.

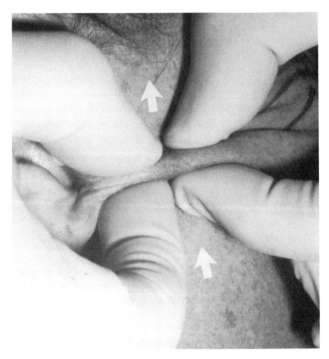

Fig. 2-3 The amount of hairline shift can be determined preoperatively by pinching up the excessive skin in the direction that it is expected to be shifted. This pinch shows the expected sideburn and temporal hairline elevation. A 3-cm pinch means the hairline will shift at least 3 cm higher.

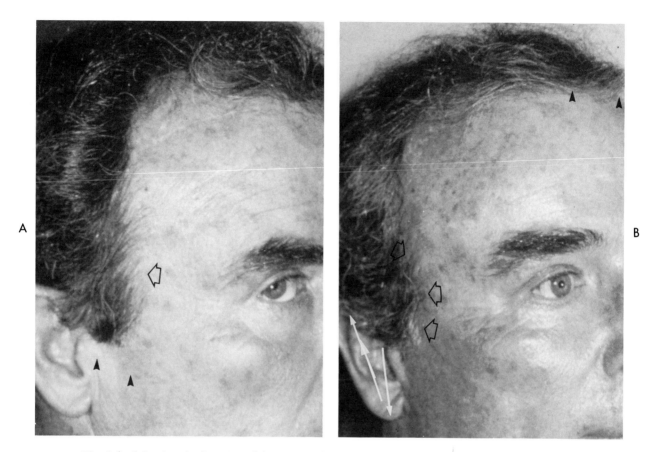

Fig. 2-4 Selecting the location of the temporal portion of the face-lift incision. **A,** Before surgery, the arrow indicates that the incision will be made along the temporal hairline to preserve the distance between the lateral canthus and the sideburn. The incision will be just inside the hairline and inclined parallel to the hair shaft. The black arrows indicate the discernable difference in color and texture of the tragal and cheek skin. The incision should therefore be made along the edge of the tragus to prevent a visible discrepancy around the scar. **B,** After surgery, scars follow the frontal hairline as indicated by the small black arrows. The open arrows in the temporal area show the course of the facelift scar, which is difficult to detect along the hairline. The lower end of the scar curves toward the ear to pass along the helix and the edge of the tragus. There is no objectionable color match or scar anterior to the tragus. The angle between the long axis of the earlobe and the long axis of the ear is greater than 12 degrees, which produces an unoperated appearance.

prevent hairline shifts, hair loss, and improve the appearance of the temporal face but may leave a telltale scar at the upper temporal hairline, where hair almost always slants posteriorly. An incision that stops at the junction of the sideburn and temporal hair will leave the entire temporal region of the face essentially untreated.

When deciding where to place the temporal incision, it is important to note the distance between the lateral canthus and the temporal hairline. This distance is usually 3 to 4 cm in youthful-appearing individuals and increases with age. Equally important is the sur-

geon's estimate of the skin shift possible in this area. This skin shift can be estimated by pinching up and measuring redundant skin in a posterior-superior direction (Fig. 2-3). If the temporal hairline will be moved more than 4 cm away from the lateral canthus or the sideburn shifted above the junction of the ear with the scalp, the surgeon should consider placing the incision a few millimeters inside the temporal hairline as illustrated in Fig. 2-4, *A* and *B*. This incision will permit large posterior-superior skin shifts and prevent objectionable relocation of the temporal hairline. If the incision is made carefully and inclined precisely parallel to

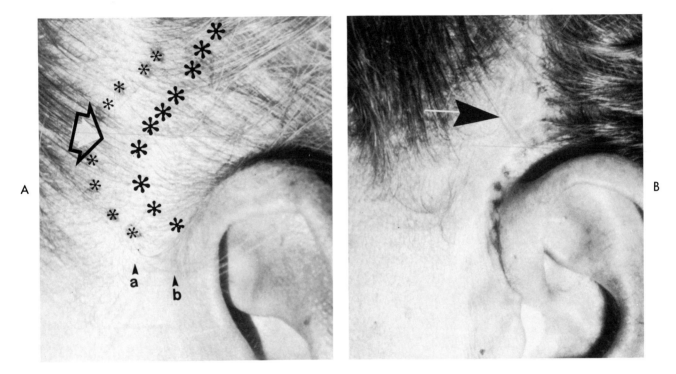

Fig. 2-5 A, The design of the basic face-lift incision should be modified to create a small hair—bearing scalp flap anterior to the ear to prevent the shift of nonhair-bearing preauricular skin into the temporal scalp. A forehead flap is easier to turn downward by designing an even wider flap *(line a),* but this is unnecessary for a standard face-lift procedure. The most frequently used incision *(line b)* is outlined by the larger asterisks. **B,** The arrow indicates nonhair-bearing preauricular skin has shifted into the scalp and is perceived as scar tissue by the patient. This deformity could have been prevented if the flap described in Fig. 2-5, A had been incorporaterd into the design of the face-lift incision.

the hair follicles and the wound edges approximated without tension, hair will grow through the resulting fine scar, which is usually well disguised by even the short hair behind it.

Placement of the temporal portion of the face-lift incision is discussed with the patient as a choice between two imperfect alternatives. A visible scar along the temporal hairline can be revised, concealed with make-up, or even tattooed. Since the scars are situated at a natural anatomical interface, they are usually only noticed by skilled observers on close inspection. A posterior-superior shift in the temporal hairline or sideburn makes the area appear aged and is sometimes considered grotesque. This deformity is difficult to conceal and almost impossible to correct.

A minimal temporal skin shift permits the temporal hairline to remain within 4 cm of the lateral canthus. The temporal portion of the face-lift incision can be placed in the "standard" location approximately 5 cm within the temporal hair, extending upward from the ear. If this incision is chosen, it is important to design a

small hair-bearing projection of temporal scalp on the posterior flap above the ear to prevent the shift of hairless preauricular skin into the temple hair (Fig. 2-5, A). This occurrence is frequently mistaken by the patient as widening of the scar (Fig. 2-5, B). It is really a transposed island of preauricular skin.

Preauricular incision

Most patients have a gradient of facial skin color with increasing redness or pigmentation from the tragus to the cheek, which is especially true in men. This color differential becomes more obvious with a standard preauricular incision as the amount of cheek skin resected anterior to the tragus increases. Most incisions should therefore be placed along the 3 mm wide edge of the tragus to avoid creating a color mismatch around the scar.

The superior portion of the preauricular incision should be marked as a soft curve paralleling the curve of the helical margin. A curved incision will produce an artistically pleasing visual width to the helix in

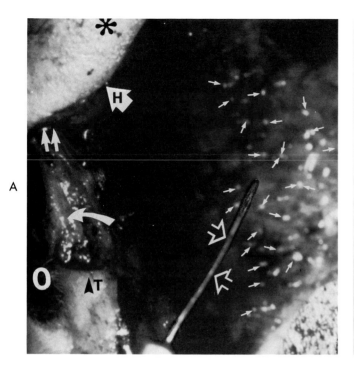

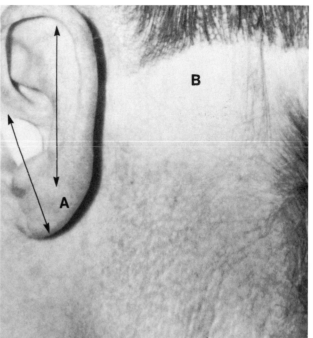

Fig. 2-6 A, Beard hair is eliminated from the skin that will cover the tragus by stretching this part of the flap over a finger, which forces hair follicles above the surrounding fat, where they can be excised or cauterized. The open arrows indicate the electrocoagulation needle. The curved white arrow indicates the tragus denuded of skin, and the asterisk indicates the skin of the helix. The "o" indicates the concha and, the arrow at the "T," the incision to delineate the inferior end of the tragus. Two solid white arrows identify the superior end of the tragus, with the *H* arrow indicating the incision along the helix. **B,** A shift of the nonhair-bearing hypopigmented skin into the occipital area prevents the patient from wearing a short hair style. The angle of the long axis of the earlobe should have been rotated 12 to 15 degrees posterior to the long axis of the ear to prevent a "face-lift" appearance.

keeping with the size of the ear. This incision should lie over the helical cartilage and should not follow its anterior border, which would make the helix appear too wide. The incision is continued into the depression superior to the tragus and then along the edge of the tragus. To define the inferior aspect of the tragus the incision must be directed perpendicularly forward (anteriorly) and then inferiorly just anterior or adjacent to the lobe. If the incision is not made with a 90-degree or less angle, skin settling will result in an irregular subtragal skin fold and an indistinct inferior tragal border.

Many surgeons once believed that incisions along the edge of the tragus could not be made on men because bearded skin would be moved into a normally hairless area. This is now prevented by excision and electrocoagulation of beard follicles on the appropriate portions of the cheek flap (Fig. 2-6, *A*). Most mature men have some hair in these areas. Consequently, the few follicles that do escape destruction produce sparse hair that is either not objectionable, easily shaved, or corrected by epilation.

Earlobe incision

With the earlobe, it is important to obtain an unoperated look. It is always preferable to preserve the natural transition of the ear/cheek sulcus by making the incision 2 to 3 mm below this junction. This maintains the natural beauty of this transition zone, which is similar to the junction of the nose with the lips and cheek. This type of incision usually looks more natural than attempts to insert the thin, soft skin of the earlobe directly into the coarse, thick cheek skin. In addition, this design avoids beard growth in an area that is difficult to shave. The long axis of the earlobe must be rotated 12 to 15 degrees posterior to the long axis of the ear when the earlobe is reset into the cheek to avoid a "face-lift look." The earlobe should not have a pulled-down, "loving cup" appearance. The proper appearance is produced when the ear is set in place as the last part of the procedure.

Postauricular incision

It is neither necessary nor desirable to place the postauricular portion of the face-lift incision over the concha to compensate for a later descent of the scar by gravity. This plan embodies several erroneous concepts that actually preclude good results.

The plan of the postauricular portion of the face-lift incision will influence the direction of neck-skin shift. Careful consideration and direct observation reveal that flap shift should be perpendicular to the neck-skin folds ("turkey gobbler" bands) in a mostly posterior, slightly superior direction. The skin pull should roughly parallel the mandibular border if an optimal result is desired in both the neck and submental areas. Tightness along the cervicomental angle and diminished effect in the submental area will occur if the skin is pulled in a more superior direction. Therefore there is never a need to shift skin directly along the long axis of the sternocleidomastoid muscle. A downward shift and widening of the postauricular scars will result. This fact must be remembered when planning the postauricular incision and directing the shift of the postauricular flap. If the incision is placed on the concha or forced too high on the mastoid in an attempt to conceal the scar, the surgeon will have to add a more anterior-superior rotation of the neck flap to close the resulting defect. This will decrease skin support in the neck and submental areas.

Occipital incision

Traditionally, this incision was placed high on the occipital scalp, usually at the level of the mid ear in the belief that this would hide the resultant scar and minimize visibility. This was indeed true in some cases when neck skin redundancy was small and occipital skin shifts were minimal. Posterior shifts of skin resulted in unnatural and objectionable displacement of occipital hair. This forced women to wear their hair down over these areas, which is an option not even available to many men (Fig. 2-6, *B*).

When deciding on occipital incision placement it is important for the surgeon to estimate the neck skin redundancy in the posteriosuperior direction of skin shift. If less than 2 cm of excessive neck skin is present, a "standard" occipital incision sweeping into the hair just above the level of the mid ear will not result in objectionable shift of the hairline in most cases. If more than 2 cm of neck skin redundancy is present, the incision should be placed along the occipital hairline but designed in such a manner that no telltale scar is left in the fine hair on the nape of the neck. This is best accomplished by curving the inferior portion of the incision posteriorly into thick occipital hair.

Submental incision

A submental incision is made only when necessary. It is indicated when a submental exposure is needed for subplatysmal sculpturing to release a submental crease for chin augmentation or platysma muscle transection at the cricoid. This incision is often erroneously placed directly in the submental crease in a well-intended but conceptually incorrect attempt to reduce its visibility. This incision should be avoided, since it will surgically accentuate the crease. In addition, exposure to the submental region will be compromised, resulting in difficulty dissecting in the anterior neck. There is less skin incision mobility when the incision is placed anteriorly, close to the chin. A more posterior placement of the incision will eliminate these problems.

The location of the submental incision is best selected while placing gentle skin traction superiorly on each cheek. It should be made approximately 2.5 cm in length and be situated posterior to the submental crease in the shadow of the chin at a point roughly half way between the anterior chin and the hyoid. This location prevents reinforcement of the submental crease and permits mobility of the incision for good exposure. It usually heals with a minimal scar.

Planning modification of the SMAS and platysma

A superior face-lift result is difficult to achieve in most patients without modifying the SMAS and platysma muscle. Traditional attempts to recontour the neck by stretching skin flaps over sagging platysma bands or bulging fat have produced disappointing results. Many surgeons in pursuit of an improved result have contributed to the extensive literature on SMAS/platysmaplasty.[4,5,9,11] For the most part, each uses a variation of the basic technique to correct various anatomical problems, but a uniform approach to deep facial rejuvenation has yet to emerge. Nonetheless, a surgeon capable of recognizing the anatomic basis of the patient's problems should, through the application of logic and careful planning, be able to select appropriate techniques that are safe, effective, and rational.

The choice of deep-layer modification to perform is dependent on the patient's deformity. Almost all patients will benefit from a posterior-superior rotation of the SMAS around a pivot point situated over the malar eminence. If the SMAS is adequately mobilized, rotation and posterior shift will provide striking support to

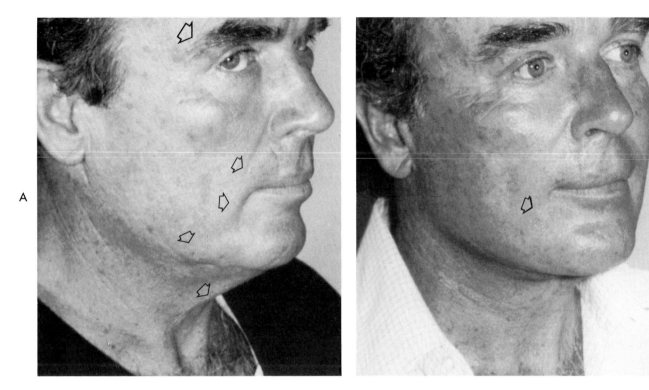

Fig. 2-7   A, The open arrows indicate areas of sagging, deep-layer subcutaneous fat and platysma muscle. This patient needs deep-layer support as well as excision of redundant skin. Correction of the eyebrow ptosis will produce a much more youthful appearance. **B,** Approximately 2 years after surgery, improvement is noted in all areas. It is most difficult to obtain a long-lasting result in the area indicated by the arrow. The incision followed the temporal hairline and passed along the edge of the tragus. SMAS rotation and full-width platysma muscle transection at the level of the cricoid cartilage was also performed.

the cheeks, improvement of the jowls (Fig. 2-7, *A* and *B*) the upper third of the nasolabial folds, and a midline submental support. The upper nasolabial fold improvement will diminish somewhat within a few months. The SMAS dissection and the direction of pull should be considered inaccurate and/or inadequate if any less effect is observed at the time of surgery.[6]

Patients with vertical platysma "shortening" and bands but no generalized muscle laxity and good definition over the lateral mandibular border are best treated by some form of localized muscle interruption and release. The result is immediate, dramatic, and long lasting. Tight anterior bands require a partial transection from jugular vein to jugular vein at the level of cricoid cartilage.[5] If lateral bands are present, the platysma transection is carried more laterally to divide these bands as well. If, in addition to anterior and

lateral bands, there is poor definition over the lateral mandibular border, the platysma transection is planned full width superiolaterally along the anterior border of the sternocleidomastoid muscle and into continuity with the SMAS incision overlying the parotid.[6] A similar full-width transection would be used to treat an obtuse neck with poor mandibular definition but no bands. In most cases *anterior submental suturing* is also performed. Wedge resections and vertical excisions of anterior bands are unnecessary when these techniques are employed.

Lateral platysma suturing is performed when there is a horizontal redundancy and maximum improvement in cervicomental obtusity is desired. In small necks the cut muscle edges are overlapped, beveled slightly, and sutured to the mastoid fascia of the immobile upper fourth of the upper sternolceidomas-

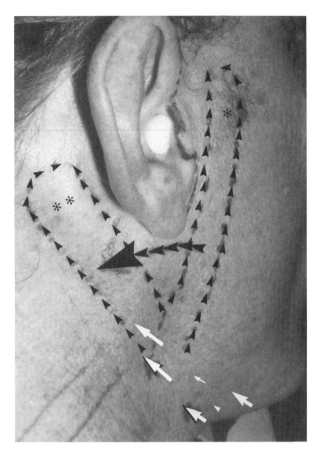

Fig. 2-8 The SMAS transposition flap is outlined on the skin. The flap with the single asterisk will be transposed from the cheek to the mastoid area indicated by two asterisks and sutured in place with the cervicomental angle at 90 degrees. The white arrows indicate the vector of support in the submental and neck areas produced by this SMAS flap. Submental support can be directed to a specific area by modification of the flap design.

toid muscle. The mobility of the sternocleidomastoid muscle in the lower half of the neck makes this area of little value as an anchor-point for the platysma. In larger necks the cut edges of the platysma muscle are trimmed and sutured edge-to-edge.[13] SMAS flaps (Fig. 2-8) are transposed from the cheek to the occipital area in patients who need increased submental support. This will tighten the neck when the patient looks down.

Extensive undermining of the SMAS across the cheek and the platysma onto the anterior neck is neither necessary or desirable. Undermining the SMAS is continued only until the desired effect, motion at the philtrum with a small tug of the flap, is achieved. Most restraining fibers of clinical significance, the anterior zygomatic ligaments, lie just anterior to the malar ori-

gin of the zygomaticus major muscle.[18] Undermining of the platysma is unnecessary because there are no ligaments to restrain it other than its attachment to the parotid gland.

CROW'S FEET CORRECTION

The results of face- and neck-lift procedures have improved rapidly over the last few years. The quest for beauty and harmony in the rejuvenated face now requires attention be given to the residual deep smile creases when they are present.[1,14] Rection, developed in the last two decades, has produced long-lasting improvement for many patients. It is difficult to accurately determine, however, the patient who will benefit from a crow's feet correction using this technique that differs from earlier methods, which elevates the lateral orbicularis muscle with the skin.[1,14]

Contraction of the orbicularis oculi muscle is the major cause of objectionable wrinkles lateral to and extending onto the eyelids and temporal and malar skin (Fig. 2-9, *A* and *B*). These wrinkles become more obvious as the person ages and subcutaneous fat thins.

All objectionable smile creases are marked with a skin-marking pen. Dermal attachments between the fascia of the orbicularis oculi muscle and the skin are then divided. This separation must be precise and requires a four-hand technique with the assistant stabilizing the skin. The depth of skin dissection is determined by local transillumination and distal palpation. Slight skin traction with a finger of one hand is helpful while dissecting with scissors in the other hand. Blunt-tipped Metzenbaum scissors are useful for this dissection. The orbicularis oculi muscle should not be elevated with the skin but permitted to remain in place. The separation of the skin creases from the underlying muscle produces much improvement. However, the best results are obtained when the orbicularis oculi is transected as well. Patients with deep smile creases often have thick muscles. The ideal location to transect such a muscle to avoid creating a deep valley is in the natural depression, which lies lateral to and in a line with the lateral canthal raphae. Transection is best accomplished with Iris scissors and should begin 3 mm anterior to the lateral muscle edge to avoid injury to the frontotemporal branch of the facial nerve. The muscle edges must be beveled to create a smooth transition into the valley and prevent sharp ridges from showing through thin eyelid skin. The lateral 3 mm of the orbicularis muscle should be carefully examined before being cut to make sure that only the muscle is transected. There is no need to suture, stretch, pull, rotate, and place the muscle in an abnormal position.

Approximately 90% of smile creases are eliminated with this technique. However, creases attributable to

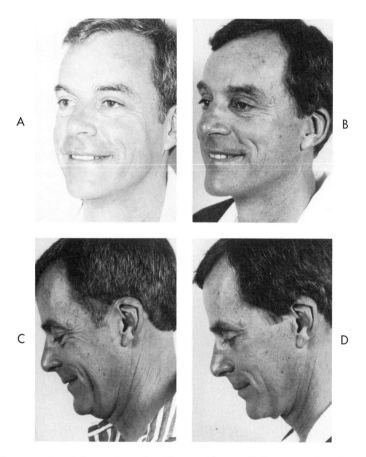

Fig. 2-9 A, Preoperative oblique view of a 48-year-old man. **B,** Postoperative view at 6 months. A striking improvement in the cervicosubmental region is evident. The earlobe is actually improved over the preoperative condition. Malar soft tissues have been elevated to a more youthful position. **C,** Preoperative lateral "looking down" view. **D,** Postoperative view at 6 months. A pleasing improvement is evident, even in this position, which is due in part to the dynamic action of the postauricular SMAS transposition flap. This flap tightens the submental region when the patient looks down. Note also the natural and unoperated look about the ear.

inelastic skin will remain. As a result, patients with sun damaged, inelastic skin will benefit less from this technique.

Preoperative preparations

All patients undergo a complete physical examination and are cleared for surgery by their internist or family physician. Each is asked to avoid agents known to cause platelet dysfunction for 1 month before surgery. A list of offending over-the-counter medications (see box on p. 20) is given to each patient. Patients are not asked to quit smoking, since they rarely quit when asked. Flap necrosis, for the most part, depends on other factors and is avoided if all tissues are handled carefully.

Men are instructed to stop shaving 1 to 3 days before surgery to aid in identification of beard pattern and beard follicle inclination. The hair is not shaved or clipped along any proposed incision site to permit pre-

cise incisions parallel to hair shafts. Rubber bands, tape, surgical lubricants, and hair clips have also been abandoned for the same reason.

Patients shower and shampoo with dilute antiseptic soaps 1 or 2 nights before surgery and receive a full surgical scrub and prep of the scalp, face, ears, nose, neck, shoulders, and upper chest the day of surgery. Colored and concentrated prep solutions that might tint the skin or obscure skin color are not used. Cotton dental rolls are cut and placed in each of the ear canals. They are changed as necessary during the procedure. The patient is draped, leaving the head and neck unobscured from the clavicles up. No head drapes are used.[15]

Anesthesia

A detailed consideration of anesthetic techniques applicable to face-lift surgery is beyond the scope of this chapter. Any skillfully administered anesthetic, lo-

List of Medications that Contain Aspirin*

Advil
Alka-Seltzer Plus Cold Medicine
Anacin
A.P.C. Tablets with Butalbital
A.P.C. Tablets with Codeine
Arthritis Pain Formula
Arthritis Strength Bufferin
Ascriptin
Ascriptin A/D
Ascriptin with Codeine
Aspirin Tablets
Aspirin with Codeine
Aspergum
Bayer Aspirin
Bayer Children's Chewable Aspirin
Bayer Children's Cold Tablets
Bayer Timed Release Aspirin
Buff-A Comp Tablets
Bufferin
Cama Inlay Tablets
Congesperin
Coricidin "D" Decongestant Tablets
Coricidin Demilets or Medilets for Children
Coricidin Tablets
Darvon with A.S.A.
Darvon N with A.S.A.
Dristan
Ecotrin
Empirin
Empirin with Codeine
Emprazil
Equagesic
Excedrin

4-way Cold Tablets
Fiorinal
Firoinal with Codeine
Goody's Headache Powder
Ibuprofen
Midol
Momentum Muscular Backache Formula
Monacet
Motrin
Norgesic Forte
Norwich Aspirin
Nuprin
Pabirin Buffered Tablets
Pacaps
Pamprin
Panalgesic
Percodan
Percodan Demi Tablets
Persistin
Quiet World Analgesic/Sleeping Aid
Robaxisal Tablet
SK-65 Compound Capsules
Sine-Off
St. Joseph's Aspirin for Children
St. Joseph's Cold Tablets
Supac
Synalgos
Synalgos-DC Capsules
Triaminicin
Vanquish
Viro Med
Zorprin

*This list is not all-inclusive. If in doubt, please check with your pharmacist.

cal or general, is adequate. Most of our face-lift procedures are performed under intravenous (IV) sedation and local nerve block. Each patient is fully monitored with ECG, automatic sphygmomanometer, and pulse oxymeter. Overly apprehensive patients, those with a history of anesthetic difficulties, or any patients with significant medical problems are provided an anesthesiologist. All local anesthestic solutions are buffered with sodium bicarbonate to a neutral pH to minimize discomfort on injection (1 mEq $NaHCO_3$ to 20 ml 0.5% lidocaine). Sensory nerve blocks are administered first, and all skin marked for incision is then infiltrated with 0.5% lidocaine with epinephrine 1:200,000. Areas of subcutaneous dissection are then injected with a solution half as strong, ensuring that the total dose of lidocaine does not exceed 7 mg/kg/4 hr. No injection

into the SMAS or platysma is necessary if the subcutaneous tissues overlying the deep layer incisions are infiltrated at the beginning of the case. The ear and other sensitive areas are then systematically reinjected every 90 minutes. This prevents loss of local block and prevents pain of reinjection.

SURGICAL TECHNIQUE
Temple dissection

When the incision is placed within the temporal hair, it is carried down through the superficial temporal fascia to the fascia of the temporalis muscle. The temporal hair-bearing fasciocutaneous flap anterior to the incision is next undermined beneath the superficial temporal fascia. At the anterior temporal hairline the dissection is brought superficially to a subcutaneous level. This procedure protects hair follicles and maintains a good blood supply to the skin. Peterson,[11] Pitanguy, and Silveira[12] have shown the frontotemporal branch of the facial nerve to lie well anterior to this transition point. Thus the dissection is safe when executed as described. The temporal skin is then undermined at a subcutaneous level, often to the lateral canthal raphae. The motor nerves remain safely beneath the undisturbed superficial fascia. This change in the plane of dissection with an anteriorly extended subcutaneous undermining results in a greater improvement in the upper lateral face and allows modification of the lateral portion of the orbicularis oculi muscle if indicated.

When an incision along the anterior temporal hairline is indicated, it is made approximately 2 mm within the hairline parallel to the hair shafts at the interface of fine and thick hair. This incision should be made no higher than the junction of the temporal and frontotemporal hairlines. The temporal skin flap is then subcutaneously undermined.

Cheek and neck dissection

Correct positioning of the operating room lights and proper retraction of the skin flaps by the assistant will greatly aid this dissection. Good light should be placed on both sides of any flap being dissected to provide simultaneous direct and transmitted illumination. Transillumination will precisely reveal flap thickness, an effect sometimes washed out by harsh light from headlights or fiberoptic retractors. The surgeon should avoid retracting for himself, since this invariably leads to rougher handling of the flap when exposure and dissection become difficult. This task should instead be entrusted to a knowledgeable assistant who with two retractors instead of one can focus on providing exposure and protecting the blood supply of the flap. All other operating room personnel must work together with the surgeon and assistant to ensure that flaps are handled gently and not subjected to pinching, excessive traction, or folding beneath instruments.

Skin flaps should be elevated sharply under direct vision, preserving approximately 3 mm of subcutaneous fat. Blind or blunt dissection, which on gross inspection may appear to produce a good flap quickly, is unacceptably traumatic to the subdermal microcirculation and may produce focal areas of raw dermis. By frequently moving from area to area and completing flap dissection in stages, the surgical team can avoid prolonged vascular compromise of any one portion of the flap.

Subcutaneous undermining, although extensive in most necks, should not arbitrarily include the entire face. If SMAS shift and rotation is planned, preservation

of the anterior platysma cutaneous ligaments[8] will produce a pleasing effect on the cheek, unobtainable by other methods. These ligaments, which are variable fascial condensations anchoring the SMAS and upper platysma to the dermis of the cheek, provide a means of creating a youthful sweep beneath the zygoma and an attractive enhancement of the malar region.

It is important that the regions over the zygoma, mandibular border, and mentum, are undermined. Traditional face-lift dissections, that avoid the vascular subcutaneous tissue over the malar bone and the anterior zygomatic ligament will produce an inferior result. Failure to undermine the skin over the mandibular border prevents needed sculpturing of subcutaneous fat in those areas and does not permit release of the mandibular skin—restraining ligaments.

Modification of SMAS/platysma

Almost all patients will benefit from a posterior shift and upward rotation of the SMAS, but treatment of the platysma depends on the deformities present.

A key step in marking the SMAS incision is selecting the malar pivot point on which the flap will rotate. This point should correspond with the high-point of cheek projection and must be chosen individually for each face and each side of the face. It will lie approximately one finger's breadth below and lateral to the lateral canthus. A Methylene blue line is drawn from this point laterally over the lower third of the zygoma and zygomatic arch to a point 1 cm in front of the tragus. This line is then turned inferiorly and carried along the sulcus in front of the ear. At the tailend of the parotid it continues anteriorly and posteriorly to the anterior border of the sternocleidomastoid muscle and the anterior border of this muscle is then followed to the level of the cricoid cartilage. The line is then passed transversely to join a line of similar design on the opposite side.

This design incorporates several important points that are worth considering. By placing the flap rotation point at the malar eminence, fullness gained during rotation is converted to a subtle but significant augmentation of this region. Likewise, overlap of the SMAS along the zygomatic arch enhances the skeletal projection there. By carrying the incision posteriorly from the tail of the parotid to the anterior border of the sternocleidomastoid muscle, a 3 to 4 cm "safety zone" from the mandibular margin is maintained. This moves the dissection well away from the marginal mandibular nerve in almost all cases. Planning the remainder of the incision, along the anterior border of the sternocleidomastoid muscle, keeps the dissection in a relatively thin and avascular area of the platysma muscle and along a line where the cut edge, if visible, would appear as sternocleidomastoid muscle border. Accentuation of the larynx is avoided by transecting the platysma low in the neck. This also preserves a smooth transition from the neck to the submental area.

Tracing the SMAS/platysma incision locations generously with Methylene blue ensures that each flap edge when cut is marked for easy identification during the procedure. The first incision is made SMAS over the zygoma beginning just anterior to the ear. Allis clamp traction placed on the SMAS layer makes dissection easier, since scissors will tend to follow the tensed plane. The vertical limb of this incision is then made in a similar manner. The SMAS flap is carefully elevated until the desired result, motion at the philtrum and upper nasolabial fold, is achieved by a small tug superiorly on the flap. Generally speaking this does not require an extended dissection across the cheek because most restraining fibers lie just anterior to the zygomaticus major muscle.

Once elevated the posterior edge of the SMAS flap is then grasped by three Allis clamps to determine the directional shift that produces the best result. The superior margin is then sutured to the superficial temporal fascia with 4-0 nylon sutures. Care is taken to avoid suturing along the course of the frontotemporal branch of the facial nerve. No trimming of the superior margin of the SMAS is performed, since overlap augments the sweep of the zygomatic arch and provides an ideal point where a secondary SMAS dissection could be performed. Some trimming of the lateral flap margin, is usually required. There is always a need to provide support to the submental area and to the submaxillary glands. When a submental incision and anterior submental platysma suturing is unnecessary, a 1 cm wide flap is cut from the posterior margin of the SMAS flap and is transposed to the mastoid area.[3,16] The flap is sutured in place to the mastoid with the cervicomental angle at 90 degrees. When the patient looks downward, submental support is increased. This postauricular transpositional flap may be designed to provide selectively directed support to specific submental areas. In most cases, support should be directed to the anterior two-thirds of the submental region. Support may also be directed along the cervicomental angle to accentuate the thyroid cartilage, if indicated. This flap produces more support than other methods such as suturing of the cut lateral platysmal edges. The amount of support produced by suturing alone is limited to the upper part of the neck where the sternocleidomastoid muscle is immobile. In addition, suturing here will produce only static support. Suturing a transposed flap of SMAS to the mastoid will provide dynamic support and reinforcement of the submental region when the patient looks down.

Appropriate division and release of the platysma is then performed according to the patient's deformity as described earlier. Wide undermining of the platysma is not necessary because there are no ligaments restraining it in the neck.

Submental dissection

Cervicosubmental lipectomy is an important step in rejuvenating the neck. Earlier attempts to compress cervical fat by tightening cervicofacial skin flaps produced uniformly poor results. Cervical fat excision should only be performed after shifting the SMAS/platysma flaps. This prevents excision of fat from neck regions that will be advanced onto the face by shifting the SMAS and avoids creating a harsh mandibular contour or fat ridges on the face. The technique of fat excision is not as important to the final result as is the amount of fat removed and the secondary contours created. It is particularly important to carefully sculpt the fat in the transition zone from the neck to the face. When fat is removed with a suction cannula, the SMAS flap should be stabilized with Allis clamps to prevent disruption of previously placed sutures supporting it. Typically, fat removal by this technique is easier in the lower and lateral neck and more difficult near the chin.

Preoperative palpation of the neck with and without platysmal action may help identify abnormal accumulations of subplatysmal fat. Typically, these collections are present in patients troubled by life-long cervical obtusity, and subcutaneous lipectomy alone may produce only modest improvement. Subplatysmal lipectomy is essential in such cases.

Significant accumulations of subplatysmal fat are identified during surgery by placing gentle superior traction on the cheeks and flexing the neck. The platysmal space is entered through a transverse submental skin incision by placing opposing traction on the medial borders of the platysma muscle and incising the fascia between them. Fat is then removed incrementally, paying close attention to the new contours created. Overresection is possible, and the fat excision can be bloody and somewhat tedious. However, the improvement is usually significant.

Reinforcement of the submental floor usually provides an improved result. This is accomplished by suturing the medial platysmal borders together from the mentum to the hyoid. Redundant muscle, when present, is trimmed and discarded. If a depression is present between large bellies of the anterior digastric muscles or if there is a need to have more fullness between large submaxillary glands, excessive platysma muscle is not trimmed but inverted in the midline with a continuous 4-0 vicryl suture in two or three layers.[7] Simple excision of redundant muscle and midline approximation is sufficient in most cases. The approximation should be made with the cervicomental angle at 90 degrees. Excessive tension may result when the patient looks straight ahead or down if closure is made with the neck extended.

Closure

The addition of the SMAS/platysmaplasty deep-layer support to the technique of modern face-lifting has made possible precision closure under minimal tension and a marked reduction in detectable scars. Nonetheless, time and attention to detail are required to obtain a good result.

Closure begins with correct positioning of the patient's head, since flexion and extension of the neck will profoundly influence the amount of skin excised over the occipital region. Hyperflexion will reduce the amount excised and compromise improvement in the neck. Hyperextension will lead to over excision, discomfort, and wide scars.

Close attention to the effect desired and that produced (and not a rigid formula) should guide the surgeon in shifting face-lift flaps. There are, however, six key suspension points that take precedence during the remainder of the closure. The first suspension suture is placed above the ear, where its superior-most part joins the scalp. Skin redundancy is gauged with a face-lift marker and a pilot incision cut to allow closure under tension slightly greater than that of normal skin. This point is secured with a half-buried vertical mattress suture of 4-0 nylon with the knot placed on the scalp side. The second suspension suture is placed behind the ear in the apex of the occipitomastoid defect. The flap is moved posteriorly and somewhat superiorly, roughly parallel to anterior neck creases and perpendicular to the anterior neck folds ("turkey gobbler"). Often no skin is trimmed from its anterior border adjacent to the postauricular sulcus. Trimming skin from these areas will compromise proper shift and yield a poor result. The third and fourth suspension sutures are placed in the midportions of the remaining temporal and occipital flaps, each a half-buried vertical mattress suture of 4-0 nylon. The temporal incision is then closed with half-buried vertical mattress sutures of 4-0 nylon and staples if located within the temporal hair or half-buried vertical sutures of 4-0 nylon and multiple simple interrupted sutures of 6-0 nylon if along the temporal hairline. A soft, round, and multiperforated silastic drain (IOF Jackson-Pratt) is then placed through a small stab wound in the occipital scalp and secured. It is then passed across the anterior neck to the opposite side of the face. No other drains are used unless the dissections on the right and left sides of the face are not in continuity. The superior portion of the occipital flap is then marked, trimmed

with 2 mm excess, inset, and sutured with half-buried vertical mattress sutures of 4-0 nylon, leaving a "dog ear" at the inferior end of the incision. Intuitively, one is tempted to eliminate this in a standard fashion, but a better result is obtained if it is inset into the occipital scalp. This moves the end of the incision into dense hair and avoids a visible scar (Fig. 2-10).

A pretragal concavity is then created by excising SMAS in the pretragal region over the parotid. This will provide a natural-appearing transition from face to ear and prevents a loss of tragal definition seen with other techniques. The skin flap is then pushed gently down into this hollow while pilot incisions are marked and cut for the suspension sutures five and six above and below the tragus. This part of the closure should not be under tension and failure to allow for skin to fill the pretragel hollow will result in a suboptimal scar and passible tragal retraction.

Before suturing around the ear, beard follicles on the tragal, preauricular, and postauricular portions of the flap should be fulgurated and/or excised. This is best done by everting these areas over a finger with a skin hook. This will protrude the follicles and separate them from more superficial portions of the flap. Most may then be excised with a small, sharp scissors. Follicles resisting excision should be cauterized. This technique produces a near-normal periauricular beard pattern and prevents hair from growing on these areas.

A final check for hemostatsis is made, and pilot incisions above and below the tragus are secured with simple interrupted sutures of 6-0 nylon. Skin abutting the anterior helix is then trimmed in a soft curve, and the incision in this region closed with simple interrupted sutures of 6-0 nylon. The tragal flap is then trimmed conservatively, leaving it intentionally redundant. It is secured with 6-0 nylon.

Dressings

The need for a face-lift dressing should be weighed against its possible drawbacks.

Surgeons who use a garment dressing claim that it prevents oozing, edema, seromas, and hematomas but when questioned more carefully openly admit this to be untrue. Still others claim their dressings provide increased comfort and improved neck contour. Experience, simple logic, and common sense all argue against these claims.

There are, however, many rational arguments against the use of face-lift dressings, the most obvious of which is the danger in confining, compressing, or placing pressure on delicate skin flaps that have been widely undermined. Dressings also limit direct observation of the face and neck and may conceal an evolving or established problem. None will reduce edema,

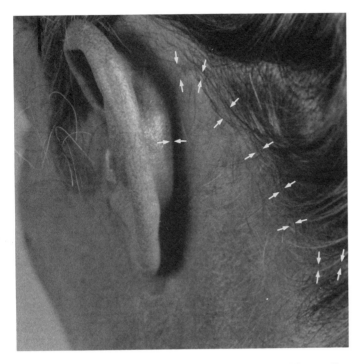

Fig. 2-10 A face-lift patient 1 year after surgery. The small arrows indicate the course of the postauricular face-lift scar. The inferior end of this scar passes into thick hair on the occipital scalp. No scar is present in the fine hair on the nape of the neck.

and most create a tourniquet effect enhancing it. Finally, face-lift dressings are uncomfortable. They are tight and confining, obstruct hearing, complicate hygiene, and attract undue attention.

If a dressing is used, no portion of it should be placed on the face or neck. A small, loose wrap that confines long hair is appreciated by most patients and is usually removed the next day (Fig. 2-11).

Postoperative care

Proper postoperative care of the face-lift patient will ensure the best result with the fewest complications. All patients are discharged to the overnight care of an aftercare specialist familiar with the postoperative plan of care used in our office. A physician is always available to answer questions or see patient if needed.

All patients return to the office the morning after surgery and are carefully examined. Drain output is checked, and, if less than 30 ml, the drain is usually removed. All sutures are then checked, and any that appear too tight are snipped and left in situ. This averts bleeding from the suture site, which occurs if the stitch is removed. All flaps are carefully inspected as well. Any signs of postauricular-flap compromise should raise suspicion that the patient has been flexing the neck and not keeping the cervicomental angle

greater than 90 degrees as instructed. Patients must rely on observers to remind them of this, since they lack proprioception about the neck. Patients are forbidden to hold a book or magazine in their hands, sit up straight without a headrest, or lay supine without a neckroll for 10 days, since these activities all result in inadvertent and counterproductive neck flexion. A good position to maintain an open cervicomental angle is having the patient sit with the elbows on the knees. This posture allows activities such as reading, writing, eating, and watching television to be performed without neck flexion. Any time postauricular-flap compromise is noted, a check should be made to ensure that a tight closure has not created tension across its base, limiting its circulation. If there is doubt, the offending sutures should be removed without hesitation, since secondary healing is always preferred to skin slough.

All postoperative instructions are reviewed at each postoperative visit, and the patient is reminded that although laughing and squinting reduce edema and relax tension along suture lines, yawning and head turning do not. Patients are also reminded that their dental occlusion may be off for 4 to 6 weeks after surgery, which sometimes results from an aggressive SMAS shift.

Sutures are removed as indicated, usually in stages, over a period of 9 to 10 days. Fine sutures are removed from areas of low tension first, usually on the third and fifth postoperative days. Half-buried vertical mattress sutures are removed later, between the fifth and tenth postoperative days. Sutures in relatively high-tension areas such as sideburns (mouth opening) and behind the ears (neck flexion) are removed last.

Complications

Experience has shown that longer and more extensive face-lift procedures have not resulted in an increased complication rate. Hematomas, the most common complication reported in our literature, are thought to be common in men. This finding has been attributed to an increased circulation in bearded skin and is supported by the experience of most surgeons. Nonetheless, in the last several thousand cases in this office, no patient undergoing a face-lift procedure has been returned to surgery for evacuation of a hematoma. Hematomas occurring on the table, requiring the removal of several stitches, rarely occur but are indeed more common in men. Because our procedures tend to outlast the effect of epinephrine, bleeding is usually discovered and corrected before wound closure. Credit should also be given to an increased sophistication in anesthetic technique and skilled postoperative care.

There has not been a case of marginal mandibular nerve palsy and only one injury to the frontotemporal branch of the facial nerve during this period. Three patients experienced temporary unilateral weakness of the frontalis muscle, but all fully recovered within 12 weeks.

Skin necrosis is extremely rare in our patients, and in only one case has it exceeded 1 cm². We attribute this to precise planning, gentle technique, and thoughtful postoperative care.

SUMMARY

It is impossible to design a universal face-lift technique applicable to all patients. Each case requires a precise anatomical diagnosis and appropriately planned repair. It is important to note the distance between the lateral canthus and the temporal hairline when planning the placement of the temporal incision. This distance is usually 3 to 4 cm in individuals who appear youthful. Consideration should be given to placing the incision at the hairline rather than within the temporal hair if the temporal hairline will be shifted more posterior.

Experience has shown that in all but the ideal candidate an excellent face-lift result is not possible without modification of the SMAS and platysma. Submental incisions should not be made in the submental crease. This surgically accentuates the double-chin deformity. Correct positioning of the patient's head is important when closing to prevent overresection or underresection of the occipital skin flap. Close observation of the effects produced, instead of a rigid formula, should be used to guide the surgeon in shifting the face-lift flaps. Correct flap movement is in a mostly posterior, somewhat superior direction toward the occiput and is perpendicular to the neck-skin folds seen when the patient is seated or standing.

Proper postoperative care is important for a good result, and, in skillfully executed procedures, the complications should be rare.

REFERENCES

1. Aston SJ: Platysma muscle in rhytidoplasty, Ann Plast Surg 3:529, 1979.
2. Camirand A: Personal communication, 1986.
3. Carlsen L: Personal communication, 1987.
4. Connell BF: Contouring the neck in rhytidectomy by lipectomy and a muscle sling, Plast Reconstr Surg 47:534, 1971.
5. Connell BF and Gaon A: Surgical correction of aesthetic contour problems of the neck, Clin Plast Surg 10:491, 1983.
6. Connell BF: Facial rejuvenation. In Brent B (ed): The artistry of reconstructive surgery, St. Louis, 1987, The CV Mosby Co.
7. Feldman J: Personal communication, 1989.
8. Furnas D: Mandibular restraining ligaments, Plast Reconstr Surg 83:1, 1989.
9. Kay B: Personal communication, 1984.
10. Mitz V and Peyronie M: Superficial musculoaponeurotic system (SMAS) in the parotid and cheek area, Plast Reconstr Surg 58:80, 1976.
11. Peterson R: Personal communication, 1974.
12. Pitanguy I and Silveira R: The frontal branch of the facial nerve: the importance of its variations in face lifting, Plast Reconstr Surg 38:352, 1966.
13. Randall P and Skiles MS: The "SMAS sling": an additional fixation in face lift surgery, Ann Pl Surg 12:1, 1984.
14. Rubin LR: The anatomy of a smile: its importance in the treatment of facial paralysis, Plast Reconstr Surg 35:384, 1974.
15. Tessier P et al: Le systeme musculo-aponevrotique superficiel de la face et ses applications chirurgicales. Paper presented at the annual meeting of the French Society of Plastic Surgeons, Paris, October 14, 1974.

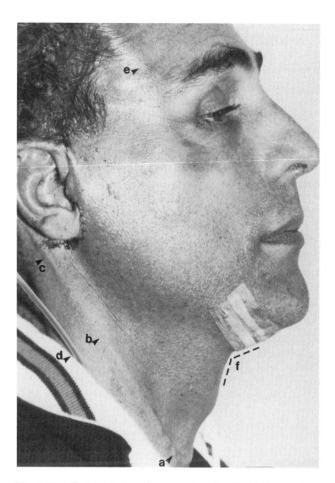

Fig. 2-11 Patient 1 day after an extensive SMAS face- and neck-lift, including full-width transection of the platysma muscle at the level of the cricoid cartilage. *a,* The small drain passes from one side of the neck to the other at the level of the cricoid cartilage. *b and c,* The course of the drain under the skin is indicated. *d,* The external portion exits a separate stab wound, higher than the postauricular incision and is connected to a compressable suction reservoir. *e,* Most patients have only one drain; however, this patient has a separate drain in the temporal area passing down to the area of his crow's-feet correction. *f,* The chin-neck angle is maintained slightly higher than 90 degrees for 10 days after surgery. No dressing was used on the face and neck other than the steri-strips reinforcing the submental incision.

16. Weisman PA: Simplified technique in submental lipectomy, Plast Reconstr Surg 48:443, 1971.

ADDITIONAL READINGS

Adamson JE, Horton CE, and Crawford HH: The surgical correction of the "turkey gobbler" deformity, Plast Reconstr Surg 34:598, 1964.

Bourguet J: La Chirurgie esthetique de la face: les rides, Le Monde Medical, 38:41-51, 1928.

Connell BF: Cervical lift: surgical correction of fat contour problems combined with full-width platysma muscle flaps, Aesthetic Plast Surg 1:355, 1978.

Connell BF: Cervical lifts: the value of platysma muscle muscle flaps, Ann Plast Surg 1:355, 1978.

Connell BF: Eyebrow and forehead lifts. In Courtiss EH (ed): Male aesthetic surgery, St. Louis, 1982, The CV Mosby Co.

Connell, BF, Lambros VS, and Neurohr GH: The forehead lift: techniques to avoid complications and produce optimal results, Aesthetic Reconstr Surg 13:217-237, 1989.

Cronin TD and Biggs TM: The T-Z plasty for the male "turkey gobbler" neck, Plast Reconstr Surg 47:534, 1971.

Davis AD: Obligations in the consideration of meloplasties, J Int Coll Surg 24:567, 1955.

Ellenbogen R: Pseudoparalysis of the mandibular branch of the facial nerve after platysmal face-lift operation, Plast Reconstr Surg 63:364, 1979.

Flowers RS: Ancho blepharoplasty, In Transactions of the International Congress of Plastic Surgery, Paris, 1976, Mason et CIE.

Gorney M and Harries T: The preoperative and postoperative consideration of natural facial asymmetry, Plast Reconstr Surg 54:187, 1974.

Gray H: Anatomy of the human body, ed 25, Philadelphia, 1949, Lea & Febiger.

Guerrerosantos J, Espaillat L, and Morales F: Muscular lift in cervical rhytidoplasty, Plast Reconstr Surg 54:127, 1974.

Loeb R: Posterior auricular nerve preservation, double chin leveling, and earlobe reimplantation during neck lifts, Clin Plast Surg 10:405, 1983.

Maliniac JW: Is surgical restoration of the aged face justified? MJ and Rec 135:321, 1932.

Marchac D: Julien Bourguet, the pioneer in aesthetic surgery of the neck, Clin Plast Surg 10:363, 1983.

Millard DR et al: Submental and submandibular lipectomy in conjunction with a face lift in the male or female, Plast Reconstr Surg 49:385, 1972.

Morel-Fatio D: Cosmetic surgery of the face (other than rhinoplasty). In Gibson T (ed): Modern trends in plastic surgery, Washington, DC, 1964, Butterworth Publishers.

Padgett EC and Stephenson KL: Plastic and reconstructive surgery, Springfield, Ill, 1948, Charles C Thomas.

Rees TD, Liverett DM, and Guy CL: The effect of cigarette smoking on skin-flap survival in the face lift patient, Plast Reconstr Surg 73:911, 1984.

Skoog TG: Plastic surgery: new methods and refinements, Philadelphia, 1984, WB Saunders Co.

Vinas JC, Caviglia C, and Cortinis JL: Forehead rhytidoplasty and brow lifting, Plast Reconstr Surg 57:445, 1976.

CHAPTER 3

Rhytidoplasty: Improving Cheek and Neck with Simplified and Refined Surgical Technique

José Guerrerosantos

It has been fascinating during the past 25 years to observe the evolution of cheek- and neck-lift as a surgical technique. The idea of rejuvenating both the face and the neck simply by undermining the skin, removing excess skin, and suturing is now out of date. Actually, a surgeon who aspires to achieve a better result must undermine and tighten the cutaneous flap aided by additional surgical maneuvers such as cervical lipectomy or liposuction, plication, and lifting of the platysma muscle and the submandibular gland, and lifting and plication of the SMAS, removal of the Bichat fat pad, and careful liposuction of the melolabial sulcus and/or the jowl fat pad.

I currently use a combination of techniques to improve the appearance of the patient with an aging face, as determined by the physical characteristics of each patient.[1] To adequately plan the surgical procedure to be used on each patient, I first do a clinical and photographic study to classify the patient and select the most appropriate surgical technique.

CLASSIFYING THE PATIENT FOR IMPROVING THE CHEEK AND NECK

It is important before planning cervicofacial rhytidoplasty to make a clinical and photographic study of the cheeks and neck.

STUDY OF THE CHEEKS

When examining a candidate for rhytidoplasty, the surgeon should carefully examine the cheeks to determine if the patient has a long, round, or broad face. The plastic surgeon must be able to detect individual minor variations in the shape of the face before surgery. Long faces generally have elongated noses, ears, or chins, while broad or round faces have square, broad, or round facial features.

Notice the characteristics of the skeletal bones and soft tissues when examining the cheek. It is interesting to observe whether the zygoma is prominent, flat, or retracted in the cheek. Likewise, the prominence of the cervicomandibular angle should be observed because these features help decide whether the contour can be corrected by altering only soft tissue or if the shape of the underlying bone must be changed. It is advisable when studying the soft tissues of the cheek to observe whether the patient is obese, slender, or of average build. Each patient should be classified into one of these three groups. We should also observe the prominence of the cheek near the melolabial sulcus and determine the size of the jowl fat pad. On the other hand, especially in slender or average patients, it is important to also look for depressions generally appearing around the masseter muscle. The observed physical findings derived from studying the facial form permit planning the operation. A patient with prominent cheeks is probably a candidate for partial resection of the Bichat fat pad or suction of the cheek and/or the prominence of the melolabial area and the jowl. If depressed areas are obvious, the patient may benefit from fat injection to restore contour.

CLASSIFICATION OF THE DEFORMED NECK

Several years ago, when classifying a patient's neck before performing a neck-lift, I only considered how flaccid the skin was in the area and therefore usually only operated on elderly patients. Now, however, with the evolution of surgical techniques and the advent of liposuction, it is practical to operate on younger people with less than ideal neck contour. I now consider two basic factors in classifying these patients: the degree of cervical soft tissue redundancy and the amount of fat present in the neck.

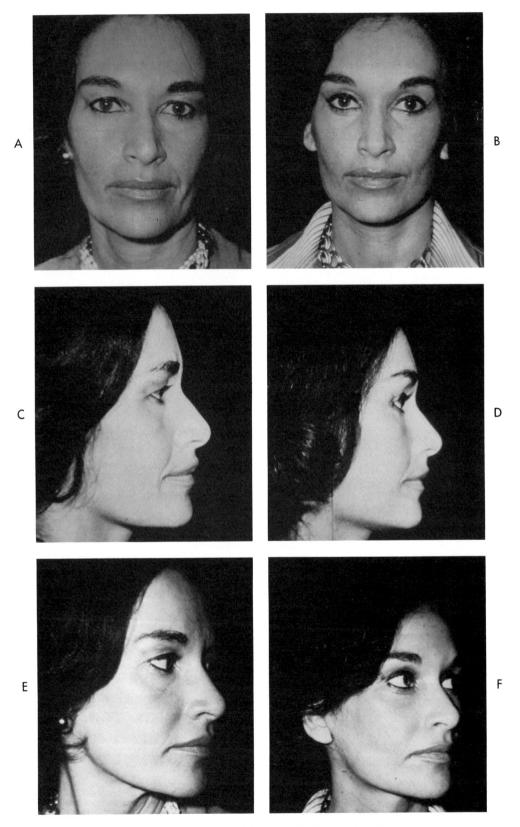

Fig. 3-1   A middle-aged woman with signs of facial senility but with little redundant neck skin. This patient has a grade 0 neck deformity. **A, C,** and **E,** The preoperative appearance. **B, D,** and **F,** The result 1 year after segmental classic rhytidoplasty.

A   B   C

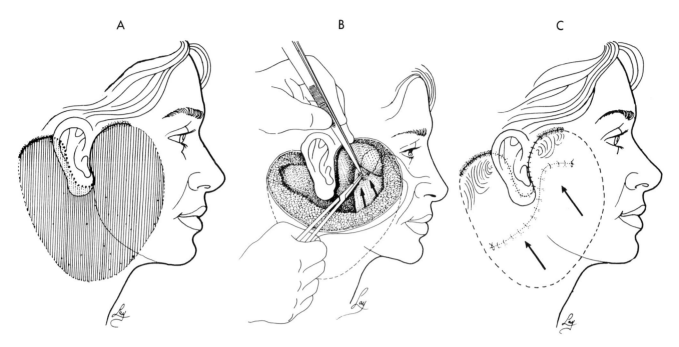

Fig. 3-2   Diagram of the surgical technique used on patients with grade 0 cervical deformity. **A,** The segmental undermining is marked with dotted lines and includes part of the cheek, neck, and the mastoid region. **B,** It is best to lift the SMAS in the cheek and the platysma muscle in the neck. **C,** After pulling the cutaneous flaps, the excess skin is trimmed and the incisions closed.

I classify the neck in our surgical unit[27] by considering the degree of cervical soft tissue redundancy as follows: grade 0, grade I, grade II, and grade III. I also take into account the amount of fat present in the neck by noting types *A* for thin neck and *B* for fat neck.

When I examine the patient's neck, I analyze the condition of the following tissues: the skin, fat, platysma muscle, and submandibular gland. It is also important to observe the aesthetic condition of the cheek. The classification I describe can be applied to both the preoperative assessment and the surgical correction of observed abnormalities.

Grade 0

Patients classified as grade 0 cervical aesthetic deformity are those with early senile changes in the face but who still appear realtively youthful and without redundant neck skin (Fig. 3-1, *A, C,* and *E*). I only include thin individuals in this grade of neck deformity. The surgical technique I use on these patients is similar to classical rhytidoplasty and consists of making a limited cutaneous undermining as part of the cheek, neck, and the mastoid region (Fig. 3-2, *A* to *C,*). After cutaneous flap undermining and hemostatsis is achieved, the SMAS is imbricated over the cheek, using a modification of the classic Aufricht maneuver.[5] The posterior border of the platysma muscle is then plicated in the neck toward the mastoid region, as suggested by Baker, Gordon, and Whetlow.[7] Finally, the cutaneous flaps are

closed after excess skin has been removed.

If the surgical technique is correctly performed on patients with prematurely flaccid facial skin and a slender face and neck, the results achieved are especially good (Fig. 3-1, *B, D,* and *F*).

Grade I

I include in grade I deformity thin patients (grade I—type A) and fat patients (grade I—type B). They are usually young with or without flaccid neck skin.

In addition to changes associated with senility, patients with grade I—type A aesthetic neck deformity may also show the following variations: mildly flaccid skin, a thin layer of subcutaneous fat in both the submental and submandibular areas, a mildly flaccid platysma muscle in the submental area, and occasional ptosis of the submandibular gland (Fig. 3-3, *A* and *C*).

The surgical technique I use on these patients includes wide undermining of the neck skin from side to side, creating a single cavity. I then imbricate the SMAS in both cheeks (Fig. 3-4, *A*) and the posterior part of the platysma muscle to lift both the cheek and the neck. I use a continuous running suture that follows the line shown in Fig. 3-4, *B* (see also Fig. 3-9). In addition, bilateral plication sutures using absorbable material are used in the platysma muscle (Fig. 3-10). The cutaneous flaps are then pulled, the excess skin is removed, and the skin flaps sutured in place. Patients with grade I—type B are young people who have an

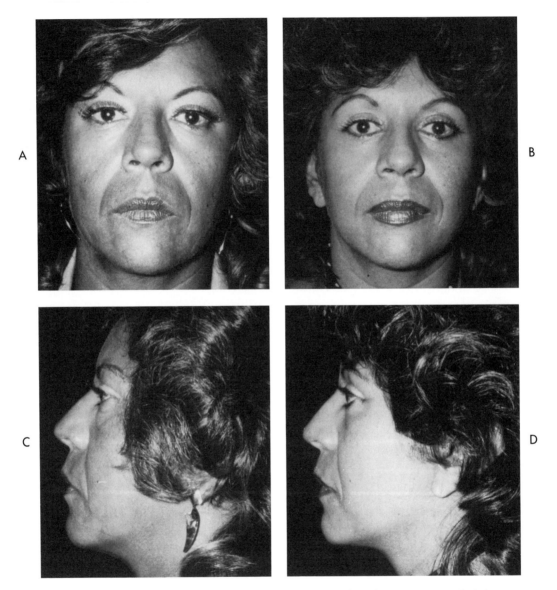

Fig. 3-3 (**A** and **C**) A woman with a senile appearing face and grade I—type A neck deformity. **B** and **D,** The result 2 years after a forehead lift, blepharoplasty, cervicofacial rhytidoplasty with imbrication of the SMAS and the posterior border of the platysma muscle and platysma plication.

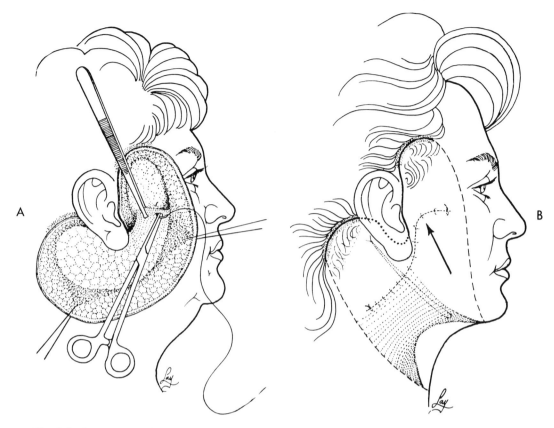

Fig. 3-4 Diagrams of the surgical technique used in patients with grade I—type A neck deformity. The cutaneous undermining is wider than that used in grade 0. **A,** The SMAS and the posterior border of the platysma muscle are imbricated. **B,** Bilateral platysmal plication sutures are used.

accumulation of fat localized in the neck. These patients have no firm neck skin with the cervical deformity formed by excess fat in the area (Fig. 3-5). These patients are treated by cervical liposuction, which I carry out through three small 1.5 cm incisions. One of these incisions is made in the submental crease and the others just below the earlobes bilaterally.

Grade II

Patients with grade II—type A neck deformity (Fig. 3-6), have moderately loose neck skin, an above average amount of subcutaneous fat, some redundant platysma muscle, and occasional ptosis of the submandibular gland. The surgical technique for aesthetic correction consists of performing a wide undermining both in the cheeks and in the neck. The two medial portions of the platysma should be sutured together in the midline with a continuous running suture in one or two layers (Fig. 3-7). If the posterolateral area of the platysma is thick and contractile, it should be thinned. I then plicate the SMAS on the cheek and the postero-

lateral part of the platysma muscle (Fig. 3-8). I then place bilateral plication sutures using absorbable material in the platysma muscle (Fig. 3-9). Careful hemostasis should be achieved before the skin flaps are trimmed and the cutaneous flaps on the cheek and neck redraped and closed.

Patients with grade II—type B deformity (Fig. 3-10) are individuals with excess fat and moderate loose cervical skin. Treatment of patients with this deformity consists of removing the fat either by the classical method (with forceps and scissors) through submental and auricular incisions or by means of liposuction. After removing the fat, I estimate the looseness of the tissues and then imbricate the SMAS on the cheek and posterior part of the platysma muscle and place the bilateral plication sutures. I then pull the cutaneous flaps, remove the excess skin in the preauricular area, and close the incisions. It is important to avoid excising skin in the submental region in 95% of patients, since it is unnecessary and can cause vertical cutaneous bands to form, which secondarily deform the neck and give it a senile look.

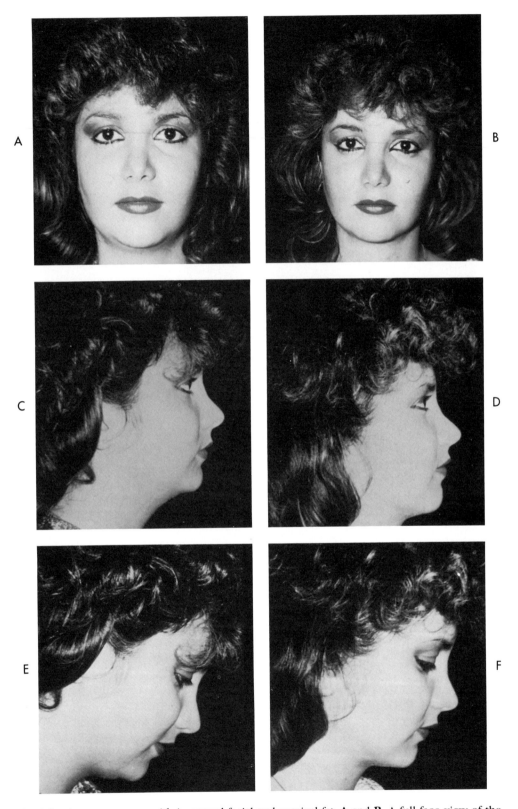

Fig. 3-5 A young woman with increased facial and cervical fat. **A** and **B,** A full face view of the patient before surgery and 1 year after suctioning the cheeks and neck and partial resection of the buccal fat pad. **C** and **D,** The side view before surgery and 1 year after surgery. **E** and **F,** The cervical profile with the neck bent.

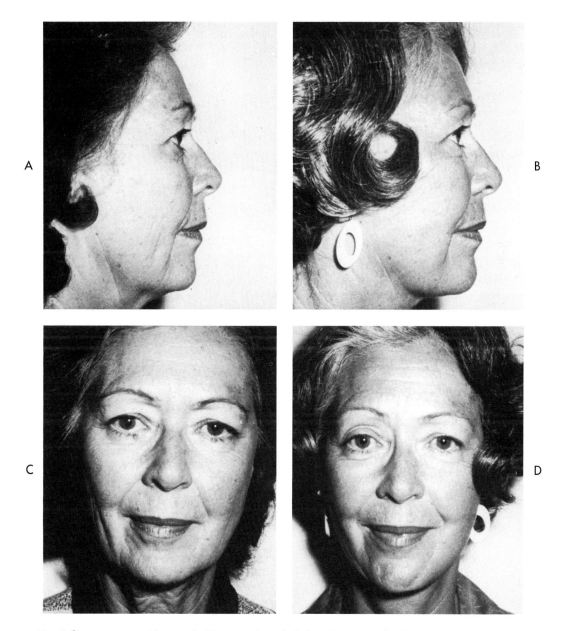

Fig. 3-6 A woman with a grade II—type A neck deformity. **A** and **C**, The patient before surgery. **B** and **D**, The patient 2 years after cervicofacial rhytidoplasty.

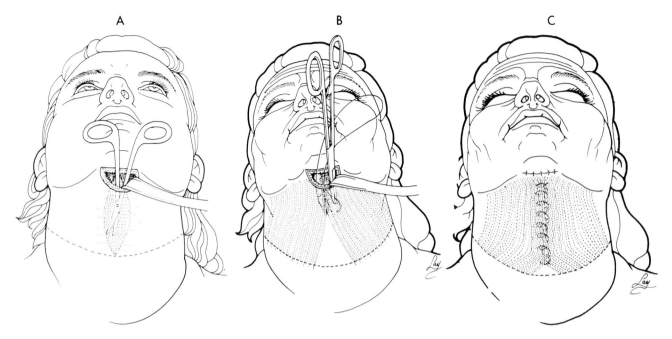

Fig. 3-7 A, Through a submental incision 2 cm long, I resect a vertical ellipse of subcutaneous fat, some medial fibers of the platysma muscle, and if necessary, a layer of subplatysmal fat. **B,** I join the paramedial borders of the platysma muscle with 3-0 dexon or vicryl after removing the subcutaneous fat layer from the platysma muscle. **C,** A continuous suture is placed in one layer, and in certain cases, in two or three layers, until the platysma muscle is well stretched.

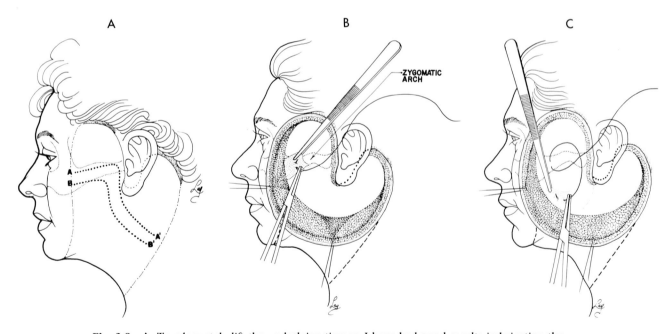

Fig. 3-8 A, To adequately lift the underlying tissues, I have had good results imbricating the SMAS and the posterior border of the platysma muscle with a continuous running suture that joins the two lines A and A′ and B and B′. **B,** The continuous running suture starts at the SMAS over the zygomatic arch, where I make the first stitch with the suturing needle. **C,** Then grasping the SMAS in the cheek at a distance of approximately 2 cm I make the second stitch with the suturing needle.

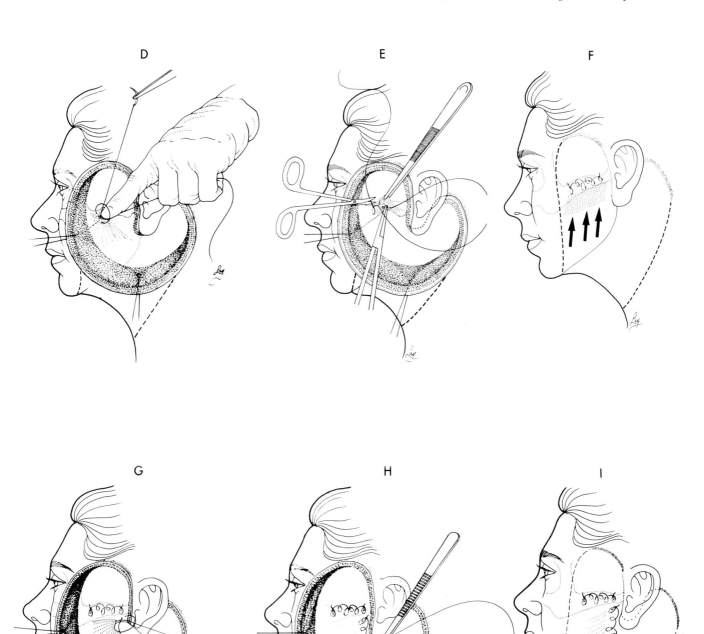

Fig. 3–8—cont. D, I then tie the thread, elevating the SMAS of the cheek. **E,** As soon as the knot is tied, I continue suturing the SMAS over the zygomatic arch. **F** I do a continuous running suture (in the cheek SMAS) ending in a point situated 1 cm in front of the tragus. **G,** The suture is continued downward and backward in front of the ear **H,** and then to the posterolateral part of the platysma. **I,** This diagram shows the finished continuous running suture with which I elevate the SMAS and the platysma upward and backward.

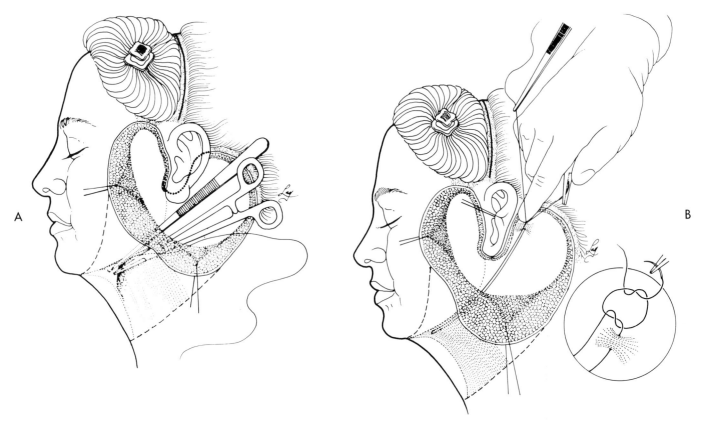

Fig. 3-9   The bilateral plication sutures are used to complete the lifting of the underlying tissues, as well as to improve the profile of the cervical angle and raise the submandibular gland to define the mandibular border. **A,** I place a stitch in the platysma in the area that corresponds to the anterior border of the submandibular gland and at a point approximately 1 cm below the mandibular border. **B,** The second stitch is taken in the mastoid fascia. Then I tie the suture, under adequate tension but without making it too tight to avoid overcorrection or tearing of the platysma muscle.

Grade III

Patients with grade III—type A deformity, have severely flaccid neck skin, moderate or little subcutaneous fat, hypertrophy and/or loose platysma muscle, and occasionally ptosis of the submandibular gland (Fig. 3-11). In this type of neck deformity, the main feature is the senile alterations in the platysma muscle that become apparent on the outside because of the presence of vertical bands of different thickness, which in most patients are located on both sides of the midline in the submental area. Some patients also have external deformity attributable to senile changes in the platysma in the posterolateral area. When examining a patient of this grade, it is necessary to look for and document in the clinical record all the alterations observed to plan the most adequate surgical technique. Usually the vertical bands of platysma muscle are asymmetrical, which is important to document and to tell the patient.

The surgical technique employed in most patients with grade III—type A deformity includes the following steps: wide undermining of both cheeks and the neck from side to side through a submental approach and laterally through preauricular incisions. In the submental region, after generously undermining and performing careful hemostasis, I make a vertical elliptical resection of soft tissues, including subcutaneous fat, cervical fascia, platysma muscle, and subplatysmal fat (see Fig. 3-7, *A*). I then proceed to approximate the platysma muscle in the midline by doing a continuous running suture in one or two layers and giving adequate tension to the tissues to improve the cervical contour in this area (see Fig. 3-7, *B* and *C*). This technique is exactly the same as that of Vistnes and Souther,[44,45] as well as that published by Feldman.[20] After undermining the cheeks and the posterolateral areas of the neck subcutaneously, I imbricate the SMAS in the cheek area to raise it both vertically and posteri-

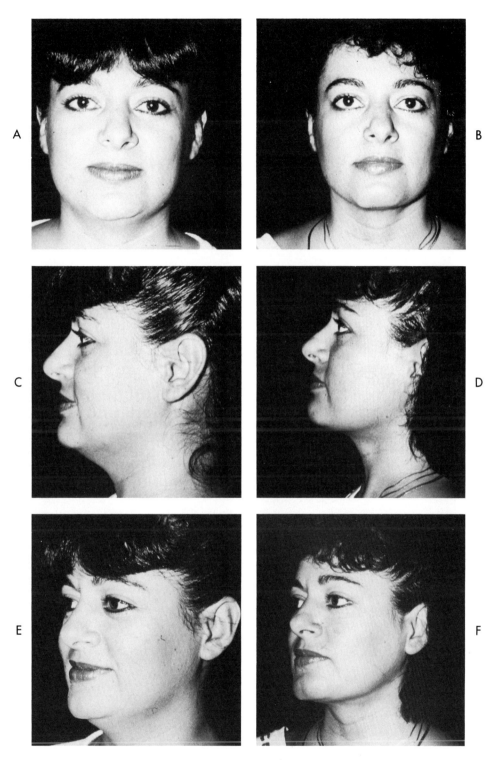

Fig. 3-10 A young woman with a grade II-type B neck deformity with very chubby cheeks because of excess subcutaneous tissue, hypertrophy of the buccal fat pad and excessive subcutaneous fat in the neck. **A, C,** and **E,** The patient before surgery. **B, D,** and **F,** The result 1 year after partial resection of the buccal fat pad and liposuction in the cheeks and neck.

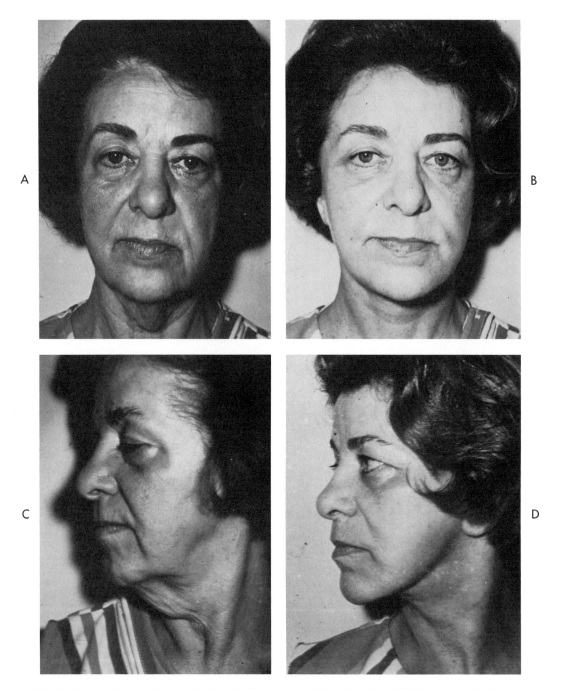

Fig. 3-11 A patient with a cervical grade III—type A deformity. **A** and **C,** The patient before corrective surgery. **B** and **D,** The patient 1 year after surgery with adequate management of the SMAS and the platysma muscle.

orly. The SMAS is anchored with a continuous running suture from above, downward in the cheek and neck, following the posterior border of the platysma muscle (see Fig. 3-8). Afterward, I place bilaterally the platysma-mastoid plication suture (see Fig. 3-9). The advantages of this plication are that it lifts the platysma muscle, improves the mandible-neck angle, lifts the submandibular gland, and defines the submandibular line. Finally, the cutaneous flaps are closed after excision of the excess skin.

Patients with grade III—type B deformity have severely flaccid skin, abundant subcutaneous and subplatysmal fat, mild or moderately flaccid platysma muscle, and frequent ptosis of the submandibular gland (Fig. 3-12). These patients usually have the typical double chin from excessive fat. We have never seen a patient with a fat neck who also had severe hypertrophy or a flaccid platysma muscle. In my opinion, this is significant in planning the surgical technique, since radical methods with complete transection of the platysma

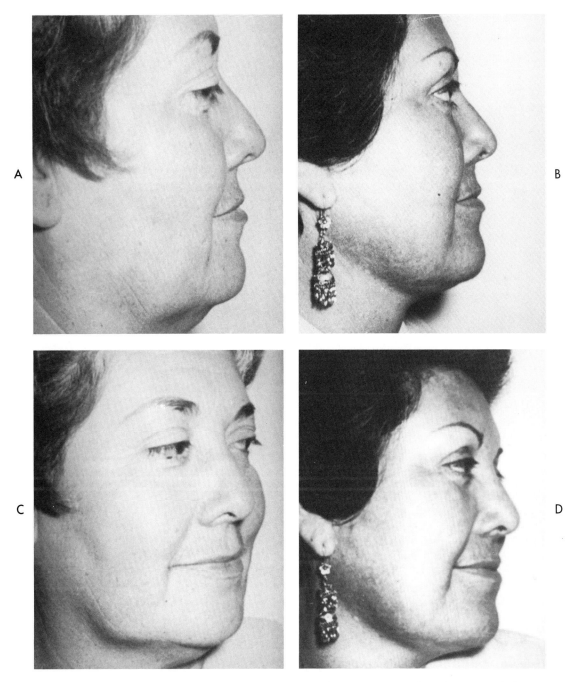

Fig. 3-12 A patient with cervical grade III—type B deformity. I operated on this patient before the advent of liposuction when we had not attempted excision of the buccal fat pad. **A** and **C,** The patient before the cervicofacial rhytidoplasty. Note the redundant facial skin, excess cheek and neck fat, jowl deformity, moderately flaccid platysma, and ptosis of the submandibular gland. **B** and **D,** The patient 3 years after cervical lipectomy, medial plication of the platysma muscle, plication sutures, and SMAS imbrication.

muscle are contraindicated, and more conservative corrective maneuvers should be performed. The secondary deformities that the surgeon can create by radical procedures to the platysma muscle in such patients create an overcorrection resulting in an angular neck with masculine features that give an inappropriate look to women patients. Overcorrection also accentuates a hanging submandibular gland, which becomes even more apparent in such patients. The surgical technique I use with these patients includes an extensive undermining of the cheeks and neck, forming a single cavity in the neck from side to side and radical cervical lipectomy, which can be done with forceps and scissors (Fig. 3-13) or by liposuction (Fig. 13-14). It is advis-

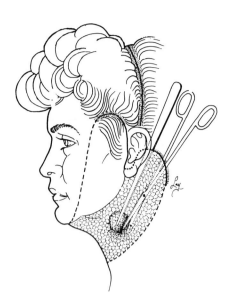

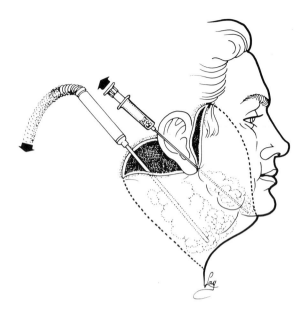

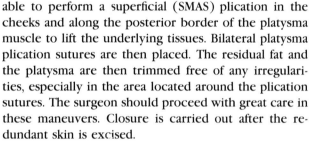

Fig. 3-13 Cervical fat can be removed carefully with scissors and a scalpel.

Fig. 3-14 Cervical fat and fat in the cheeks can also be removed by liposuction.

able to perform a superficial (SMAS) plication in the cheeks and along the posterior border of the platysma muscle to lift the underlying tissues. Bilateral platysma plication sutures are then placed. The residual fat and the platysma are then trimmed free of any irregularities, especially in the area located around the plication sutures. The surgeon should proceed with great care in these maneuvers. Closure is carried out after the redundant skin is excised.

The conservative classical cervicofacial rhytidoplasty removing only skin was commonly performed two decades ago and gave a good immediate result. Within 1 or 2 years however, the results were often disappointing in patients with grades I, II, and III neck deformity or those with severely flaccid cheek tissues. Such results should have been expected because the procedure failed to correct the shift that occurs in relation to the underlying tissues, especially in the areas beyond the limited area of undermining.

To obtain the best result the surgeon must plan the treatment of each patient on an individual basis, first by making an accurate diagnosis. The suggested classification in this chapter may be useful in this respect. The surgeon can use either the classic procedure with skin undermining only in patients with thin cheeks and grade 0 neck-skin redundancy or more modern and sophisticated methods in patients with chubby cheeks and grade I, II, and III neck skin.

I studied two groups of patients in 1979. In group A, I made incisions and undermined the SMAS and the platysma.[4,14,15,31,38] In group B, I only imbricated the SMAS and the platysma as described by Aufricht.[5] The

final results in both groups with regard to the appearance of the neck, cheeks, and jowl were similar over the short and long term. The group that had undermining of the SMAS, however, had two cases of transitory upper-lip paresis. Patient improvement was similar in both groups and after this experience I decided to use only a modification of the Aufricht maneuver, i.e., the simple imbrication of the SMAS and platysma. The complications I[28] and other authors[6] have observed when undermining and sectioning the SMAS and the platysma were much more common than when doing only plications of these structures.

Plastic surgeons now have at their disposal a great many surgical maneuvers for aesthetically improving the face and neck in patients with loose skin or excess fat. Moreover, surgeons should use the maneuvers that work best for them and give the best results. All patients should be studied carefully before surgery and their deformity classified. The surgeon can then plan and carry out the surgical procedures that will result in the best overall improvement in facial appearance.

REFERENCES

1. Adamson JE, Horton CE, and Crawford HH: Surgical correction of the turkey gobbler deformity, Plast Reconstr Surg 34:589, 1964.
2. Appiani E: Observations on cervical rhytidectomy—platysmaplasty, Clin Plast Surg 10:479, 1983.
3. Aston SJ: Platysma muscle in rhytidoplasty, Ann Plast Surg 3:529, 1979.
4. Aston SJ: Platysma—SMAS cervicofacial rhytidoplasty, Clin Plast Surg 10:507, 1983.
5. Aufricht G: Surgery for excess skin of the face. In Transactions of the Second International Congress of Plastic Surgeons, Edinburgh, 1960 E&S Livingstone.

6. Baker DC: Complications of cervicofacial rhytidectomy, Clin Plast Surg 10:543, 1983.

7. Baker TJ: Sectioning and plication of flaccid cervical bands. Presented at the First Congress of the Iberolatin-American Federation of Plastic and Reconstructive Surgery, Quito, Ecuador, 1976.

8. Baker TJ, Gordon HL, and Whitlow DR: Our present technique for rhytidectomy, Plast Reconstr Surg 52:232, 1973.

9. Biggs TM and Koplin L: Concepts of neck lift, Clin Plast Surg 10:367, 1983.

10. Bourguet J: La chirurgie esthetique de la face: les rides, Le Monde Medical 38:41, 1928.

11. Cannon B and Pantazelos HH: W-plasty approach to submandibular lipectomy. In Transactions of the Fifth International Congress of Plastic and Reconstructive Surgeons, Melbourne, 1971, Butterworths.

12. Cardoso de Castro C: Extensive mandibular and cervical lipectomy, Aesth Plast Surg 5:239, 1981.

13. Cardoso de Castro C: The value of anatomical study of the platysma muscle in cervical lifting, Aesth Plast Surg 8:7, 1984.

14. Connell BF: Cervical lifts: the value platysma flaps, Ann Plast Surg 1:34, 1978.

15. Connell BF: Contouring the neck in rhytidectomy by lipectomy and muscle sling, Plast Reconstr Surg 61:376, 1978.

16. Connell BF: Neck contour deformities, Clin Plast Surg 14:683, 1987.

17. Connell BF and Gaon A: Surgical correction of aesthetic contour problems of the Neck, Clin Plast Surg 10:491, 1983.

18. Cronin TD and Biggs TM: The T-Z plasty for the male turkey gobbler neck, Plast Reconstr Surg 47:534, 1971.

19. Ellenbogen R and Karlin JV: Visual criteria for success in restoring the youthful neck, Plast Reconstr Surg 66:826, 1980.

20. Feldman JJ: Corset plastysmoplasty, Plast Reconstr Surg 85:333, 1990.

21. Furnas DW: The restraining ligaments of the cheek, Plast Reconstr Surg 83:11, 1989.

22. Guerrerosantos J et al: Correction of cervicofacial rhytidoplasty, Rev Lat Amer Cir Plast 14:31, 1972.

23. Guerrerosantos J, Morales F, and Spaillat L: Muscular lift in cervical rhytidoplasty, Plast Reconstr Surg 54:127, 1974.

24. Guerrerosantos J: Extensive rhytidoplasty. In Instructional Course Summaries for the Educational Foundation of Plastic and Reconstructive Surgeons, Chicago, 1977.

25. Guerrerosantos J: The role of the platysma muscle in rhytidoplasty, Clin Plast Surg 5:29, 1978.

26. Guerrerosantos J: Surgical correction of the fatty fallen neck, Ann Plast Surg 2:389, 1979.

27. Guerrerosantos J: Simplified surgical technique, refinements, and clinical classification, Clin Plast Surg 10:379, 1983.

28. Guerrerosantos J, Sandoval M, and Salazar J: Long-term study of complications of neck lift, Clin Plast Surg 10:563, 1983.

29. Guy CL, Converse JM, and Morello DC: Aesthetic surgery for the aging face. In Converse JM (ed): Reconstructive Plastic Surgery, ed 2 Philadelphia, 1977, WB Saunders Co.

30. Kaye BL: Facial rejuvenative surgery, New York, 1987, Gower Medical Publishing Ltd.

31. Lemmon ML: Superficial fascia rhytidectomy: a restoration of the SMAS with control of the cervicomental angle, Clin Plast Surg 10:449, 1983.

32. Loeb R: Surgical elimination of the retracted submental fold during double chin correction, Aesth Plast Surg 2:31, 1978.

33. Loeb R: Posterior auricular nerve: preservation, double chin leveling, and earlobe reimplantation during neck lifts, Clin Plast Surg 10:405, 1983.

34. Marchac D and Bourguet J: The pioneer in aesthetic surgery of the neck, Clin Plast Surg 10:363, 1983.

35. Marino H, Galeano EJ, and Gandolfo EA: Plastic correction of the double chin, Plast Reconstr Surg 31:45, 1963.

36. Millard DR, Pigott RW, and Hedo A: Submandibular lipectomy, Plast Reconstr Surg 41:513, 1968.

37. Millard DR, Garst WP, and Beck RL: Submental and submandibular lipectomy in conjunction with a face lift in the male or female, Plast Reconstr Surg 49:385, 1972.

38. Owsley JQ: SMAS—platysma facelift: a bidirectional cervicofacial rhytidectomy, Clin Plast Surg 10:429, 1983.

39. Padgett EC and Stephenson KL: Plastic and reconstructive surgery, Springfield, Ill, 1948, Charles C Thomas.

40. Pennisi VR and Capozzi A: The transposing of fat in cervicofacial rhytidectomy, Plast Reconstr Surg 49:423, 1972.

41. Peterson R: Cervical rhytidoplasty: a personal approach, Presented at the Annual Symposium of Aesthetic Plastic Surgery, Guadalajara, 1974.

42. Skoog T: Plastic surgery: new methods and refinements, Philadelphia, 1974, WB Saunders Co.

43. Snyder GB: Submental rhytidectomy, Plast Reconstr Surg 62:693, 1978.

44. Vistnes LM and Souther SG: The anatomical basis for common cosmetic anterior neck deformities, Ann Plast Surg 2:381, 1979.

45. Vistnes LM and Souther SG: The platysma muscle: anatomic considerations for aesthetic surgery of the anterior neck, Clin Plast Surg 10:441, 1983.

46. Weisman PA: Simplified technique in submental lipectomy, Plast Reconstr Surg 48:443, 1971.

47. Weisman PA: One surgeon's experience with surgical contouring of the neck, Clin Plast Surg 10:521, 1983.

48. Wilkinson T and Swarts BE: Expanded applications of platysma surgery, Clin Plast Surg 10:573, 1983.

CHAPTER 4

Cartilage Grafting

Samuel Stal
David Netscher
Melvin Spira

Cartilage, which is a phylogenetic tissue, is essential to bony skeletal formation in early fetal life. The ability of the human body to regenerate lost cartilage is minimal, since it is usually replaced by fibrous tissue. The three varieties of cartilage include the following[3]:

1. *Hyaline cartilage* has a firm consistency and blue color and tends to calcify with age. The costal, nasal (including septum), tracheobronchial, and xiphoidal are body tissues composed of hyaline cartilage.
2. *Elastic cartilage* comprises a matrix with a network of elastic fibers. The external ears, corniculate cartilages of the larynx, epiglottis, and apices of the arytenoids are examples of elastic cartilage.
3. *Fibrocartilage* has great tensile strength. The intervertebral disks and the articular surfaces of the mandible consist of fibrocartilage.

Cartilage, a specialized form of connective tissue, comprises cells, chondrocytes, and extracellular fibers embedded in an amorphous gellike matrix. Intercellular components predominate over the cells, which are isolated in small lacunae within the matrix. Unlike other connective tissues, cartilage has no primary nerves or blood vessels.[3]

The colloidal properties of its matrix are therefore important to the nutrition of its cells, which survive by passive imbibition from adjacent tissue. Except where it is exposed to the synovial fluid in joints, cartilage is invariably enclosed in dense, well-vascularized fibroconnective tissue called *perichondrium.*[3]

PROPERTIES OF CARTILAGE GRAFTS

Elves[12] noted that cartilage is immunologically protected from the host immune environment by a mucopolysaccharide matrix surrounding the chondrocytes. However, the protein and polysaccharides of cartilage matrix contain at least two measurable antigenic determinants. An immunological response occurs with allograft and xenograft cartilage, but this rejection process is cell mediated locally rather than humorally.[13] Chondrocytes are therefore antigenic but cannot get in contact with lymphocytes because they are surrounded by the weak, antigenic, cartilage matrix, which prevents release of antigens.[6] Exposure of the antigenic chondrocytes and breakdown of the matrix barrier probably explains why crushed allograft is more quickly reabsorbed than block allograft, since the matrix barrier is destroyed in crushed specimens. The protective matrix barrier also explains the slow but nonetheless continuous resorption seen in cartilage allografts. More rapid resorption and greater inflammatory response are seen in xenografts. Preservation of allografts decreases their antigenicity.

Accepted terms for the various grafts include the following:

1. *Autografts* are free grafts that are transferred from one site to another in the same individual.
2. *Allografts* (homografts) are transferred from one site to another of different genetic make-up but within the same species.
3. *Xenografts* (heterografts) are transferred from a member of one species to a member of a different species.
4. *Alloplasts,* "biologically inert" foreign materials, are used for implantation.

Shape, biocompatibility, availability, and minimal donor-site morbidity are important criteria for selecting autologous implant material. The advantages cartilage has over free-bone grafts are as follows:

1. Cartilage is easily carved and shaped.
2. It does not require functional use to retain bulk. Thus survival in both orthotopic and heterotopic sites is essentially the same.
3. Cartilage does not require as vigorous a vascular supply for survival.

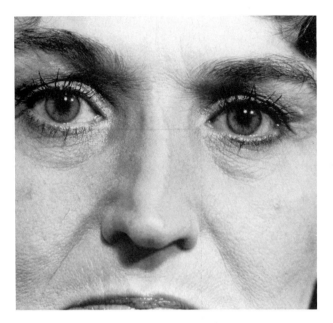

Fig. 4-1 Warping 3 months after insertion of rib-cartilage graft to dorsum.

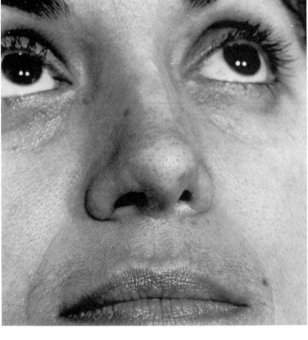

Fig. 4-2 Migration of a dorsal graft placed in a large pocket without fixation.

4. It has a lower absorption rate after implantation.
5. Cartilage is superior for onlay grafting and contour restoration.
6. Several sites have less donor site morbidity (e.g., nasal septum and ear concha).
    However, cartilage grafts have several disadvantages, which include the following:
1. There is a tendency to warp (Fig. 4-1).
2. Cartilage cannot support weight or bear stress.
3. It can migrate (Fig. 4-2).
4. Dissolution is possible, especially if exposed to external pressure or infection.
5. Incidence of infection and exposure is fairly low but is nonetheless a recognized complication.

It is difficult to establish from the literature the true resorption rate of various types of cartilage grafts, since different workers have used different preservatives. In addition, placement of an allograft in the abdominal wall of a rabbit must react differently than allograft placement to restore human facial contour as in the nose. Various methods have also been used to assess cartilage viability.[6] The most commonly used method is simple histological presence or absence of chondrocytes, which can be refined by electron microscopic study to assess the degeneration of intracellular organelles. Craigmyle[7] has also used an autoradiographic method to assess viability. Purified chondroitin sulfate alone will not incorporate SO_4 in vitro, but use of SO_4 is dependent on the presence of living cells and does not occur in cartilage killed by heat or chemicals.[7] The amount of resorption in various studies has been assessed in different ways, from questionnaires to clinical examinations using weight and surface area determinations of removed implants. The latter, however, may be influenced by the amount of soft tissue that adheres to the cartilage graft when it is removed. Despite these variations, review of the literature is included, but the methods of reporting must be considered when judging the results.

HISTORY

Autogenous cartilage grafts were used experimentally by Best in 1865, and its use in humans was reported by Konig in 1896.[2,23] Survival of rib and septal cartilage grafts was demonstrated by Peer in 1911.[35] Gillies was the only investigator before that time who had actually removed a cartilage graft and examined it under a microscope, showing that 18 months after transplantation the cartilage cells and matrix appeared normal.[17] The clinical application of septal grafts was proposed in 1929 by Metzenbaum[28] and has subsequently found more extensive use in rhinoplasty as attested by the impressive results achieved by Aufricht[1] and later by Ortiz-Monasterio et al.

In 1902 Konig[24] reported the first composite auricular graft for nasal reconstruction. In 1912, Joseph[21] described the use of a composite graft from the ala nasi to repair deformities of the contralateral side.

In 1943, Peer[36] described reconstruction of contour depressions using multifaceted diced cartilage. The perichondrial potential for cartilaginous regeneration was first alluded to by Skoog, Ohlsen, and Sohn.[41] Perichondrial small joint arthroplasty has since been described, but generally the regeneration of cartilage from perichondrium in the head and neck region has been clinically unsatisfactory, except in eyelid reconstruction, where the support and rigidity of perichondrocutaneous grafts and newly formed cartilage are beneficial.[4,20] The results of autografts, allografts, and xenografts depend on the methods of preservation.

Use of preserved cartilage

Donald and Col[9] did a national survey on cartilage implantation in head and neck surgery in 1981. Among those using preserved cartilage, alcohol (55%) and Methiolate (20%) were the most common preservatives. There was a similar infection rate between autologous (16%) and preserved cartilage grafts (19%). However, the mean absorption rate for autologous grafts was 23.7%, which was significantly lower than for preserved grafts. Preservation with Methiolate or alcohol resulted in higher overall resorption rates than irradiation.

Viable cartilage seems to undergo less resorption than cartilage in which the chondrocytes are nonviable. Consequently, attempts have been made to effect long-term storage in the viable state. The following box summarizes the methods of storage of viable cartilage.

Long-term storage of residual cartilage is feasible by "banking" the fragments in deep subcutaneous pockets in the postauricular scalp. Cartilage banked this way may retain its form when harvested years later.

Cartilage may survive for up to 72 hours at room temperature and can be stored for longer periods in a viable state at lower temperatures. Thus chondrocytes remain viable for the time it takes to carve an ear during total ear reconstruction. Mikhelson[29] reported that cartilage restored at 4° C retains some metabolic activity for at least 6 weeks. When cooled to below 0° C, the chondrocytes die and do not regenerate. Smill dissected chondrocytes from their matrix and treated them with dimethyl sulfoxide (DMSO). He found that they survived temperatures of 0 to 79° C and reconstituted their matrix after transplantation.[42]

Although viable cartilage is preferred for transplantation, it does have several disadvantages, which include the following:

1. A tendency to warp when removed from preservation.

Storage of the Viable Cartilage

SUBCUTANEOUS POCKET "BANKED" CARTILAGE

Room temperature
Refrigeration
Dimethyl sulfoxide

Methods of Cartilage Preservation

Alcohol
Methiolate
Irradiation
Antibiotic solutions
Freeze-drying (lyophilization)
Formalin
Aqueous zephiran
Cialit
Freezing

---

2. Temporal limitations of storage in a viable state.
3. Limited availability when large amounts are needed.
4. Donor-site morbidity when autogenous cartilage is used.

Preservation generally kills the chondrocytes but may have the advantage of decreasing the antigenicity of allograft material. Several methods have been devised for preserving cartilage indefinitely (see box above).

Cartilage xenografts have traditionally been deemed inferior to both autografts and allografts because they are capable of evoking an immunological reaction even after preservation and extraction, leading to excessive resorption. In 1947, Wardill and Swinney[44] described the use of bovine cartilage preserved in Methiolate.[25] In 1951, Gillies and Kristensen[18] published their experiences with 144 of these grafts. Of these, 22 "minced" grafts were found to be totally unsatisfactory. Patients were followed for up to 2½ years, and solid grafts were found to be satisfactory in 95% of cases involving the nose, 50% involving the ear, and 80% involving other facial sites. Gibson and Davis published their own reservations about the survival of preserved bovine cartilage and, in a series of 205 solid preserved bovine cartilage grafts, became totally disenchanted with the use of xenografts. They wrote, "Though the early results may appear promising, the chances of later disappointment for both patient and surgeon are such that the use of bovine cartilage as a routine material for the restoration of contour should be discontinued."[16] Recent developments may, however, discourage the use of homografts and suggest a return to xenografts, especially with recent reports of transmissible diseases in stored graft materials. Ersek reports both animal and clinical studies in which bovine cartilage was prepared by combined irradiation and chemical cross-linking.[14] This results in stabilization of the collagen molecule, making it antigenically inert and dimensionally stable. He reported on 28 patients, who were followed for up to 3 years with no evidence of cellular reaction or resorption, provided the procedure was not complicated by infection.

The use of stored allografts is currently more common than the use of xenografts.[9] Cadaver cartilage should be harvested within 24 hours of death, and donors should be under 40 years old because hyaline cartilage ossifies after that time. They should be free of malignant disease and infections, especially syphilis and acquired immune deficiency syndrome (AIDS). The lyophilization technique has been developed under the direction of Sailer.[38] It is known that fast freezing erythrocytes with liquid nitrogen results in an 80% cell survival rate. However, if protective solutions are added, slow freezing yields an even larger number of viable cells. The most commonly used protective solution for blood storage is glycerine. Tissue thickness should not exceed 1 mm or the cells will be destroyed by freezing. Therefore it is technically possible to use deep freezing to preserve the viability of large portions of tissues but may be undesirable, since foreign tissue increases the risk of rejection. The freeze-dried lyophilized material is stored in vacuum containers at room temperature. The major advantage of freeze drying is that the material is not temperature sensitive and can be stored for almost an unlimited period. The material is rehydrated before use simply by placing it in distilled water or Ringer's solution that preferably contains antibiotics. We use 1 million units of penicillin G and 2 gm of streptomycin per liter. Lyophilized cartilage grafts have an extremely low infection rate. This may be due to the use of antibiotics in the rehydration solution. The infection rate reported by Kole[22] using Methiolate was 6% and for preserved refrigerated cartilage, 4.3%. The overall incidence of infectious complications in his Zurich clinic was only 2.7%. It appears that dried lyophilized cartilage is capable of absorbing large amounts of antibiotics from the hydration solution. For this reason, cartilage grafts for malar contouring inserted using external or intraoral incisions show no difference in the rate of infection. The extent of resorption with lyophilized or deep-frozen cartilage is reported to be 20%, requiring some overcorrection in clinical cases.[22]

Methiolate preservation is accomplished by placing the graft in a solution of one part aqueous Methiolate (1:1000) to four parts normal saline and then refrigerating at 4° C. The solution is changed twice weekly for 2 weeks and then weekly. The graft is good for up to 2 years. Before implantation, the graft is washed in normal saline solution to remove the Methiolate. Muhlbauer, Schmidt-Tintemann, and Glaser[30] used homologous rib cartilage preserved in Methiolate for correction of saddle-nose deformity. There was no evidence of resorption in 75% of cases, moderate absorption was seen in 20%, and 5% had almost total resorption. The majority of implants demonstrated progressive calcification, beginning at about 1 year after insertion. Rasi[37] reported that in long-term follow-up, Methiolate-preserved cartilage showed sufficient loss of bulk in 13.6% of cases, giving a poor result.

Meanwhile, in Glasgow, McGlynn and Sharpe[27] had developed Cialit cartilage preservation. Cialit is an organic mercurial compound that has good bactericidal and fungicidal properties with low toxicity. Unlike Merthiolate, it is not light sensitive and has less risk of losing its efficacy. The cartilage is placed in a 1:1000 Cialit solution for 24 hours and then transferred to Cialit 1:5000. Cartilage and preserving solution are refrigerated at 4° C and the solution changed every 6 weeks. Frequent samples are taken for bacteriological examination. The cartilage is washed in sterile saline solution before use. Good clinical results were reported in 80% of cases.

Sterilization

Dingman and Grabb[8] developed a method of sterilizing human cartilage by exposure to 3,000,000 rads of gamma radiation from a cobalt source. The technique involves sealing the cartilage in a glass jar in saline and placing it in a Cobalt source for 15 hours. The cartilage may then be stored in the sealed jar of saline at room temperature. Lynch, Ashbury, and Dingman[25] compared irradiated cartilage and Methiolate preserved cartilage in a dog model. Their study indicated that irradiated cartilage had significantly less absorption than Methiolate-sterilized cartilage. It is believed that cartilage preserved in Methiolate, alcohol, or formalin may cause a more pronounced local tissue reaction that increases the rate of absorption when compared with tissue stored in isotonic saline. Sterilization by irradiation not only renders the tissue immunologically inert, but, with storage in saline, there is less chance of local reaction after implantation. Schuller, Bardach, and Krause[39] reported the results of a 3-year study of 145 implants of irradiated homologous costal cartilage used in facial contour restoration. The overall infection rate was 4.1%. There was no statistically significant difference in

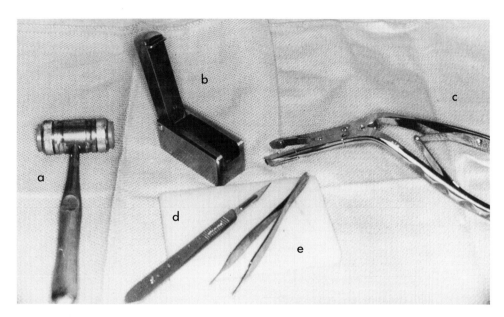

Fig. 4-3 The instruments used to modify cartilage. *a*, Mallet; *b*, Cottle bone crusher; *c*, Ruben morselizer *d*, no. 11 blade *e*, Brown Addison Forceps.

the rate of infection for implants inserted intraorally onto the maxilla from the rate for the entire series. The partial resorption rate was only 1.4% and the frequency of the graft loss only 2.8%. Lynch, Ashbury, and Dingman[8,25] reported on 600 patients over a 15-year period, using irradiated cartilage with overall excellent results.

Prevention of warping

One of the reasons that cartilage allografts and xenografts were preferred during the 1940s and 1950s was that preserved cartilage in which the chondrocytes were killed did not have a tendency to warp. Some workers believed that the effect of warping could be overcome if all the perichondrium were removed.[17,39] They found that if fresh autogenous cartilage was carved so that the perichondrium remained on one side only, the graft would curve toward that side and it was the perichondrium that acted like a bowstring. Despite wide adoption of this principle, fresh autogenous cartilage continued to behave unpredictably. Thus although dead cartilage was known to undergo inevitable, slow dissolution, it was still favored over autogenous cartilage.

Gibson and Davis[15,16] finally resolved the issue of warping. These workers came to two important conclusions. The first was that when warping occurred, it was an early phenomenon. In the majority of patients, it occurred within just 10 days of implantation and in most of the remaining within 3 months. The second more significant finding was that it was not the peri-

chondrium that was important but the outer layer of cartilage. Only the outer layers that contain flattened chondrocytes bend when carved. They compared rib cartilage with a "tight-skinned sausage" and described four basic "balanced cross-sections" for carving cartilage that would prevent warping[15]:

1. Intact surface layer surrounding the cartilage.
2. Surface layers removed from two opposite sides, leaving the remainder balanced.
3. Surface layers removed from all four sides.
4. Cartilage removed from only one side of the rib graft, leaving a deep "D." At least one half of the cross-section may be removed before bending occurs.

Another method of obtaining a balanced cross-section, especially when using conchal ear cartilage, is to cross-hatch the curved part. Cross-hatching may also be used when the objective is to induce a curvature to the opposite side (Fig. 4-3).

A third way to overcome warping when using autogenous ear cartilage is simply to roll the cartilage like a cigarette and stitch it in position. This not only prevents warping, but also enables conchal cartilage to provide more rigid support, as when used for a columellar strut graft.

Survival of cartilage grafts

Having already established that dispensing with the outer layers of cartilage helps overcome the difficulty of warping, there remains the problem of whether intact perichondrium may play a role in actual cartilage

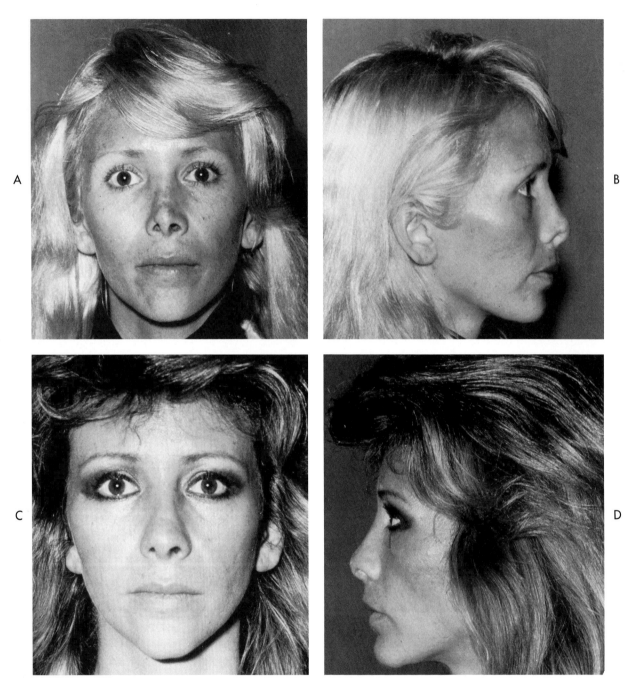

Fig. 4-4   A patient who had multiple previous rhinoplasties. She underwent nasal reconstruction using composite cartilage grafts covered with temporalis fascia. **A,** Preoperative AP view; **B,** preoperative lateral view; **C,** postoperative AP view after 1 year; **D,** postoperative lateral view after 1 year.

survival. This debate, at least as far as elastic cartilage is concerned, seems to have been settled by Zalzal, Cotton, and McAdams.[46] They found good survival of autograft elastic cartilage in a study on New Zealand rabbits. There was similarity in survival between bare cartilage and perichondrial-covered cartilage, either one-sided or two-sided, proving that perichondrium did not have either a beneficial or detrimental effect on graft survival. They were unable to determine if perichondrium had a protective role against infection. Growth of transplanted autogenous cartilage has been shown to occur in both the perichondrial level, as well as within the cartilage matrix.[11] Zalzal, Cotton, and McAdams[45] did not believe the neochondrogenic potential was significant enough for dependable clinical use.

The use of diced or crushed cartilage has been well described by Peer.[36] His studies were stimulated by the observation that intact rib cartilage used for forehead reconstruction often produced a corrugated effect. He then used crushed cartilage to reconstruct facial defects to give a smoother contour. He found that the cells in crushed autologous cartilage remained viable and that there was complete absence of invasion or absorption. However, when preserved allografts were used, the diced cartilage grafts showed definite invasion and partial absorption.[36]

Breadon, Kern, and Neel[5] similarly found that chondrocytes in crushed cartilage remained viable, while osteocytes in crushed bone did not remain viable. They also found crushed cartilage to be very suitable for subcutaneous augmentation. Thus perichondrium is not required for maintenance of cartilage graft viability. Gunter[19] has used diced autologous cartilage to correct enophthalmos. He described a method of using a trochar and cannula to introduce the crushed cartilage. This is obviously used only in patients with a blind eye or an exophthalmic prosthesis. A small incision is made in the inferior orbital margin and a subperiosteal route then dissected along the orbital floor to introduce the trochar into the orbital apex. Cartilage fragments can then be easily introduced down the cannula. Migration of the graft material has not been a problem with this technique.

Crushed allografts do, however, undergo significant resorption. It appears that intact perichondrium does play an important role in decreasing the immunogenicity of allograft cartilage and therefore decreases the amount of resorption. Another disadvantage is that crushed allograft cartilage stimulates the immune response, resulting in an increased fibrous reaction. Grafts placed in superficial locations, such as in a rhinoplasty, may form visible lumps.

An additional layer of tissue, such as temporalis fascia or lyophilized dura, has been used to wrap cartilage grafts. This helps smooth the graft contour and may be useful in secondary rhinoplasty cases where the dorsal nasal skin is particularly thin (Fig. 4-4). Palpable step-off deformities may be avoided by beveling the graft edges with a fine blade or by gentle morselization with the teeth of a Brown-Adson forceps.[14]

CARTILAGE GRAFTING TECHNIQUES
Fixation

It is important to properly fix cartilage grafts to minimize their dislodgement. Autogenous tissue becomes incorporated, unlike smooth, synthetic materials such as silicone, which become surrounded by a capsule. Late migration is unlikely to occur if the initial fixation is secure. Tardy, Denneny, and Fritsch[43] avoid suturing implants and advocate dissecting precise subcutaneous pockets. If the host pocket is too small, however, it can distort the implant, whereas one that is too large may allow the graft to shift. Accurately mark the extent of the pocket on the external skin before anesthetic infiltration. Sheen also emphasizes accurate placement of the pocket for columellar-tip grafts to achieve maximal nasal tip projection.[40] Peck[34] uses an absorbable suture through the skin to hold cartilage grafts in place and often sutures two or more pieces of cartilage together when doing complex onlay grafting procedures.

Tissue glues, which look promising, are another way to achieve cartilage fixation. Cyanoacrylates, in particular histoacryl R, have been used in experimental animals without demonstrable cartilage damage or local tissue toxicity.[7] We have used this method to secure cartilage for onlay nasal tip and maxillary grafting with good initial success. Autologous blood must be obtained 5 days before surgery to accumulate sufficient fibrin to produce the tissue glue. Pooled autograft thrombin commonly used in Europe has not been cleared by the FDA in this country.

Common donor sites

Donor-site sources will vary depending on the degree of the deformity and the patient's individual history (previous surgery, age, trauma). Each site has its own advantages and disadvantages, as well as particular morbidity. The costal chondral rib cartilage, concha of the ear, and nasal septum are the most commonly used donor sites.

Rib cartilage

Rib cartilage is a favored donor site when large quantities of graft material are required. This is often the case when performing augmentation of maxillary hypoplasia, total ear reconstruction, or major nasal reconstruction. The seventh, eighth, and ninth ribs are

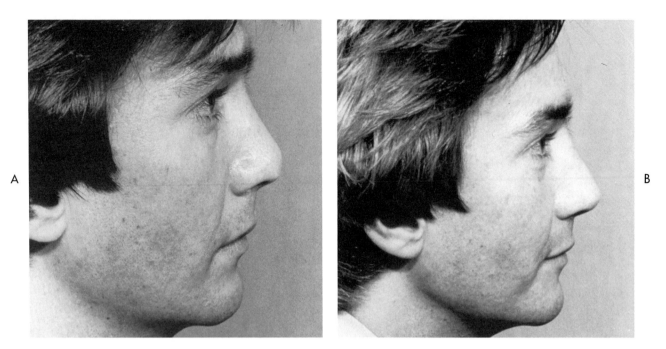

Fig. 4-5 A patient who had onlay tip grafting to improve tip projection. **A,** Preoperative view; **B,** postoperative view after 1 year.

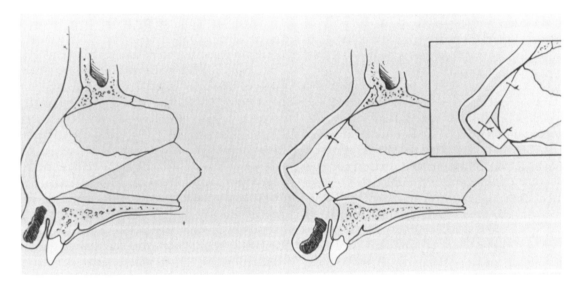

Fig. 4-6 Solid pieces of rib cartilage were used to augment the premaxilla.

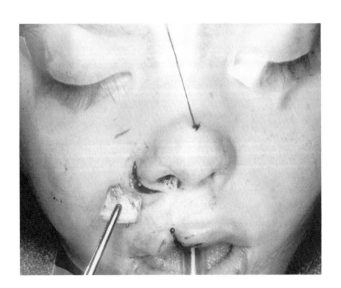

Fig. 4-7 A patient with residual nasal deformity after bilateral cleft-lip repair, including a depressed septum. Figures on right show reconstruction with cartilage grafts extending the septum to maintain support and increase projection.

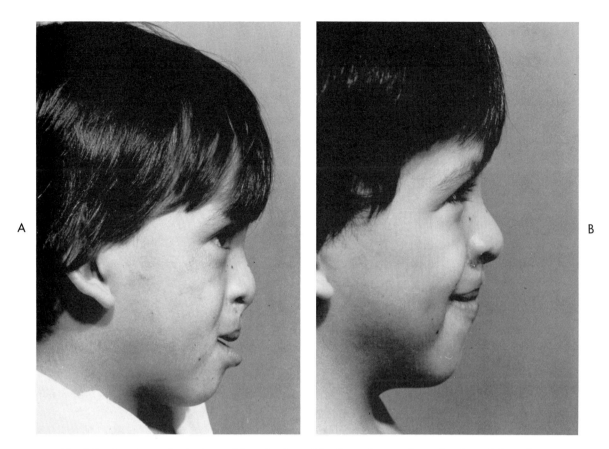

Fig. 4-8 A patient who had septal lengthening with rib-cartilage grafts at the time of the soft tissue columella lengthening procedure. **A,** Preoperative view of a 4-year-old child with bilateral cleft; **B,** postoperative view at 9 months.

easily accessed through a modified inframammary incision. This cartilage is the rigid hyaline type and is especially useful in maintaining support to the tip of the nose and for large onlay grafts to the maxilla. Careful selection of the appropriate recipient shape is necessary to compensate for the stresses inherent within the cartilage and to minimize the problems of warping when the cartilage is carved or shaped. The seventh rib cartilage is relatively straight and is appropriate for nasal dorsum augmentation, while the eighth is slightly curved and ideal for use as a malar maxillary onlay. The large amount of cartilage in this area makes it an ideal donor site in patients whose cartilage is not available or has already been used from other sources. This is also an acceptable donor site in a growing child, where harvesting septal cartilage would be unacceptable.

Rib cartilage is the graft of choice and should be used when rigid support is desired such as maintaining tip elevation with a columellar strut. Patients with a severe bilateral cleft lip often have a depressed, tethered nasal tip with absence of the nasal spine and caudal septum. Rib cartilage can be fashioned to extend the

septum after soft-tissue-columella lengthening (Fig. 4-6). The addition of cartilage helps support the tip and results in a more favorable environment for normal growth and development. Solid pieces of rib cartilage are ideal for patients with good occlusion but who have maxillary hypoplasia. They are superior to smaller plumping grafts in this area (Fig. 4-7). Bone grafts placed on the anterior maxilla undergo marked resorption, while the cartilage grafts maintain reasonable size and form.

Many people avoid this technique because with increased operative time, a large and unsightly scar, and the potential morbidity of a pneumothorax it seems like a lot of work. These objections may be true, especially when near total removal of the rib chondral cartilage is necessary such as for an ear reconstruction. However, by modifying the technique, adequate amounts of cartilage can be harvested in a safe, effective manner with minimal complications. We have used this donor site over the past 4 years in approximately 150 cases when more cartilage was needed than we could safely obtain from the nose or ear. The

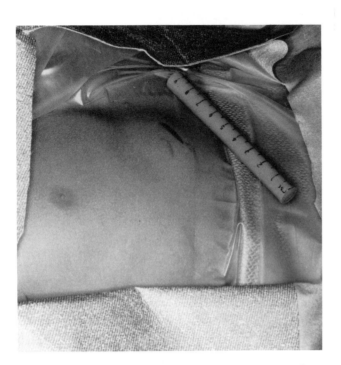

Fig. 4-9   Access incision to harvesting ventral portion of the rib cartilage at the anterior border of the costal-chondral junction.

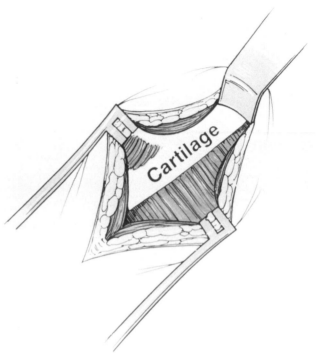

Fig. 4-10   Schematic drawing showing self-retaining retractor helping to achieve access to the cartilage.

patients ranged in age from 2 to 60, with the majority having a cleft lip or craniofacial or traumatic facial deformity (Fig. 4-8).

Surgical technique

The cartilage can be approached through a small 3- to 4- cm oblique incision directly over the seventh and eighth cartilaginous ribs, approximately 6 cm from the midline (Fig. 4-9). This is safely done with minimal disturbance of the underlying rectus muscle while a second surgeon simultaneously dissects a soft-tissue pocket in the face. Rib access is made easier by using a self-retaining retractor, with one assistant moving the retractor to facilitate exposure (Fig. 4-10). The parietal pleura is intimately attached to the deep or ventral perichondrium. It is therefore easier to remove subtotal portions of the rib cartilage, including the anterior or dorsal perichondrium. A no. 66 Beaver blade is useful to create a right-angle cut and helps dissect only the outer or ventral three fourths of the cartilage (Fig. 4-11). The appropriate amount of cartilage is removed, and the wound closed anatomically in three layers without the use of a drain. A light pressure dressing is applied.

The cartilage has already been sheared of its dorsal perichondrium and the ventral or anterior layer is then removed using a no. 11 blade. The middle portion, which is relatively straight, is then used for the shaft

(Fig. 4-12). The removed shavings make excellent filler for soft-tissue defects. They can also be used as onlay grafts for the alar cartilages because they assume a configuration and thickness similar in appearance. These shavings, when crushed in the Cottle bone crusher, also make an excellent overlay for camouflage. Large pieces can be used relatively unmodified in static areas such as the premaxilla, by feathering the edges to improve contour. The Cottle bone crusher or the Rubin morselizer are useful instruments to help shape the cartilage grafts.

We have experienced the most difficulty when rib cartilage was used to graft a large area on the nasal dorsum. Even after complete cross-sectional carving of relatively straight middle portions, we have found early warping of large grafts to be the rule rather than the exception. We routinely use cranial or rib-bone grafts for patients with severe hypoplasia or saddle-nose deformity. Bone grafts are placed in intimate contact with the proximal nasal bone and fixed with interosseous wires. Cartilage grafts can be used to enhance the bony nasal reconstruction by augmenting and increasing tip projection and allowing the creation of a contoured double break and supratip concavity. The subtotal approach of harvesting rib cartilage takes approximately 20 to 25 minutes to obtain the graft and close the wound. Unused cartilage may be banked in the original wound. Postoperative discomfort in our series was

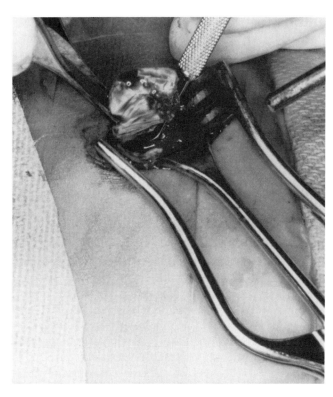

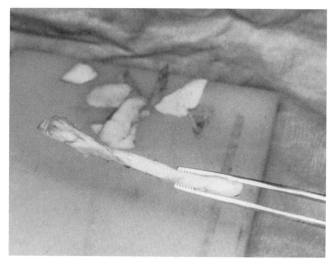

Fig. 4-12 Example of using the midline portion of the cartilage to achieve the straightest piece possible.

Fig. 4-11 Use of a right-angle Beaver blade to remove the ventral surface of the cartilage only.

minimal, with no evidence of hematoma. This is significant, since 46 of our patients were 5 years old or younger. All scars seen were acceptable, and there were no cases of pneumothorax when the subtotal approach was used. Removing a full-thickness piece of rib cartilage increases postoperative pain and the chances of complications.

Septum

There is often residual cartilage after a reduction rhinoplasty from the caudal and dorsal septum resection, as well as the cephalic alar cartilage margins. The surgeon cannot rely on these areas as a primary source because the amount of cartilage that can be obtained is often unpredictable or lacks rigidity. Septal cartilage, on the other hand, remains an excellent anatomical area for graft harvesting. Generous amounts may be harvested from the quadrangular cartilage posterior to an imaginary line connecting the osteocartilaginous junction with the nasal spine without jeopardizing septal support. Care must be taken to preserve at least a 1- to 1.5-cm strut of dorsal and caudal margins to maintain a supporting structure. Sufficient amounts may be conservatively removed during a primary rhinoplasty to create a reasonable onlay dorsal graft (4 × 1 cm) and tip grafts (0.1 × cm). A review of the operative re-

port for patients who have had a previous septoplasty might give some clue as to the extent of the septal resection that was performed. The patient must understand that cartilage may have to be obtained from another source if it is not available in the septum.

The nasal septum is composed of the rigid hyaline cartilage and is ideally suited for use as a graft in the nose. A large (4 × 1 cm) fusiform-shaped graft can be modified to distend the skin and create the illusion of a straight smooth dorsum. This is especially helpful after a reduction rhinoplasty to help restore dorsal continuity by covering the open roof and overlying any irregularities. In some cases, it can be used flat after modifying or feathering the edges. The overlying skin thins over time, exposing any edges that were left too sharp. Accurate placement and fixation is essential to minimize movement. A groove can be cut in the posterior or ventral side of the cartilage, causing it to bend into an A or a U shape as described by Gunter,[19] which is compatible with the patient's own aesthetic lines and dorsal nasal width. It is sometimes helpful to introduce these grafts with a suture that is brought out through the skin with a large Keith needle. The suture may be left in place for another week, tied over a Telfa bolster to help maintain the graft in position.

Cartilage can also be used to create tension on the overlying skin in patients with a rounded, drooping, or poorly defined nasal tip. Increased nasal-tip projection can be achieved by placing the graft over the lower lateral cartilages along the most anterior leading edge. This cartilage must be shaped and placed carefully into a predetermined position. The rectangular-shaped Peck graft increases tip projection by suturing two or more pieces of cartilage together.[34] The larger shield or

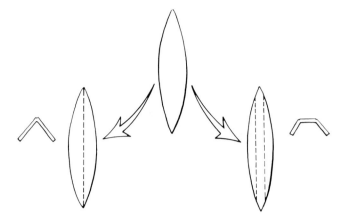

Fig. 4-13 Example of Jack Gunter's dorsal onlay with incision through anterior surface to simulate a more natural dorsum. *Left,* An A-frame graft; *right,* U-frame graft. The U-frame graft may be performed with two or three incisions and maintains a nice tension simulating a natural appearance.

Sheen graft is placed in a slightly different plane, not only enhancing projection, but creating aesthetic high points for definition[40] (Fig. 4-14).

The septal cartilage, accessed through a transfixation incision, is also a good source of sturdy material to act as a batton or strut in the columella. This can be inserted in a retrograde fashion through the transfixion incision and placed between the feet of the medial crura. The strut can also be simply inserted through a small labial-sulcus stab incision after creating a midline pocket. This is a helpful technique, used **not** to *create* projection, but to *maintain* it. It is ideally suited for patients with a lack of tip support, as commonly seen in the cleft nose, the noncaucasian nose, and the older patient with tip laxity.

The ideal material to correct an acute nasolabial angle is rib cartilage. However, when only a small amount of augmentation is necessary, layered pieces of septal cartilage will allow a modest volume increase in this area. The strut may also be anchored to the septum to augment the retruded or "hanging columella." Composite grafts have historically been taken from this area, but with the paucity of lining primary closure is difficult and should be considered only rarely.

Surgical technique

First, the mucosa is topically anesthetized using cotton saturated with 4 ml of 4% cocaine. Zylocaine (0.5%) and 1:100,000 units of epinephrine are then injected using a 25-gauge, 2½-inch needle with the bevel end down. The local anesthetic should be injected into the subperichondrial plane, forcing the fluid to hydraulically separate the perichondrium from the cartilage. It is possible to elevate the mucosa from the entire area of dissection without risk of ischemic necrosis. The subperichondrial plane is identified by using a sharp Cottle elevator, an excellent instrument for beginning the dissection. A blunt-edged Freer elevator is then used for the remainder of the dissection to prevent perforation of the mucoperichondrial flap. It is helpful to first dissect from anterior to posterior, then sweep posteriorly, dissecting forward under direct vision. The mucoperichondrium is bluntly teased away while cutting the decussating fibers found along the anterior inferior borders of the septum and vomer. The mucosa is elevated on the contralateral side only from the graft to be removed. This can be achieved by placing the fifth digit of the left hand in the contralateral nostril to exert stabilizing pressure. The cartilage is cut with a scalpel and the blunt end of an elevator used to further transect the cartilage without going through the mucosa on the other side. The septal cartilage can be removed separately or in conjunction with the perpendicular plate of the ethmoid using a serrated cartilage scissors. The mucosal flaps must be carefully delineated with a Freer elevator before removing the cartilaginous segment to avoid perforation. Interrupted mattress sutures of 4-0 plain catgut help hold the mucoperichondrial flaps together and close the incisions. This is necessary to avoid a septal hematoma by closing the dead space. The use of Teflon or Silicone septal splints (Xomed) are also an excellent way to apply additional gentle pressure to co-apt the mucoperichondrial flaps, as well as to maintain septal support.

External ear

The external ear cartilage is the elastic type and is somewhat different from the hyaline cartilage found in the nose and rib. A sturdy graft can be created to give effective form and support by appropriate carving or sculpting, stacking of the cartilage, or simply rolling the cartilage on itself.[34,40] As long as the antihelical fold is not transgressed, minimal changes occur in the ultimate appearance of the ear even after removal of the entire cymba and cavum concha. Cartilage graft segments of up to 4 cm long can be obtained from one ear. The precise area of the ear to be used as the graft donor site should be selected to resemble as much as possible the recipient part to be reconstructed. The curved concha, with slight modification, resembles the lower lateral cartilage but is too thin to be used as a columella strut without appropriate layering. Single pieces of cartilage are best used as camouflage or overlay grafts. If these grafts are to be used for support, then multiple layers must be used. It is difficult to create a large dorsal graft that will maintain its shape using ear cartilage. The ear should be considered a second-

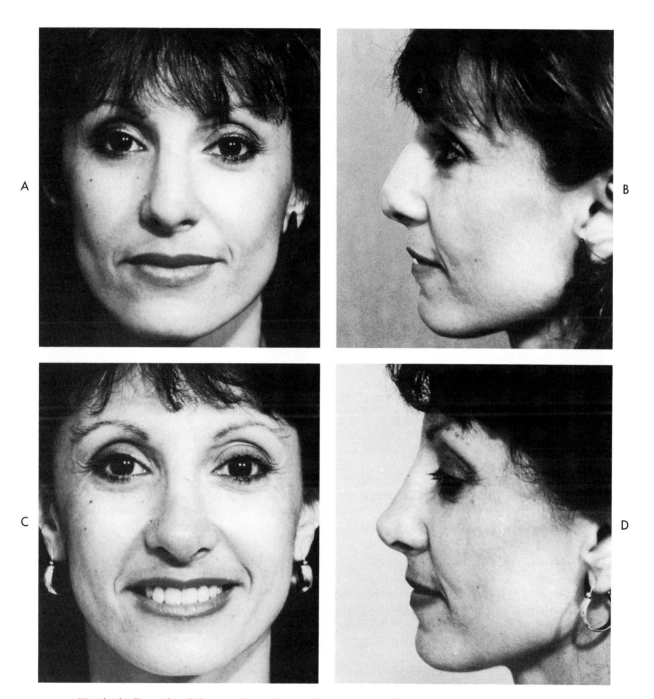

Fig. 4-14 Example of Sheen onlay grafts to achieve improved lines of the nose and increased tip projection. **A,** Preoperative AP view; **B,** preoperative lateral view showing blunted tip with loss of projection and aesthetic contours; **C,** 1 year after surgery with multiple layer Sheen graft both solid and crushed; **D,** postoperative lateral view 1 year later.

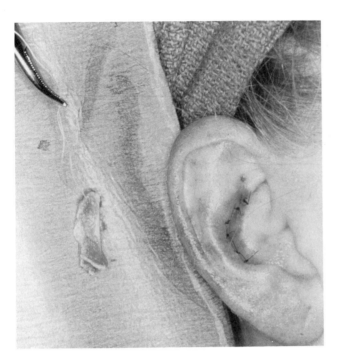

Fig. 4-15 Harvesting cartilage from the anterior surface of the ear.

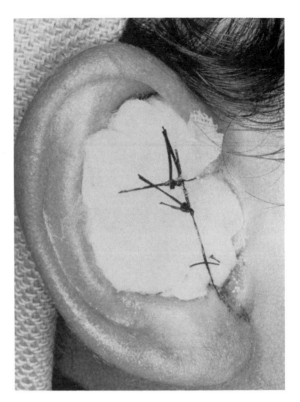

Fig. 4-16 Simple bolster tie over dressing using Vaseline gauze and an eye pad.

ary donor site for this purpose. Ear cartilage is probably more important for filling in small contour irregularities and as filler or camouflage overlay grafts in conjunction with larger septal grafts.

It is important when harvesting grafts from the ear to minimize oral and nasal contamination by using separate instruments and changing gloves when dissecting the ear. This decreases the chances of developing a donor-site wound infection.

Surgical technique

Grafts can be easily harvested through an anterior or posterior incision. When the maximum amount of cartilage is needed, an anterior incision placed at the base of the antihelix is preferred (Fig. 4-15). The anterior skin and underlying soft tissue are infiltrated with 0.5% lidocaine and epinephrine. The incision is carried down to a subperiosteal plane separating the anterior perichondrium from the cartilage. This helps preserve at least one layer of the perichondrium to maintain support in the donor site. The Cottle elevator is a useful instrument with which to elevate the perichondrium from the cartilage. The cartilage is then incised full thickness through and through, including the posterior perichondrium over the proposed area of resection. A Brown-Adson forceps is useful to grasp the cartilage and avoid a traumatic laceration. After meticu-

lous hemotasis is achieved, the skin is reapproximated with a 6-0 plain suture. A pressure dressing is applied to compress the ear and prevent accumulation of fluid. Mini-flap drains and mastoid dressings work well, but a simple bolster type of dressing using vaseline gauze and 2-0 silk sutures can be used for 3 to 5 days and is more tolerable to the patient (Fig. 4-16). The anterior scar in most patients is generally obscured in the shadow at the base of the antihelix.

Ear cartilage can also be accessed through a posterior incision (Fig. 4-17). This is ideal when small pieces are needed for onlay grafting. The natural curvature of the concha makes it an excellent choice for obtaining multiple small onlay grafts for the tip or nasal dorsum.

The ear remains the primary donor site for composite grafts of skin and cartilage. These grafts are ideal for correcting defects of the eyelid, nasal lining, and alar rim. Grafts as large as 2 × 1.5 cm can be removed safely from the root of the helix or concha and still achieve primary donor-site closure.

If excess cartilage is removed, it can be banked beneath the hair-bearing skin in the postauricular area. A small area of scalp is shaved, and a 1-cm incision is made to develop a superficial pocket, and, the wound is closed with a 4-0 plain catgut. This is helpful in cases of secondary and tertiary reconstruction.[41] Rib carti-

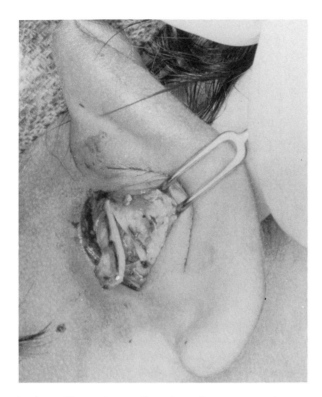

Fig. 4-17 Harvesting cartilage through a posterior skin incision.

I. Nose
   A. Dorsum
      1. Saddle-nose
      2. Contouring
      3. Spreader grafts (Fig. 4-18)
      4. Noncaucasian nose
   B. Tip
      1. Onlay and tip projection
   C. Columella
      1. Strut grafts
      2. Contouring
   D. Nasolabial angle (plumping) (Fig. 4-19)
   E. Alar contouring
   F. Nasofrontal angle
   G. Septal perforations
   H. Composite grafts for full-thickness defects of alae, upper lateral cartilages, columella
II. Eye
   A. Orbital repair
      1. Orbital augmentation
      2. Orbital floor for enophthalmos and blow-out fractures
      3. Tarsal plate repair and full-thickness lid defects using composite grafts
III. Tracheal repair
IV. Total ear reconstruction
 V. Ear ossicles
VI. Malar and facial contouring
VII. Joint replacement

lage can also be banked in its original position without making an additional incision.

Additional sources

Finally, various methods have been attempted to reconstruct hyaline articular cartilage.[10,11,26,31] Nonvascularized, autoplastic, total-joint transfer has been performed experimentally in dogs. The joint cartilage in adult animals generally necroses, producing a charcot joint. Cryopreservation of osteochondral grafts has also had only mixed success. The bone regenerates, but the cartilage undergoes degeneration, especially when weightbearing is initiated. The results of small joint reconstruction by perichondrial arthroplasty, demonstrating the potential for perichondrial cartilage regeneration, was initially reported with some enthusiasm by Skoog, Ohlsen, and Sohn.[42] However, the results cannot equal those achieved by total joint replacement using alloplastic material.

The temporomandibular joint (TMJ) has also received attention by workers attempting to use autogenous material. Successful treatment of TMJ ankylosis was reported in a child, using an osteochondral-iliac-crest graft fixed to the zygomatic portion of the temporal bone. Rib osteochondral grafts have been used in severe forms of hemifacial microsomia to restore mandibular continuity and TMJ congruity.[26,31]

Autogenous cartilage remains a versatile material for facial augmentation. Careful preoperative planning and sound basic surgical techniques yield good results when used appropriately. Additional time spent in harvesting the appropriate graft minimizes morbidity both in the donor and the recipient site. Problems of warping, displacement, infection, and extrusion can be minimized by careful attention to detail.

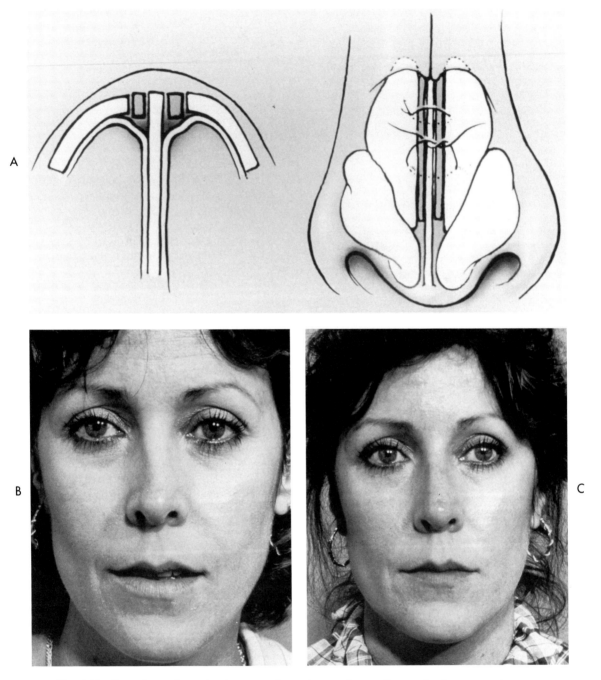

Fig. 4-18   Spreader graft used to improve airway by opening up the nasal valve area or to reposition the collapsed middle vault. **A,** Schematic showing placement of spreader graft; **B,** Preoperative patient status after rhinoplasty with nasal middle vault collapse on inspiration and
concavity in the right middle side; **C,** Postoperative position spreader graft on the left side.

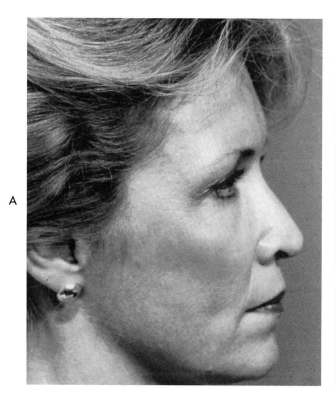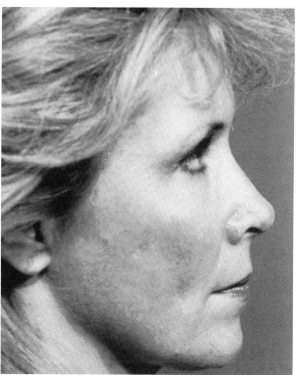

Fig. 4-19 Example of cartilage graft to nasal labial fold to increase the angle and give a more youthful look. **A,** Preoperative AP view; **B,** postoperative view 1 year later.

REFERENCES

1. Aufricht G: Rhinoplasty and the face, Plast Reconstr Surg 43:219, 1969.
2. Best P: Sur la greffe animal, Compt Rend Acad DSC 61:587, 1865.
3. Bloom W and Fawcett DW: A textbook of histology ed 9, Philadelphia, 1968, WB Saunders Co.
4. Brent B and Oh R: Perichondro-cutaneous graft, Plast Reconstr Surg 62:1, 1978.
5. Breadon GE, Kern EB, and Neel HB: Autografts of uncrushed and crushed bone and cartilage, Arch Otolaryngol 105:75, 1979.
6. Craigmyle MBL: Antigenicity and survival of cartilage homografts, Nature (London) 182:1248, 1958.
7. Craigmyle MBL: An autoradiographic and histochemical study of long-term cartilage grafts in the rabbit, J Anat 2:467, 1958.
8. Dingman RD and Grabb WC: Costal cartilage homografts preserved by irradiation, Plast Reconstr Surg 28:562, 1961.
9. Donald PJ and Col A: Cartilage implantation in head and neck surgery: report of a national survey, Otolaryngol Head Neck Surg 90:85, 1982.
10. Dupurtuis SM: Actual growth of young cartilage transplants in rabbits, Arch Surg 41:32, 1941.
11. Eisemann ML: The growth potential of autograft cartilage, Arch Otolaryngol 109:469, 1983.
12. Elves MW: Newer knowledge of the immunology of bone and cartilage, Clin Orthop 13:44, 1984.
13. Erdelyi R: Experimental autotransplantation of small joints, Plast Reconstr Sur 31:129, 1963.
14. Ersek RA, Rothenberg PB, and Denton DR: Clinical use of an improved processed bovine cartilage for contour defects, Ann Plast Surg 13:44, 1984.
15. Gibson T, and Davis WB: The distortion of autogenous cartilage grafts: its cause and prevention, Br J Plast Surg 10:257, 1957.
16. Gibson T and Davis WB: The encapsulation of preserved cartilage grafts with prolonged survival, Br J Plast Surg 12:22, 1959.
17. Gillies HD: Plastic surgery of the face, London, 1920, Oxford University Press Inc.
18. Gillies HD and Kristensen HK: Br J Plast Surg 4:73, 1951.
19. Gunter J: Personal communication, 1988.
20. Johansson SH and Engkvist D: Small joint reconstruction by perichondrial anthroplasty, Clin Plast Surg 8:107, 1981.
21. Joseph J:
22. Kole H: Isrfahringen mit der Verwendung von homogenem konserviertem Knorpel in der Kiefer-Gesichtschirugie, Langenbecks Arch Klin Chir 299:737, 1962.
23. Konig F: Zur Zeckung von Defecten in der vorderen Tracheal Wand, Berl Klin Wochenschr 33:1129, 1896.
24. Konig F: Zur Deckung von Defecten der Nasenflugel, Klin Wochenschr 7:137, 1902.
25. Lynch ID, Ashbury RB, and Dingman RD: The effectiveness of sterilization of canine costal cartilage by cobalt-60 irradiation and its fate when used in homografts, Surg Forum 6:581, 1955.
26. Matukas VJ, Szymela VF, and Schmidt JF: Surgical treatment of bony ankylosis in a child using a composite cartilage-bone iliac crest graft, J Oral Surg 38:903, 1980.
27. McGlynn MJ and Sharpe DT: Cialit preserved homograft cartilage in nasal augmentation: a long-term review, Br J Plast Surg 34:53, 1981.
28. Metzenbaum M: Replacement of the lower end of the dislocated septal cartilage versus submucous resection of the dislocated end of the septal cartilage, Arch Otolaryngol 9:282, 1929.

29. Mikhelson NM: Homogenous cartilage in maxillofacial surgery, Acta Chir Plast 4:3, 1962.

30. Muhlbauer WD, Schmidt-Tintemann U, and Glaser M: Long-term behavior of preserved homologous rib cartilage in the correction of saddle nose deformity, Br J Plast Surg 24:325, 1971.

31. Munro VJ, Szymela VF, and Schmidt JF: Surgical treatment of bony ankylosis in a child using a composite cartilage bone iliac crest regeneration, Scand J Plast Reconstr Surg 6:123, 1972.

32. O'Conner BG and Pierce GW: Refrigerated cartilage isografts, Surg Gynec Obstet 67:796, 1938.

33. Ortiz-Monasterio F, Olmedo A, and Oscoy LD: The use of cartilage grafts in primary aesthetic rhinoplasty, Plast Reconstr Surg 67:596, 1981.

34. Peck GC: The onlay graft for nasal tip projection, Plast Reconstr Surg 71:27, 1983.

35. Peer LA: Fate of autogenous septal cartilage after transplantation in human tissues, Arch Otolaryngol 34:696, 1911.

36. Peer LA: Diced cartilage grafts: new method for repair of skull defects, mastoid fistula, and other deformities, Arch Otolaryngol 38:156, 1943.

37. Rasi HB: The fate of preserved human cartilage, Plast Reconstr Surg 24:24, 1959.

38. Sailer HF: Experience with the use of lyophilized bank cartilage for facial contour correction, J Maxfac Surg 4:149, 1976.

39. Schuller DE, Bardach J, and Krause CJ: Irradiated homologous costal cartilage for facial contour restoration, Arch Otolaryngol 103:12, 1977.

40. Sheen JH: Achieving more nasal tip projection by the use of a small autogenous vomer or septal cartilage graft: a preliminary report, Plast Reconstr Surg 56:35, 1975.

41. Skoog T, Ollsen L, and Sohn SA: Perichondral potential for cartilaginous regeneration, Scand J Plast Reconstr Surg 6:123, 1972.

42. Smill AU: Survival of frozen chondrocytes isolated from cartilage in adult mammals, Nature (London) 205:782, 1965.

43. Tardy ME, Denneny J, and Fritsch MH: The versatile cartilage autograft in reconstruction of the nose and face, Laryngoscope 95:523, 1985.

44. Wardill WEM and Swinney J: Bovine cartilage in plastic surgery, Lancet 253(2):389, 1947.

45. Zalzal GH, Cotton RT, and McAdams AJ: Cartilage grafts: present status, Head Neck Surg 8:363, 1986.

CHAPTER 5

Aesthetic Surgery of the Facial Skeleton

Linton A. Whitaker

The techniques of craniofacial surgery have become increasingly routine in the past decade. Surgeons now recognize the capacity to change the skeletal framework of the face as a frequent consideration for both the aging and youthful face.* The appearance of a normal face can be improved by aesthetic procedures that change the basic form by permanently altering the skeletal contour. This contrasts with aesthetic surgery specifically to reverse the aging process and mandates more psychological certainty that the patient desires a specific change rather than a procedure to simply "turn back the clock." The desired results are similar to those of routine aesthetic procedures at this time in the development of the field, and highly predictable outcomes have become routine.†

Aesthetic procedures should change form without altering function. Although function may be an important element in jaw osteotomies or osteotomies around the orbit, these are not frequent considerations in skeletal contouring procedures. Many of the procedures were originally performed on patients with borderline craniofacial abnormalities. The techniques were subsequently used when their safety and predictability had been established, to improve the appearance of patients with totally normal faces. The surgery has since been called *interface surgery* because it functions at the interface between aesthetic and reconstructive facial surgery.

The surgeon must understand the aesthetics of human facial form in detail, the accepted standards of beauty, and the procedures that are possible to achieve these standards. Knowledge of physical anthropology and a sense of aesthetics as developed by the study of the human facial form are essential to understanding the aesthetics of the human face. The surgeon who wishes to alter the bony structure of the face must understand when osteotomies are essential, when soft tissue shifts can be achieved to create enhanced bony architecture, and when contouring with onlay grafts or by osteoplasty is indicated. The procedures have become more frequent in recent years, and the public has begun to accept them, but there is a more limited understanding of their potential than with routine aesthetic procedures. Consequently, it is important for the surgeon to combine physical anthropology and aesthetics to properly counsel the patient as to what may be achieved in light of known surgical techniques. The surgeon must evaluate the face for symmetry of its two sides, highlight areas, length, width, and depth of the various parts.*

For the past 10 years, Fernando Ortiz-Monasterio and I have given this course on aesthetic surgery of the facial skeleton. When we began, most of the patients had borderline craniofacial abnormalities, and many of the procedures were osteotomies. The course evolved over the years to reflect increased patient demands and expectations. Most procedures are now performed for contouring, using more synthetic materials; osteotomies are being performed less frequently.

FACIAL EVALUATION
Historic perspective

The face has three highlight and four lowlight areas important for defining the aesthetically pleasing face. The three highlight areas are the supraorbital and temporal ridges, the malar-midface ridges, and the jaw ridges defined by the mandible. The lowlight areas are above and between these ridges, with the forehead sloping away from the supraorbital and temporal ridges. The orbit, lateral orbital rim, and temporal fossa are above the malar-zygomatic ridge and below the supraorbital ridge. The soft tissue of the cheeks are between the malar-zygomatic ridge and the mandibular

*References 6, 9, 17, 21, 24, 35, 39, 41.
†References 27, 30, 31, 45, 48, 54, 57.

*References 2-4, 7, 8, 16, 18, 46, 51, 52, 60.

ridge, and the neck is below the mandibular ridge. These general highlight and lowlight areas can be seen historically and are depicted in today's fashion magazines in models with prominent supraorbital ridges, tilted palpebral fissures, accentuated cheek bones, and extremely well-defined jaw and neck lines. They are also clearly visible in aesthetically ideal faces from the past, including photographs of Greta Garbo, paintings by Leonardo da Vinci, the sculpture of Nefertiti and a *National Geographic* (October 1988) cover illustration depicting the oldest human portrait, almost surely an ideal face, with exaggerated highlight and lowlight areas.

Fashions and fads can change the emphasis of these highlight and lowlight areas. The Rubenesque-Renoir ideal had a fleshier look, while today, a more slender, face and body is considered ideal. Nevertheless, both eras still emphasize the highlight and lowlight areas, with clear-cut jaw lines and facial features, and well-defined bony architecture. These ideals represent the goal for aesthetic skeletal changes but are rarely achieved. This must always be emphasized to patients.

Variations in facial structure

Facial structure can be divided into three categories: deformity, borderline deformity, and normal. Examples of these categories at the interface level abound with borderline examples of each of the known and described syndromes. For example, mild hemifacial microsomia may show very slight manifestations of palpebral fissure, inferior tilt, zygoma retrusion, oral commissure upward tilt, weak jaw-neck definition, and inferior ear positioning on the affected side. This may be simply an exaggeration of normal facial asymmetry.

In fully developed hemifacial microsomia these features are present in extreme cases. In each of the other major syndromes, similar variability is also present. For example, severe mandibulofacial dysostosis is characterized by total absence of the zygomas. In the microform, hypoplasia is present along with minimal pseudocolobomas with increased scleral show, minor nasal deformity, and mild hypoplasia of the chin-mandible. In orbital hypertelorism, there may be more soft tissue than bony spread with mild telecanthus and slightly increased bitemporal distance. In full-blown orbital hypertelorism, there may be an extreme spread between the eyes in addition to an exaggerated forehead and mild facial abnormalities.

Crouzon's disease in its microform may appear as a minimal protrusion of the eyes, midface hypoplasia, and mild forehead deformity. In fully-developed Crouzon's disease these stigmata are exaggerated. The spectrum of deformity ranges from an almost unrecognizable microform to the grotesque.

In addition to the syndromic microform variations, there are basic facial shapes that people seek to change, including short, long, wide, narrow, formless, and exaggerated individual proportions. The short or long face may be the result of changes in the upper middle or lower third. These may be measurable differences or abnormal differences only in relation to the width of the face. For example, the bigonial distance may be either narrow or grossly exaggerated. For example, other individual disproportions may include excessive anterior protrusion of the chin, underprojection or overprojection of the cheek bones, frontal sinus hyperpneumatization, and inferior tilt of the palpebral fissures.

Physical examination

Careful physical examination of the facial features is the first step in surgical planning.* The examiner should proceed from superior to inferior and consider the symmetry of the face, noting individual proportions and disproportions. If pathology is present, as in a progressively developing syndrome such as Romberg's disease, the timing of the surgical procedure must be taken into account. Satisfactory results in aesthetic surgery of the facial skeleton are achieved by incorporating the patient's wishes and physical findings along with anthropomorphic and aesthetic ideals. To this end, the use of PA and lateral cephalometric x-rays, panorex x-rays, computed tomography (CT), and magnetic resonance imaging (MRI) scans, as well as appropriate dental and opthalmological examinations, are frequently required.[16,61] The need for all of these tests may diminish with experience.

Gonzalez-Ulloa's standard profileplasty is a starting point for examining any face.[18] The vertical orientation consists of a line from the deepest point of the nasofrontal angle that passes through the lower lip and chin in profile with the upper lip, projecting slightly beyond this vertical line. In the horizontal orientation the line passes from the superior tragal notch through the inferior orbital rim. This line transects the vertical line at a 90 degree angle, thus providing ideal reference points. In the full-face view, symmetry is determined by the aesthetic features of the face. Physical anthropological measurements are used to confirm that the bitemporal, bimalar, and bigonial distances are approximately equal (105 to 109 mm each). The same measurements are used to assess whether the bizygomatic distance is the widest point of the face. These measurements provide a reference point in determining the need for and type of skeletal manipulation that is required (Fig. 5-1). The anthropomorphic standards

---

*References 2, 4, 8, 44, 47, 48.

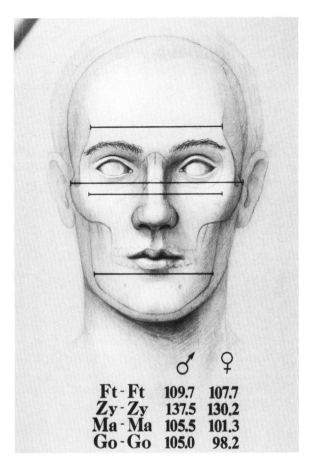

	♂	♀
Ft-Ft	109.7	107.7
Zy-Zy	137.5	130.2
Ma-Ma	105.5	101.3
Go-Go	105.0	98.2

Fig. 5-1 The bitemporal *(Ft-Ft)*, bimalar *(Ma-Ma)*, and bigonial *(Go-Go)* are approximately equal in the ideal face, while the bizygomatic distance *(Zy-Zy)* is the widest point of the face.

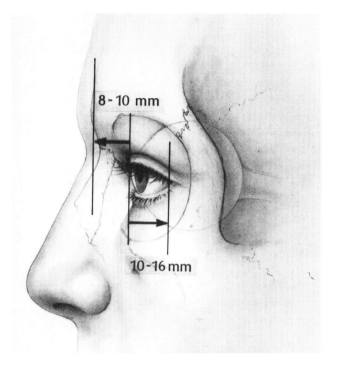

Fig. 5-2 The bony supraorbital ridge protrudes 8 to 10 mm beyond the anterior surface of the cornea, and the bony lateral orbital rim sits 12 to 16 mm posterior to the anterior surface of the cornea in ideal, normal eye-to-orbit relations. From Whitaker LA, Morales L, and Farkas LG: Plast Reconstr Surg 78:23, 1986.

of eye to orbit, and the maxillary-mandibular relationships are the prime determinants of the need for osteotomies.

The supraorbital ridge normally projects 8 to 10 mm beyond the anterior surface of the cornea in profile. The anterior surface of the cornea normally projects 12 to 16 mm beyond the anterior surface of the lateral orbital rim in profile (Fig. 5-2). The maxilla sits slightly anterior to the mandible in a Class I dental relationship. If these measurements are not within the range described, osteotomies may be advisable. At the least, if the jaw relations are not normal, orthodontic consultation may be required. Other measurements, including the slope of the forehead (approximately −10 degrees in men), the interorbital distance (11 to 15 mm between superior and inferior orbital rims), the nasofrontal angle, the cervicomental angle, and the mandibular angle must be considered. These measurements are detailed in *Anthropometric Facial Proportions in Medicine* by Farkas and Munro, in a chapter I wrote on facial proportions in aesthetic surgery.[44,47]

Aging face

Finally, the aging craniofacial skeleton should be considered when a person is to undergo a face-lift procedure to change the bony volume. There may be a salutory effect on the soft tissue adaptation to bone. In a study done by Bartlett, Grossman, and Whitaker[3] there were specific changes noted in the aging facial skeleton. These included the following objective measurable changes:

1. A slight decrease in mid-face and lower-face height greatly exaggerated in the presence of edentulous jaws.
2. No change in orbital dimensions and height of the mandibular ramus.
3. A slight increase in facial width.

The net change is one of either no loss or an actual gain in the bony architecture of the face, unless teeth are lost.

Subjective observations of the skulls showed the following:

1. Coarsening of the major eminences, especially at the frontal sinus, zygomatic, and chin areas.

2. Relative protrusion of the bony chin, especially with loss of teeth.
3. Heterogeneity that increases with bony prominence changes.[3,4]

Surgical possibilities

In considering the possibilities for surgical change, all areas must be taken into account, even when only one area is to be altered, since the other areas relate indirectly to the area undergoing surgical modification. The possibilities for change include:

1. Supraorbital ridge–temporal restructuring.
2. Lateral canthal-palpebral fissure repositioning and shaping.
3. Malar-midface reshaping, including the highlight and lowlight areas.
4. Paranasal and nose-lip angle changes.
5. Genioplasty.
6. Mandibular body and angle changes and cervical soft tissue alteration.

SURGICAL PROCEDURES
Choice of materials and methods

In condsidering surgical changes, the procedures of choice are listed in decreasing order of preference:

1. Segmental osteotomy.
2. Onlay bone grafting with cranial bone, rib, and iliac crest bone grafts listed in order of preference.
3. Soft tissue alteration.
4. Synthetic material implantation.

A number of synthetic materials may be employed with relative success. These inlcude Proplast,* Silastic, hydroxyapatite, and methylmethacrylate. Although it would be ideal to use no synthetic materials, in practice, implantation of these materials is often the procedure of choice, since segmental osteotomies work effectively only at the chin, while soft tissue alterations are useful only in the lowlight areas. Onlay bone grafting using autologous tissue shows a less predictable final outcome. It is desirable but not always possible to use autogenous materials.† In this context, a concept of "biological boundaries" has been developed.[49]

Biological boundaries concept

The concept of biological boundaries is an extension of Moss's functional matrix concept[31] and Wolfe's law.[59] It is a concept based on the observations that although bone grafts reabsorb unpredictably, they demonstrate some degree of predictability. In certain areas of the face, bone grafts survive to a greater degree than in other areas. This process appears to be linked either directly or indirectly to the following factors: the na-

ture of the soft tissue cover and vascularity of the surfaces, the type of bone graft, the degree of immobilization of the bone graft, and the depository and resorptive surfaces of the bones.* Within the biological boundary concept, the face has a genetically predetermined limit, which will tend to make onlay bone grafts reabsorb, unless that specific limit or boundary has been disturbed. If the boundary has been disturbed, it can be restored with the expectation that bone grafts of virtually any kind will survive. However, if the boundary is to be extended, as in making cheek bones more prominent, then a segmental osteotomy or synthetic onlay should be considered. Since segmental osteotomies have not been shown to be aesthetically acceptable anywhere but in the chin and in rhinoplasty, currently these are the only two places where they should be considered for aesthetic contouring. Thus in restoring biological boundaries, as an onlay, any type of bone will suffice. In general, however, the most readily available graft with the least morbidity should be used. Most often this means cranial bone, with rib being the second most frequent choice. In restoring a boundary or replacing material, "like" tissue should be used whenever possible. Therefore bone should be used to replace bone, membranous bone to replace membranous bone, cartilage to replace cartilage, and soft tissue to replace soft tissue.[24,39,50,62]

In extending biological boundaries, segmental osteotomies are the method of choice. The chin is generally the only area where osteotomies should be considered, except when orthognathic surgery or craniofacial surgery with maxillary-mandibular osteotomies or with orbital-forehead osteotomies are the procedures of choice. Therefore in extending biological boundaries, synthetic materials, notably Proplast, hydroxyapatite, Silastic, and methylmethacrylate, are the materials of choice.* Each of these has inherent advantages and disadvantages that must be considered on a case-by-case basis.

Proplast has proved to be a versatile and highly effective implant material for augmenting any area that is not in contact with the sinus, nasal, or oral cavities.† It is approximately one third the weight of Silastic, easily carved, and is immobilized to some degree by tissue ingrowth. It is sufficiently pliable to allow for contouring along the curving planes of the face. Consequently, it is the material of choice for contouring small areas on the forehead, supraorbital ridge, temporal fossa, malar-midface region, and along the posterior mandible. When segmental osteotomies of the nasal dorsum are

---

*Novamed, Houston, Tex.
*References 11, 26, 28, 32, 37, 39, 61, 62.
†References 24, 26, 28, 32, 35, 37, 39, 61, 62

on the bone of the zygoma. At this point the malar implant is inserted and held in position laterally with its extension onto the zygomatic arch. To achieve symmetry, it is necessary to insert one finger into the mouth to ensure that the implant has reached the same point medially just lateral to the pyriform as on the opposite side. A permanent suture around the zygomatic arch holds the lateral extension a measured amount beyond the lateral orbital wall so that the amount of extension laterally on both sides can be determined and equalized.

Malar-midface complex

The malar-midface complex should be evaluated with reference to the amount of projection and highlighting of this middle ridge of the three important highlight areas of the face. The malar-midface complex can be divided into outer, middle, and inner thirds. Each of these divisions must be considered in determining how much augmentation is desirable (Fig. 5-10). The inner or medial third lies just lateral to the nasolabial fold and superiorly and laterally extends up to the juncture with the middle third, which is the normal highlight area of the malar eminence. The lateral third is the end of the malar eminence and extension onto the zygomatic arch. Each of these thirds may need augmentation or reduction. The amount of augmentation or reduction is determined after examining the patient and according to the patient's wishes. Generally, the lateral and medial thirds will need to be augmented less than the middle third.

Various types of implants have been used and generally provide reliable results.[7,17,20,37,41] The anatomical concept of malar-midface structure, extending from the paranasal area onto the zygomatic arch, is important. Therefore regardless of implant type, this concept should be remembered when evaluating this area of the face. Proplast is my material of choice because of the previously described characteristics. It can be individualized to the patient's face. The implant is of standard length (60 mm) and width (10 mm on the lateral end and 16 to 18 mm on the medial end). Its thickness, 4, 6, or 8 mm, is the major variable (Fig. 5-11). The 6-mm implant is standard, and variations are determined from that thickness. In an individual with thicker soft tissues and more hypoplasia, a thicker implant will be necessary. In individuals with thinner soft tissues and/or less hypoplasia, a thinner implant, such as 4 to 5 mm, will be necessary. The implants may be trimmed as needed, but size determination should be made before the procedure.

Acceptance of synthetic implants has developed gradually. Problems with autogenous tissues, i.e., rib graft absorption, cranial bone graft irregularity, and poor contouring and asymmetry following osteotomies have tipped the balance in favor of synthetic materials. Thus the Proplast implant was developed into the size and shape that is currently used, based on the amounts of autogenous material being inserted. After preoperative determination of the required implant thickness, the implant is carved at the time of surgery but before the incision is made. The implant is then soaked in an antibiotic solution according to the manufacturer's instructions so that its pores are entirely permeated with antibiotic solution.

The implant may be inserted either through a coronal incision or through a lower-eyelid incision. However, the lower-eyelid incision may create temporary ectropion because of poor implant pliability and considerable stretching of the skin necessary to position the implant. Thus the upper buccal–sulcus incision is used most frequently.

A throat pack is inserted, and the upper buccal sulcus is irrigated with dilute Betadine solution and injected with ½% lidocaine with 1:200,000 epinephrine. The incision is made on only one side if both sides are to be done. Using a no. 10 blade, the incision is made from the lateral edge of the lateral incisor to the medial edge of the first bicuspid and is approximately 2 cm long. It is carried to bone midway between the mucosa of the upper buccal sulcus and the infraorbital nerve. The soft tissue between the mucosa and bone is then reflected downward to create a ledge of soft tissue for implant seating. The dissection is carried laterally, beneath the infraorbital nerve, over the malar eminence, and onto the zygomatic arch. At the malar eminence, osteocutaneous ligaments will make the dissection more difficult and must be elevated from the bone, removing all soft tissue from the malar eminence and onto the zygomatic arch, past the zygomatic temporal suture.

Once the bone has been adequately cleared of soft tissue throughout the entire tunnel, the area is inspected visually to make sure there is no soft tissue left on bone, especially medially. A long Langenbeck retractor is inserted, and then the implant is inserted. Insertion of the implant is performed by grasping it with a standard straight hemostat at its distal end, with the end of the implant sitting within the jaws of the hemostat. It is inserted along the undersurface of the retractor, out to the most lateral extent of the dissection, and the hemostat grasping the implant is then removed. The implant should sit freely in the pocket with no tendency to buckle and should be lateral to the anterior projection of the pyriform (Fig. 5-12).

Symmetry and positioning of the implant is achieved by correct dissection of the pocket. This re-

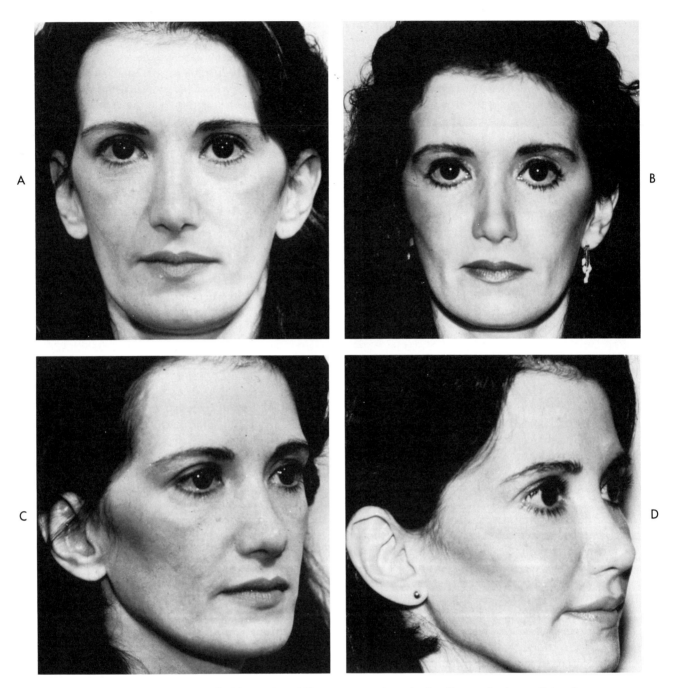

Fig. 5-13 **A,** A patient desiring malar-midface augmentation who has flatness in the medial and middle zone. **B,** The patient after augmentation with 6-mm thick malar implants, with the lateral third trimmed to maximum thinness so as to decrease the amount of augmentation of the zygomatic arches. **C,** Preoperative view. **D,** Postoperative view. From Whitaker LA: Plast Reconstr Surg 80:337, 1987.

quires precise subperiosteal dissection. If the medial positions of the implant match on the two sides as seen by direct visualization, and there is no folding of the distal end, symmetry will be achieved. The pocket is then closed in a single layer using 3-0 vicryl running suture on one side before proceeding to the opposite side where the same procedure is performed. Consistently excellent results with minimal morbidity can be achieved with this procedure (Fig. 5-13).

Problems with the procedure and implant consist

primarily of initial lack of mobility of the upper lip and frequent lip hyposensitivity. These almost invariably disappear, although in two or three patients in my series of approximately 350 implants, one side has remained hyposensitive in spotty areas of the upper lip for more than 1 year after surgery. Normal sensation usually returns within 3 months after surgery, and the stiffness of the lip usually disappears within 6 to 12 weeks. When the series was evaluated, 288 implants had been inserted; 3.4% of patients or 2.1% of implants developed infections requiring removal. Two implants extruded in patients who had radiation or inadequate soft-tissue coverage, and eight implants were removed because the patients did not like them. Fourteen patients had implants revised, making them smaller or larger. Consequently, the overall implant revision rate is 11% of implants in 14% of patients. This number has decreased as experience has increased. Approximately one third of the 288 implants have been inserted through a coronal or lower-eyelid incision, and none have become infected. Problems with malar augmentation have been discussed by others.[25,56]

Infraorbital rim augmentation

Hollowness along the infraorbital rim may result after lower-lid blepharoplasty with exaggerated excision of fat, an exaggerated lower eyelid skin-cheek juncture, or an excessive infraorbital rim protrusion. Augmentation of this area is the newest application of skeletal contouring. Experience thus far is limited to only 10 patients.

At present, the procedure is done by marking the exact area requiring augmentation. This is done with the patient in a sitting position. The bone of the infraorbital rim is approached through a standard lower blepharoplasty incision. The incision is made and carried beneath the orbicularis muscle, down to the orbital rim. The rim is exposed subperiosteally, from medial to the infraorbital nerve and laterally out to the lateral orbital rim and zygomatic arch. No standard implants have yet been devised for the rim. The 4-mm malar implant has been used, carving the 10-mm wide tail-end extension to fit precisely onto the rim above the infraorbital nerve, tapering medially, laterally, and superiorly to a fine edge that is not palpable. It is held in place by passing a drill hole through two points of the infraorbital rim and a suture through the implant. Postoperative corrections have been satisfactory in every instance except with two patients who had palpable implant extension laterally. In neither instance did the patients desire to have anything done. There have been no postoperative infections, displacement, or other problems.

Posterior mandible

The posterior mandible involves the ramus, angle, and posterior body of the mandible to the level of the inferior alveolar nerve. The current ideal of the exceptionally clean-cut jaw-neck line seen in fashion models can be achieved in many instances by augmentation. The muscle and bone can be reduced where there is too much fullness, especially with masseter muscle hypertrophy common to Asiatic races in which there is often lateral mandible angle flaring.

Reduction

If the patient wishes to undergo mandible reduction, this can be achieved with a contouring burr. More anteriorly, the inferior edge is best approached through a submental incision, which tunnels posteriorly and laterally, raising the edge by contour reduction. The anterior and posterior tapering must be sufficiently fine so that the inferior length projection is adequately corrected, and the transitions are not palpable.

Reduction of excess width is performed through an intraoral approach. A throat pack is inserted, and the mouth irrigated thoroughly with half-strength Betadine solution. A vertical incision is made lateral to and paralleling the ramus of the mandible and is carried to the anterior edge of the ramus. The masseter muscle is elevated from its fossa. Inferiorly, it is elevated below the inferior border, superiorly to the fixed gingival mucosa, along the posterior mandibular body.

For masseter and bony-angle reduction, the contouring burr is used to reduce the laterally flaring bone. This bone should be visualized by panorex and cephalometric x-rays and the amount of reduction determined. Typically, 5 to 6 mm of bone is removed. The most important area for reduction is along the posterior edge of the mandible at the ramus, especially at the angle. The posterior edge can be contoured so that a full-thickness reduction shifting the posterior edge anteriorly is accomplished. More anterior to that, the lateral or inferior cortices of the mandible can be reduced. In addition, approximately half the width of the masseter muscle on its medial or bony surface can be removed by direct excision, going inferiorly and extending near the zygomatic arch. Afterward, the wound is closed using a single layer running 3-0 vicryl suture.

After reduction all patients experience transient but problematic trismus, which may persist for 6 to 12 weeks before returning to normal. There is also often massive swelling after this procedure, and there has been one instance of infection but no significant asymmetry. Thus masseter and bony-angle reduction is a highly effective procedure.

MANDIBULAR ANGLE IMPLANT and POSTERIOR MANDIBULAR IMPLANT*

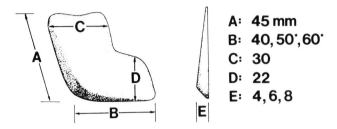

A: 45 mm
B: 40, 50°, 60°
C: 30
D: 22
E: 4, 6, 8

Fig. 5-14 Dimensions of the mandibular angle implant. From Whitaker LA: Plast Reconstr Surg (in press).

Augmentation

For augmentation of the posterior mandible, sagittal splitting of the lateral cortex of the ramus was initially attempted using interposition bone grafts after onlay bone grafts proved ineffective. Since symmetry was impossible to achieve with this procedure, a Proplast posterior mandibular implant was designed. Again, other materials could readily be used in this area, but for reasons previously described, Proplast is the material of choice.[53]

The angulation of the patient's mandibular angle and the amount of lateral projection desired is determined by direct examination, including panorex and cephalometric x-rays. The standard mandibular-angle implant, which is 45 mm long vertically along the ramus, extends 40 to 60 mm anteriorly, has a width of 30 mm at the ramus and 22 mm along the posterior mandible, and is 4, 6, or 8 mm thick (Fig. 5-14). Furthermore, it is tailored precisely to the individual posterior mandible. With the patient on the operating table, the pattern is cut to the patient's sterile face using a template of exposed x-ray film. It is then matched against the panorex and cephalometric x-rays. The implant is thus carved to the individual mandible in every instance. Fine tapering is most essential anteriorly, since the skin becomes thinnest in that area, and the implant may show as it emerges from beneath the masseter muscle. It is also extremely important that the implant not be too wide at any point so that it does not overhang the edges of the bone.

After carving the implant, the incision and approach to the posterior mandible are performed as previously described. The incision must be sufficiently long so that the L-shaped implant can be inserted without buckling. Thus the incision typically extends from just below the zygomatic arch through the lateral buccal mucosa posteriorly and around the angle of the mandible. The soft tissue is then elevated from the entire ramus and posterior portion of the mandible.

In theory, the entire posterior mandible can be augmented. However, my experience has been that the augmentation does best when kept confined to the area covered by the masseter muscle. After elevating the soft tissue, the carved implant is carefully inserted, while ensuring that it is not buckling. The implant must sit comfortably in place, especially along the posterior body of the mandible.

It should have no buckles or folds and be sufficiently tapered so that its transition into bone is imperceptible (Fig. 5-15). The masseter muscle layer is closed with 3-0 vicryl, then a running 3-0 vicryl is used to close the mucosa.

After surgery the patient is treated with a 5-day course of antibiotics, a liquid diet for 5 days and a semi-solid diet for an additional 5 days.

In the 22 patients, there have been two infections, both from an excessively large implant with extrusion. In one patient, the implant overlapped the mandibular border, causing a perceptible edge (Fig. 5-16).

Genioplasty

There are many variations in chin contour that can be improved by a genioplasty procedure. I believe a segmental osteotomy is the procedure of choice for chin augmentation.* A properly performed sliding genioplasty is natural looking. It probably achieves better tightening of the submental area in the aging face and avoids the long-term uncertainties of synthetic material.

Synthetic materials

Silastic implants are the best synthetic material to use in the chin.[30] The porous nature of Proplast makes it more susceptible to infection when subjected to pooled saliva in the anterior buccal sulcus. My experience has been that Silastic chin implants are extremely effective, although bony erosion can occur. I have performed several hundred anterior chin implants with few complications, including the extended chin implants as described by Terino[38] and Flowers.[13] This is an excellent procedure with a highly predictable outcome. In addition, when there is a distinct chin-jowl juncture, the implants can fill that juncture if the patient or physician prefers to avoid an osteotomy.

Horizontal ostetomy

A sliding genioplasty should be done in virtually all circumstances. It is essential in a vertically short chin, since implants do not effectively lengthen the chin, except when used as an interposition material. The relative indications for a sliding genioplasty include young

*References 9, 21, 29, 33, 36, 49, 57, 58.

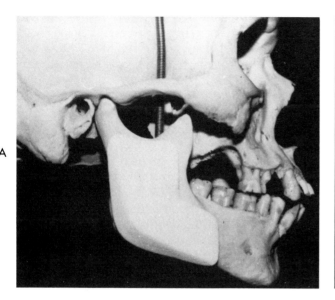
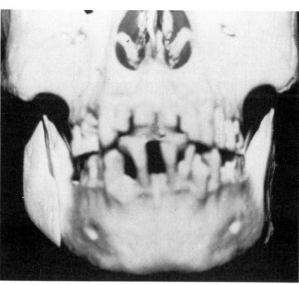

Fig. 5-15 **A,** The mandibular angle implant as seen in the lateral view must closely follow the posterior and inferior borders of the mandibular ramus and posterior body. **B,** The taper of the implant anteriorly should be extremely fine to avoid any bulges. From Whitaker LA: Plast Reconstr Surg (in press).

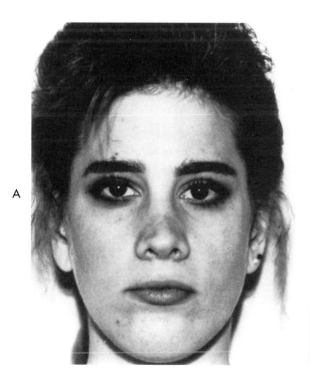
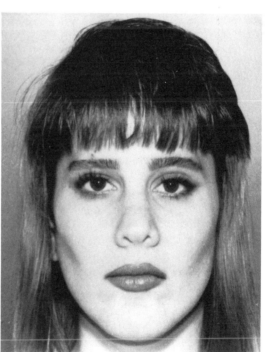

Fig. 5-16 **A,** Preoperative view of a patient desiring posterior mandibular augmentation. **B,** The patient after bilateral posterior mandibular augmentation, malar-midface augmentation, and secondary rhinoplasty. From Whitaker LA: Plast Reconstr Surg 87:229, 1991.

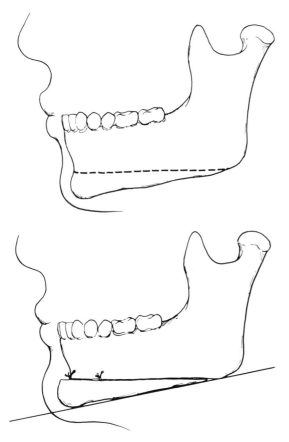

Fig. 5-17 The horizontal osteotomy for a sliding genio-plasty should be tapered as far posteriorly as reasonably pos-sible to minimize the step off of the juncture of the free segment. From Whitaker LA and Bartlett SP (eds): Perspect Plast Surg 2:23, 1988.

patients, patients who do not wish to have artificial ma-terial implanted, patients with long retroinclined chins, or to achieve an optimal chin/neck angle. In the young patient, where the artifical material may be in place for 50 or 60 years, a sliding genioplasty should strongly be considered.

Genioplasty, which is performed as an outpatient procedure, produces about the same morbidity as a rhinoplasty. It can be accomplished in about 30 min-utes when only the inferior border of the anterior man-dible is cut.

The procedure is performed with the patient un-der general anesthesia. The throat is packed, and the buccal sulcus exposed by lifting the lower lip with the surgeons nondominant hand. The area is injected with 0.5% lidocaine with 1:200,000 of epinephrine. The buccal sulcus is irrigated with Betadine solution. The incision is carried through the mucosa, from lateral in-cisor to lateral incisor, about 1 cm superior to the at-tached gingival mucosa. The soft tissue is elevated off

the underlying bone, often with some difficulty be-cause of attachments of the mentalis muscle. A tunnel is created laterally beyond the mentalis muscle be-neath the inferior alveolar nerve. Soft tissue is elevated off the inferior border of the mandible and up to the mentalis nerve on either side. The tunnel is carried back near the angle of the mandible on either side.

A right angle saw blade is then used to score the midline of the mandible corresponding to the midline of the incisors. A reciprocating saw is fitted into the tunnel of soft tissue laterally below the alveolar nerve. The cut is angled to taper finely into the mandible, emerging posteriorly one half or two thirds of the way back toward the angle. The saw is inserted over the in-feriolateral edge of the mandible posteriorly and held there until the cut through three surfaces is complete. It is then carried anteriorly, staying below the mental nerve, across the midline. The same is then done on the opposite side. The segment is thus freed. Wires are used for stabilization via drill holes, and position is de-termined by the desired advancement. One is placed in the midline of the tooth-bearing segment and another, ½ to 2 cm on either side of the midline. Drill holes are placed just anterior to the posterior cortex of the freed segment. The wires are passed through a 19-gauge nee-dle from the skin surface through the hole in the freed segment of bone; one end is passed through, then the opposite end is passed through the same hole in the skin beneath the chin and sawed down to bone. The wires are then brought through the tooth-bearing seg-ment, and the free chin segment is advanced the prede-termined amount (Fig. 5-17).

Typical amounts of advancement are small (5 to 7 mm), moderate (7 to 9 mm), and large (9 to 11 mm). At 10 to 11 mm, the posterior edge of the free segment usually comes in contact with the anterior edge of the tooth-bearing segment. If the chin is to be lengthened, bone or hydroxyapatite is interposed between the tooth-bearing segment and the free segment. The wires are then secured. If there is chin asymmetry because of shortness on one side compared with the other, that side can be further lengthened. The wound is closed in two layers using 3-0 vicryl, positioning the mentalis muscle back into place and closing the mucosa with a running continuous 3-0 vicryl. If the chin is to be shortened, a wedge of bone should be removed and the free segment set upward. If an excessively anterior projecting chin is to be set back, this also should be done by a wedge segment removal.

Problems after a sliding genioplasty are few (Fig. 5-18). There is lower lip stiffness and often hypesthesia for several weeks after surgery. Occasionally, patients note a slight difference in lower lip contour. However, normally it returns to its preoperative condition. Palpa-

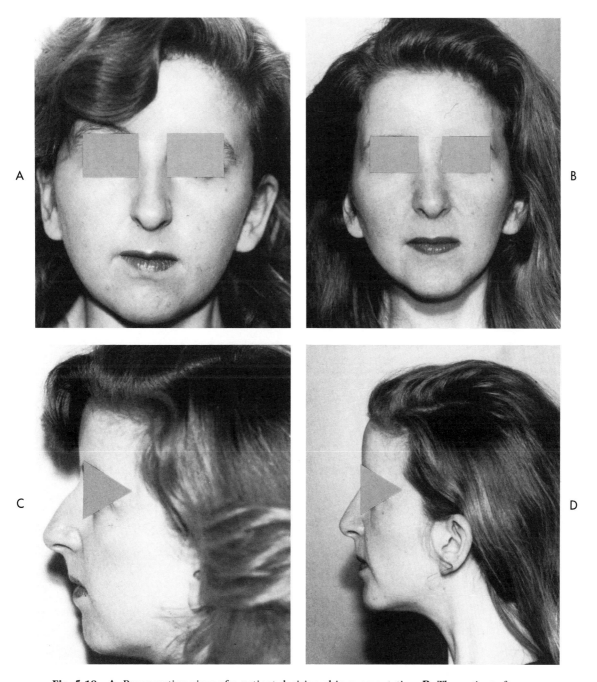

Fig. 5-18   A, Preoperative view of a patient desiring chin augmentation. **B,** The patient after sliding genioplasty. **C,** Preoperative view. **D,** Postoperative view after sliding genioplasty and rhinoplasty.

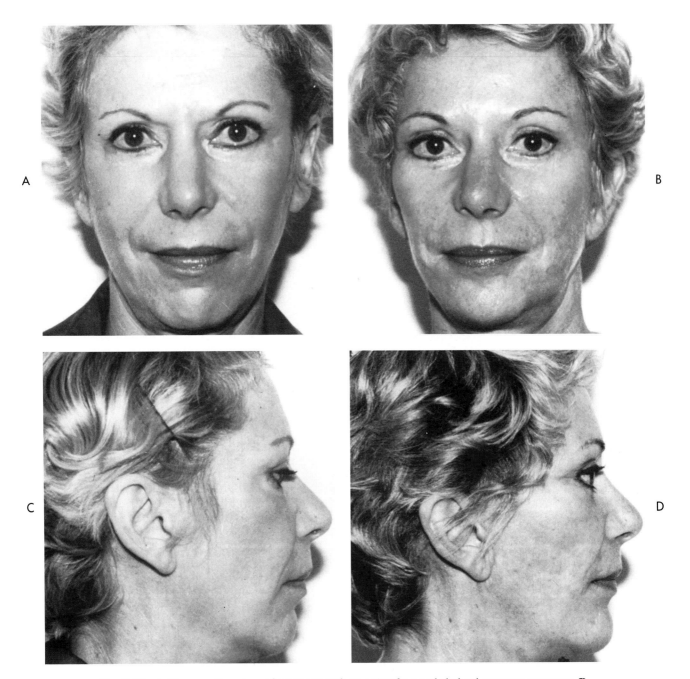

Fig. 5-19 **A,** Preoperative view of a patient with an aging face and skeletal contour concerns. **B,** The patient 3 years after a brow-lift, bilateral lateral canthopexies, bilateral malar augmentation, rhinoplasty, face-lift, and augmentation genioplasty. **C,** Preoperative profile view. **D,** Postoperative profile view. **A,** From Whitaker LA and Pertschuk M: Plast Reconstr Surg 69:245, 1982.

ble edges at the posterior extent of the bone cut may be detectable, but this can usually be avoided by a finely tapered, long posterior extension of the osteotomy along the inferior border of the mandible. Infections are rare, and in my experience there has been only one infection where hydroxyapatite was used for chin lengthening. The results are highly satisfactory and consistent.

Aging face

All of the procedures described can be used in patients with an aging face.* The soft tissue should be considered as the envelope surrounding the underlying bony foundation. With aging the envelope becomes too large in proportion to the bone. This may be true even with youthful faces when premature aging occurs, which is especially notable in the submental area beneath the supraorbital ridges or beneath the malar-midface ridge. In these areas, soft tissue sag may occur, giving the appearance of bony hypoplasia. With aging, this pattern occurs, and an expansion of the bone volume with or without reduction of the soft tissue volume can be performed to counterbalance the ongoing process.

Augmentation of the supraorbital ridges, tightening of the palpebral fissures with a lateral canthopexy, malar augmentation, and sliding genioplasty, or chin augmentation, are useful in connecting soft tissue laxity. These procedures may sometimes substitute for soft tissue tightening and thus may delay the need for a face-lift, blepharoplasty, or brow-lift. Most often soft tissue tightening and bone expansion are used in combination. The previously described surgical approaches can produce dramatic changes. Again, the patient with an aging face should desire a specific change in the shape of the face rather than the need to take the face "back in time." If the patient has always desired to have stronger cheek bones or a stronger chin, then it is safe to do the procedure. If, however, the surgeon perceives some deficiency of bone structure and suggests augmentation to the patient, it can be a problem for the patient who has not noticed nor desired that correction. When combining a bone change procedure with soft tissue changes, the temporary morbidity is increased, but the actual length of time to complete healing and permanent morbidity are probably no different, and the results can be striking (Fig. 5-19).

Recently, subperiosteal face-lift procedures have been the topic of much discussion. These procedures, however, have limitations. The subperiosteal face-lift procedure is really an extended brow-lift, and it is performed as one would approach the zygomatic arch. A coronal incision is made, and the soft tissue mass is

*References 3, 4, 13, 17, 27, 33, 48, 55.

then elevated, overlapping the cut edges of the temporal fascia and holding them with vicryl sutures. The plane of dissection is safe but probably does not get at the most dominant area of soft tissue sag. The osteocutaneous ligaments may be altered in their position and changed as a result of the procedure, which slightly benefits the nasolabial and submalar areas.

REFERENCES

1. Arem AJ, Rasmussen D, and Madden JW: Soft-tissue response to Proplast: quantitation of scar ingrowth, Plast Reconstr Surg 61:214, 1978.
2. Barnett A and Whitaker LA: Facial form analysis of the lower and middle face, Plast Reconstr Surg 78:158, 1986.
3. Bartlett SP, Grossman R, and Whitaker LA: Age related changes of the craniofacial skeleton: an anthropometric and histologic analysis, Plast Reconstr Surg (in press).
4. Bartlett SP, Whitaker LA, and Wornum I: Evaluation of facial skeletal aesthetics and planning. In Whitaker LA (ed): Aesthetic surgery of the facial skeleton, Clin Plast Surg, Philadelphia, 1991, WB Saunders Co.
5. Belinfante LS and Mitchell DL: Use of alloplastic material in the canine fossa-zygomatic area to improve facial aesthetics, J Oral Surg 35:121, 1977.
6. Bell WH, Proffit WR, and White RP: Surgical corrections of dentofacial deformities, Philadelphia, 1980, WB Saunders Co.
7. Brennan HG: Augmentation malarplasty, Arch Otolaryngol 108:441, 1982.
8. Broadbent TR and Matthews VI: Artistic relationships in surface anatomy of the face: application to reconstructive surgery, Plast Reconstr Surg 20:1, 1957.
9. Converse JM and Wood-Smith D: Horizontal osteotomy of the mandible, Plast Reconstr Surg 34:464, 1964.
10. Deeb ME and Holmes RL: Zygomatic and mandibular augmentation with proplast and porous hydroxyapatite in Rhesus monkey, J Oral Maxillofac Surg 47:480, 1989.
11. Enlow DH: Facial growth, Philadelphia, 1982, WB Saunders Co.
12. Epstein LI: Clinical experiences with proplast as an implant, Plast Reconstr Surg 63:219, 1979.
13. Flowers R: Chin and anterior mandibular augmentation: alloplastic. In Whitaker L (ed): Aesthetic surgery of the facial skeleton, Clin Plast Sur, Philadelphia, 1991, WB Saunders Co.
14. Freeman BS and Weimer DR: Clinical uses of proplast: expectations and results. In Rubin LR (ed): Biomaterials in reconstructive surgery, St. Louis, 1983, The CV Mosby Co.
15. Freeman BS: Proplast: A porous implant for contour restoration, Br J Plast Surg 29:158, 1976.
16. Friedland JA, Coccaro PJ, and Converse JM: Retrospective cephalometric analysis of mandibular bone absorption under silicone rubber chin implants, Plast Reconstr Surg 57:144, 1976.
17. Gonzalez-Ulloa M: Building out the malar prominences as an addition to rhytidectomy, Plast Reconstr Surg 53:293, 1974.
18. Gonzalez-Ulloa M: A quantum method for appreciation of the morphology of the face, Plast Reconstr Surg 34:241, 1964.
19. Halstead A, Jones CW, and Rawlings RD: A study of the reaction of human tissue to Proplast, J Biomed Mater Res 13:121, 1979.
20. Hinderer U and del rio Legarretta O: Aesthetic surgery of the malar region. In Regnault P and Daniel RK (eds): Aesthetic plastic surgery: principles and techniques, Boston, 1984, Little, Brown & Co Inc.
21. Hinds EC and Kent JN: Genioplasty: the versatility of the horizontal osteotomy, J Oral Surg 27:690, 1969.
22. Holmes RE and Hagler HK: Porous hydroxyapatite as a bone graft

substitute in mandibular contour augmentation: a histometric study, J Oral Maxillofac Surg 45:421, 1987.

23. Holmes RE: Bone regeneration within a coraline hydroxyapatite implant, Plast Reconstr Surgery 63:626, 1979.

24. Ivy RH: Bone grafting for restoration of defects on the mandible, Plast Reconstr Surg 7:333, 1951.

25. Kent JN, Westfall RL, and Carlton DM: Chin and zygomaticomaxillary augmentation with Proplast: long-term follow up, J Oral Surg 39:912, 1981.

26. Kusiak JF et al: Early revascularization of membranous bone grafts, Surg Forum 76:510, 1985.

27. Lassus C: Ostectomy of superior orbital rim in cosmetic blepharoplasty, Plast Reconstr Surg 63:481, 1979.

28. Lin K et al: An experimental study on the effect of rigid fixation on the developing craniofacial skeleton, Plast Reconstr Surg 87:229, 1991.

29. McCarthy JG: Microgenia: a logical surgical approach, Clin Plast Rurg 8:269, 1981.

30. Millard DR: Augmentation mentoplasty, Surg Clin North Am 55:333, 1971.

31. Moss ML: Facial Growth: the functional matrix concept. In Grabb WC, Rosenstein SW, and Bzoch K (eds): Cleft lip and palate, Boston, 1971, Little, Brown & Co Inc.

32. Reichman JH, Kerr LP, and Whitaker LA: Rib grafting in facial reconstruction: an experimental approach, Surg Forum 28:535, 1977.

33. Rosen H: Surgical correction of the vertically deficient chin, Plast Reconstr Surg 82:247, 1988.

34. Rosen H: A porous block hydroxyapatite as an interpositional bone graft: substitute in orthognathic surgery, Plast Reconstr Surg 83:985, 1989.

35. Salyer KE and Taylor DP: Bone grafts in craniofacial surgery, Clin Plast Surg 14:27, 1987.

36. Spear SL, Mausner ME, and Kwamoto HK: Sliding genioplasty as a local anesthetic out patient procedure: a prospective two-center trial, Plast Reconstr Surg 80:55, 1987.

37. Stalnecker MC, Whitaker LA, and Brighton CT: Electrical stimulation of onlay bone grafts, Plast Reconstr Surg 82:580, 1988.

38. Terino E: Personal communication, 1987.

39. Tessier P: Autogenous bone grafts taken from the calvarium for facial and cranial applications, Clin Plast Surg 9:531, 1982.

40. Tessier P: Osteotomies totales de la face: syndrome de Crouzon d'Apert: oxycephalies, scaphocephalies, turricephalies, Ann Chir Plast 12:273, 1967.

41. Waite PD and Matukas VJ: Zygomatic augmentation with hydroxyapatite: a preliminary report, J Oral Maxillofac Surg 44:349, 1986.

42. Whitaker LA: Aesthetic augmentation of the malar-midface structures, Plast Reconstr Surg 80:337, 1987.

43. Whitaker LA, Morales L, and Farkas LG: Aesthetic surgery of the supraorbital ridge and forehead structures, Plast Reconstr Surg 78:23, 1986.

44. Whitaker LA: Facial proportions in aesthetic surgery. In Farkas LG and Munro IR (eds): Arthopometric facial proportions in medicine, Springfield, Ill, 1987, Charles C Thomas Publisher.

45. Whitaker LA: Interface surgery. Paper presented at the Science Writers' Symposium, Rockefeller University, New York, September, 1982.

46. Whitaker LA: Selective alteration of palprebral fissure form by lateral canthopexy, Plast Reconstr Surg 74:611, 1984.

47. Whitaker LA and Bartlett SP: Aesthetic surgery of the facial skeleton, Persp Plast Surg 2:23, 1988.

48. Whitaker LA and Pertschuk M: Facial skeletal contouring for aesthetic purposes, Plast Reconstr Surg 69:245, 1982.

49. Whitaker LA: Biological boundaries: a concept in facial skeletal restructuring, Clin Plast Surg 16:1, 1989.

50. Whitaker LA: Traumatic craniofacial deformity: late treatment, Scand J Plast Reconstr Surg 15:307, 1981.

51. Whitaker LA: Aesthetic contouring of the facial support system in orthognatic surgery, Clin Plast Surg 16:815, 1989.

52. Whitaker LA: Aesthetic alteration of the malar-midface structure. In D Ousterhout (ed): Aesthetic contouring of the craniomaxillofacial skeleton, Plast Reconstr Surg 87:268, 1991.

53. Whitaker LA: Aesthetic augmentation of the posterior mandible, Plast Reconst Surg 87:229, 1991.

54. Whitaker LA (ed): Aesthetic surgery of the facial skeleton, Clin Plast Surg 18:1, 1991.

55. Whitaker LA: Skeletal alterations in facial aging, Clin Plast Surg 18:197, 1991.

56. Wilkinson TS: Complications in aesthetic malar augmentation, Plast Reconstr Surg 71:643, 1983.

57. Wolfe SA: Application of craniofacial techniques to the everyday practice of aesthetic surgery. In Caronni EP (ed): Craniofacial surgery, Boston, 1984, Little, Brown & Co Inc.

58. Wolfe SA: Chin advancement as an aid in correction of deformities of the mental and submental regions, Plast Reconstr Surg 67:624, 1981.

59. Wolfe J: Uber die inueve Architectur der Knochen und ihre Bedeutung fur die Frage von Knocherwachstum, Virchows Ach (Path Anat) 50:389, 1970.

60. Zide B, Grayson B, and McCarthy JG: Cephalometric analysis for mandibular surgery, part 3, Plast Reconstr Surg 69:155, 1982.

61. Zins JE et al: The influence of the recipient site on bone grafts to the face, Plast Reconstr Surg 73:371, 1984.

62. Zins JE and Whitaker LA: Membranous versus endochondral bone: implications for craniofacial reconstruction, Plast Reconstr Surg 72:778, 1983.

PART TWO

RECONSTRUCTIVE SURGERY

CHAPTER 6

Refinements in Breast Reconstruction with Tissue Expansion

Jack Fisher

Plastic and reconstructive surgery is a constantly evolving field. By the time the literature has been printed, the information has either changed or become outdated. Specifically, advances in breast reconstruction with tissue expansion have occurred rapidly over the past several years.[1,2,15-17] There are now many devices on the market available for this purpose.[4,5,11,19] Today's expanders come in various shapes and proportions, and several different types of surface texturing are available. With all the technological advances, it is easy to assume that one particular expander will automatically give the ideal result. However, such logic is akin to believing that using a specific pair of scissors will always give an excellent result when performing a rhytidectomy. Although the tools are important, there is no magic in achieving good results with tissue expansion. Attention to detail and logical thought processes are imperative, and surgical skill remains the most important variable.

These basic principles and refinements of tissue expansion will enable the surgeon to obtain a contoured and symmetrical breast reconstruction. There will be complications and ultimately some failures using this technique, but it is important to deal with these problems logically. Plastic surgeons take great pride in their results, and it is easy to minimize less than optimal outcomes. Understanding why some of these reconstructions end up poorly is the first step toward improved results. Breast reconstruction with tissue expansion is a procedure with a significant learning curve. However, once one is proficient with the technique, the complication rate is low.[3,7]

The expectations for breast reconstruction have increased markedly over the past decade. No longer is the desired result simply a normal, clothed appearance. Today, the shape, contour, and symmetry of the patient's unclothed breast are the important aesthetic parameters of successful reconstruction. These stringent criteria require careful evaluation of the mastectomy defect and realistic appraisal of the reconstructive goals. Tissue expansion is not for all patients who wish to have breast reconstruction, and proper patient selection is a key factor.

PATIENT SELECTION

Today there are multiple techniques available for breast reconstruction, including autogenous tissue transfer, both pedicled and free, as well as expansion. Familiarity with these techniques is essential, since proper procedure selection requires the surgeon to be versatile. Not all patients are candidates for tissue expansion, and it is critical to identify those factors that work against an optimal result. In my practice, approximately 60% of patients are reconstructed with tissue expansion and 40% with autogenous tissue. These figures could easily change pending further developments in expander technology.

The most important physical finding related to tissue expansion in breast reconstruction is the status of the tissues that cover the expander. Any situation in which these tissues are compromised represents a relative contraindication to tissue expansion. Postoperative irradiation treatment can adversely affect the soft tissues of the chest wall.[9,10] Depending on the type of irradiation, the dose, and the individual patient response, these tissues can become scarred, indurated, and nonexpansile. Expansion under these circumstances generates high-tissue pressures and proceeds slowly. Despite reports of successful expansion of irradiated skin, there is a significant chance of tissue breakdown and exposure of the expander. Similarly, patients who have undergone a radical mastectomy or a modified radical mastectomy with a large excision of skin will have tight, relatively nonexpansile skin over the defect,

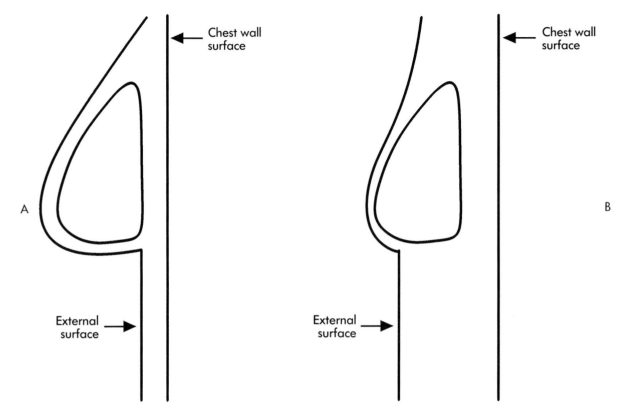

Fig. 6-1   A, The difference between the external surface and the chest wall on which the implant rests is minimal in the thinner patient. **B,** In heavier patients these surfaces are far apart, reducing implant projection and obscuring the inframammary fold.

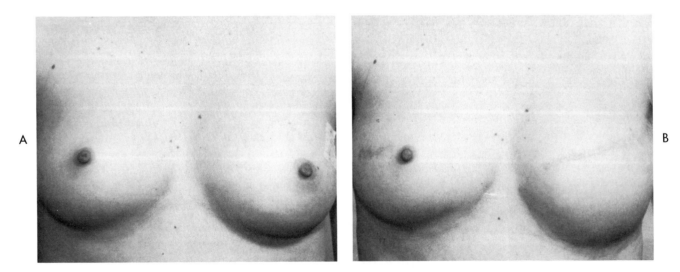

Fig. 6-2   A, A 23-year-old patient with breast cancer in the upper outer quadrant of the left breast. Biopsy site covered with tape. **B,** The patient underwent immediate reconstruction with a round long-term expander. The inframammary fold was maintained at the time of the mastectomy. In this patient, a round expander gave appropriate restoration of the preoperative contour.

which is resistant to expansion. In both of these situations, I prefer to use autogenous tissue with either a TRAM flap or a latissimus dorsi myocutaneous flap. The cutaneous paddle of both of these flaps releases the skin tension across the defect and provides a healthy, soft-tissue cover should an additional expander or implant be required.

Alternatively, breast reconstruction in obese patients is difficult using any technique, but this is especially true for tissue expansion. The excess tissue surrounding the mastectomy site tends to obscure the projection created by the expander, blunting the inframammary fold. Extremely large devices are sometimes necessary to overcome the thickness of the surrounding tissue, and prolonged expansion time may be required. This is in contrast to endomorphic patients in which reasonable expander volumes produce adequate projection and well-formed inframammary folds (Fig. 6-1).

A common misconception of expansion is that it is the simple alternative for breast reconstruction. Therefore a thorough discussion with the patient is critical. Although the initial procedure may seem uncomplicated to the patient, it is important for her to understand the more protracted course of follow-up with this technique and the necessity of a second procedure. Thus an important component of patient selection is motivation on the part of the patient to undergo a reconstructive "process" over time.

SELECTION OF THE TISSUE EXPANDER
Shape and dimension

Tissue expanders are currently available in many different sizes and shapes, as well as smooth and textured surfaces. Although each device may have a separate real or presumed advantage with regard to the final result, it is important to emphasize that tissue expanders do not create breasts, surgeons do. The expander that independently creates an optimal result has yet to be developed. Thus surgical judgment in expander choice requires a well-informed surgeon and a well-stocked central supply.

Excellent results can be obtained in thin patients by using a round expander to create a small, nonptotic breast with centrally located nipples. This is especially true when the remaining breast already has a rounded, hemispherical shape (Fig. 6-2). Placing an implant on the nonmastectomy side can then adjust for any size discrepancy while maintaining the rounded shape to the breast to ensure symmetry (Fig. 6-2).

When a larger breast is required or when greater fullness and projection are needed inferiorly, a simple round expander is inadequate. Several devices designed to satisfy these requirements are available, in-

cluding stacked expanders and differential expanders, which reportedly expand more in the lower pole because of a specific manufacturing method. Others have used oval and elliptical expanders oriented both in a horizontal and transverse plane.[12] Both stacked and oval expanders are useful when a simple round device is unsatisfactory (Fig. 6-3). Results with expanders that reportedly overexpand the lower pole because of a weakened or thinner surface in this area of the device, have been less than exciting, especially when placed in a totally submuscular pocket.

Base diameter

One of the most important criteria in selecting an appropriate expander is choosing the correct base diameter. In the past the prevailing attitude was to simply insert an expander, stretch the tissue as much as possible, and then do a lot of work at a second operation to refine the shape of the reconstructed breast mound.

Today, by selecting the appropriate expander of adequate base diameter and correctly positioning it on the chest wall, an optimal initial result can be obtained, thereby minimizing revision at the second procedure. Selecting an expander with too narrow a base diameter can create deformity that is difficult to correct at a later date. Division of the capsule medially or laterally to correct a breast mound that is too narrow can result in loss of contour and symmetry with disruption of the inframammary fold.

Choosing the correct base diameter is best performed with the patient sitting upright (Fig. 6-4). Using prefabricated templates, a base diameter is chosen to match that of the unoperated breast. In bilateral mastectomy patients, a base diameter is chosen to accommodate the patient's anatomy, and the same measurement is used on both sides. In the ideal situation, with appropriate selection of the expander and with respect to volume and base diameter, no revision would be necessary at the second procedure, which would allow for simple exchange of the expander for the implant (Fig. 6-5).

Textured and smooth walled tissue expanders

Tissue expanders were once all manufactured with a smooth surface. Recently several different textured surface expanders have become available, including the Biospan (McGhan)* device with the Biocell-textured surface (Fig. 6-6) and the MSI (Dow Corning)* textured surface (Fig. 6-7). It is important to understand the differences between these surfaces and how they act in the wound. The only textured expander that adheres to and becomes incorporated in the capsule is the Biocell-surfaced expander.[14] The other tex-

Text cont'd on p. 87.

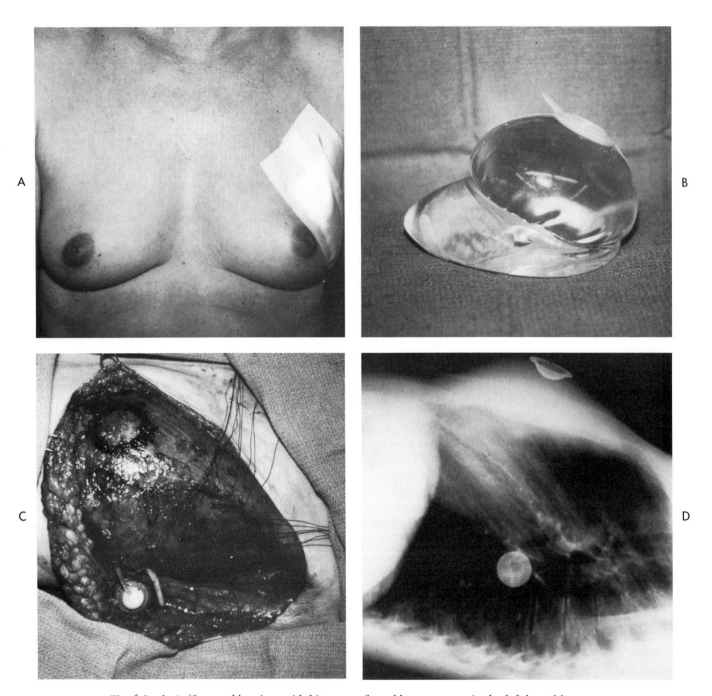

Fig. 6-3 A, A 43-year-old patient with biopsy confirmed breast cancer in the left lateral breast. **B,** Stacked double-chamber expander. **C,** The expander placed in a submuscular pocket. **D,** A postoperative chest x-ray showing the position of a self-contained anterior chamber valve and the remote port of the posterior chamber on the lateral chest wall.

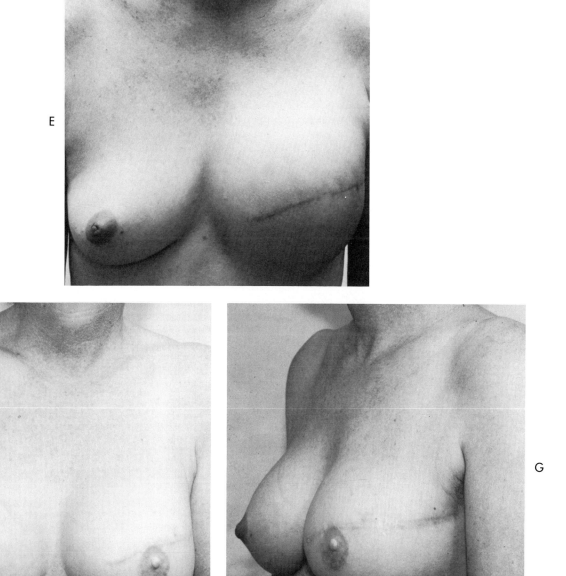

Fig. 6-3, cont'd.   E, The appearance near completion of expansion. **F** and **G,** The expander has been replaced with a smooth-walled implant. To obtain symmetry, an implant was placed beneath the patient's right breast, creating similar base diameters.

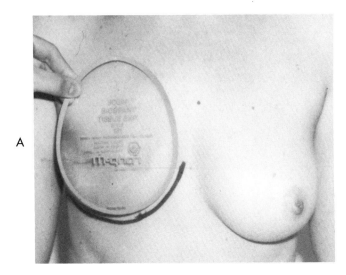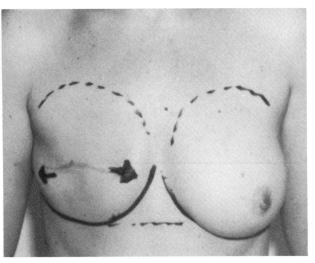

A

B

Fig. 6-4 A, The patient is marked in the upright position to determine which expander has the correct base diameter to match the remaining breast. **B,** The exact position for placement of the expander is marked on the chest wall, using the opposite inframammary fold as a reference.

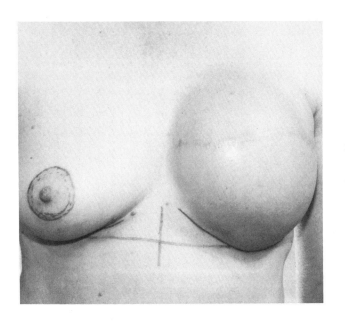

Fig. 6-5   A 39-year-old patient after expansion. The expander is in the correct location for creation of the inframammary fold and of the correct base diameter. The patient's right breast, however, needs an implant to give it a fuller, rounder shape for symmetry.

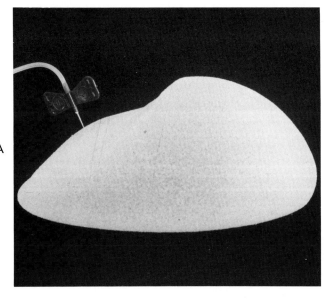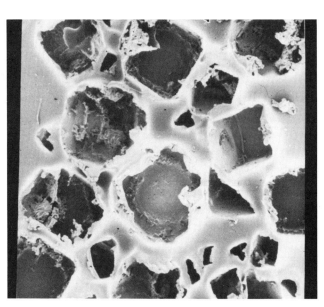

A

B

Fig. 6-6   A, An oval Biospan expander with a self-contained filling port. **B,** A photomicrograph of the Biocell-textured surface (22×).

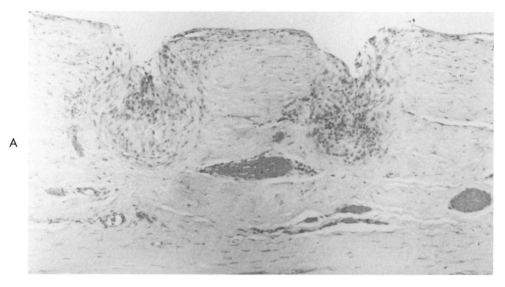

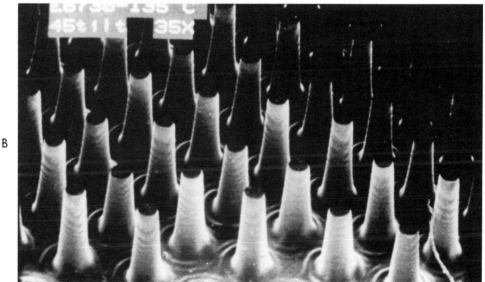

Fig. 6-7 A, A photomicrograph of the capsule surrounding an MSI-textured silicone expander 4 months after placement (10×) Showing the effect of the pillars on the MSI capsule surface. **B,** A high-powered photomicrograph of the silicone pillars on the surface of an MSI-textured expander.

tured surfaces, although they may alter the capsule and potentially reduce contracture, do not adhere to the surrounding capsule. One benefit of adherence is that the expander becomes fixed in position. Therefore it is critical to position it correctly at the time of initial placement, since it will not move later. This fixation has particular application in creating the inframammary fold. As the expander stretches the surrounding tissue, it tends to create the fold in a more defined manner, which is due to its fixation to the capsule (Fig. 6-8).

The expander does not change location, rather the force vectors stretch and push the surrounding tissue anteriorly and inferiorly over the newly created inframammary fold. The incidence of capsular contracture also appears to be diminished using the textured expander. It is important to remember that smooth-walled expanders can work well and produce thin capsules. However, the textured expander seems to be more consistent and reliable, especially when there is associated tissue fixation. Recent experience using MSI-textured expanders has revealed similar good results

*McGhan Medical Corp., Santa Barbara, Calif 93111.

*Dow Corning Wright, Arlington, Ten 38002.

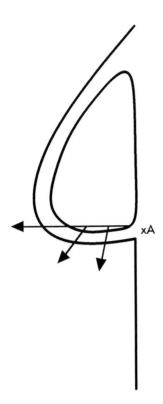

Fig. 6-8 Fixation of a textured expander to the surrounding tissue appears to facilitate creation of the inframammary fold. Point A is relatively fixed, and the vectors of force that are directed anteriorly and inferiorly help delineate the inframammary fold.

with capsular contracture control. However, this surface does not adhere to the surrounding tissue. It is likely that textured expanders will be used more frequently over the next few years.

Other textured silicone surfaces are available for tissue expansion, and, although they may reduce or control capsular contracture, they do not appear to adhere to the surrounding tissue as does the Biocell surface.

PLACEMENT OF THE EXPANDER: "THE FIRST OPERATION"

Attention to detail at the initial placement of the expander will minimize the refinements necessary at the second stage. However, even when using long-term expanders the patient must be made aware that not all patients respond well to expansion, and significant alteration at the second operation may be necessary to refine the result.

Using a totally submuscular pocket for immediate reconstructions and placing the expander partially submuscular with the lower pole of the expander in a subcutaneous plane on delayed reconstructions is effective.

Immediate reconstruction

Working closely with the general surgeon facilitates immediate reconstruction with expansion and in no way compromises the extirpative procedure. The first step is designing the mastectomy incision in an appropriate manner for an adequate resection and a well-located scar. Except in the case of a deep tumor, the underlying muscle can be spared. I prefer total submuscular coverage of the expander in immediate breast reconstruction. If there is secondary skin loss after a mastectomy, a submuscular expander is protected. Also a superficial infection does not mean the submuscular expander has to be removed if the infection can be controlled with appropriate antibiotic therapy. Certainly, the muscle may not always be totally intact after a mastectomy, and adjustments are made accordingly in expander placement.

The submuscular pocket can completely cover the tissue expander.[8] To get total submuscular coverage the pectoralis major, pectoralis minor, serratus anterior, and rectus abdominous muscles are all used, as well as a small portion of the external oblique. This latter fact is rarely discussed, but if one carefully examines the anatomy, a small portion of the external oblique muscle is actually elevated between the lower edge of the serratus anterior and the superior-lateral margin of the rectus abdominous muscle in creating a submuscular pocket.

The first step in immediate breast reconstruction is elevating the pectoralis major along its lateral margin. The pectoralis major is elevated off the anterior chest wall, freeing its attachments from the ribs and sternum. To make the pocket low enough, the dissection proceeds deep to the rectus abdominous fascia or muscle inferiorly. If the dissection stops at the inferior margin of the pectoralis major muscle, the expander will be sitting too high on the chest wall.

The lateral half of the pectoralis minor is elevated in continuity with the serratus anterior muscle. This dissection continues to the mid-axillary line. Raising the lateral half of the pectoralis minor in continuity with the serratus anterior provides extra muscle coverage for closure over the expander. The steps in creating the submuscular pocket with this technique have been described in specific detail.[8]

Once the pocket has been created, it is important to confirm the proper dimensions of the submuscular space. Putting the expander in the correct location is critical, especially when trying to minimize the need for secondary refinements. At this point, I place small lap pads submuscularly along the inferior aspect of the dissection, temporarily close the skin, and sit the patient upright. This allows assessment of the dissection of the submuscular pocket along its inferior aspect. This is a difficult step. Patience and exacting dissection are required to avoid placing the expander too high or low. I will also at this stage place a temporary sizer implant in the submuscular pocket, close the skin temporarily, and sit the patient upright. These maneuvers are necessary to confirm proper positioning of the expander during surgery. An operating table that allows the patient to be placed in a sitting position is a necessity.

The position of the expander is carefully checked to ensure proper alignment within the pocket. An error in placement is difficult to correct secondarily by manipulating the expander, especially when using the Biospan device. The textured Biocell surface "locks" the expander into position as it is incorporated into the capsule, preventing postoperative alteration of expander location. Once proper submuscular pocket dissection has been completed, the appropriate base diameter expander is placed in the pocket and the wound closed. The need to position the expander correctly at the initial operation cannot be overemphasized (Fig. 6-9).

Secondary reconstruction

In secondary breast reconstruction with a well-healed wound, placing the superior portion of the expander under the pectoralis major allows the inferior portion to lie in a subcutaneous plane. This allows for better lower pole expansion and facilitates creation of the inframammary fold.

CREATING THE INFRAMAMMARY FOLD

The importance of the inframammary fold was not recognized early in the evolution of breast reconstruction with tissue expansion. If a well-formed fold fortuitously developed, this was considered an added benefit, and if it did not, there was little to do about it. Today a properly located and symmetrical inframammary fold is an important aesthetic component of breast reconstruction, which often distinguishes the excellent result from the mediocre one.

Previously the fold has been approached as a secondary component to be created after removal of the expander. Experience has since demonstrated that the most aesthetic and permanent folds are those produced as a result of the expansion process itself. This is best accomplished with exacting attention to detail and symmetry at the first operation with the initial placement of the expander.

The contralateral fold is often the main guideline to symmetry. The expander pocket is extended to or just below the level at which the fold is to eventually lie. To accomplish this, it is necessary to sit the patient upright on the operating table to confirm proper placement (Fig. 6-10).

It has been recommended in the past to dissect several centimeters below the proposed fold when placing the expander. This applies only in cases where subsequent external or internal fixation techniques are to be employed. Creating the fold with the expander demands placement of the device at or just below the proposed fold.

The textured Biocell expander has proved to be an important adjunct in the creation of an inframammary fold. It adheres to the capsule, and precise placement of the fold on the chest wall is possible because the expander remains in a fixed position. Tissue expansion then proceeds outward from a fixed point, providing for a well-delineated fold (Fig. 6-8).

Regardless of the type of expander used, the overriding principles are unchanged and include proper placement of the expander and expansion with a device of the correct base diameter. Expanding with a textured device that is too narrow or wide and located incorrectly will require revision, which may destroy the fold created by the expander. Therefore with any expander it is important to take the time to place it correctly and choose the correct base diameter.

During immediate breast reconstruction, preservation of the original inframammary fold during the mastectomy ensures correct placement of the expander. In this situation the chances of recreating the fold with the expander are excellent. Working closely with the general surgeon facilitates this process. The markings for both the mastectomy and location of the fold are to be made preoperatively with the patient in the upright position. Once the patient is asleep, several sutures can be placed through the skin into the rectus fascia. In most patients, saving the inframammary fold at the time of the mastectomy does not compromise the extirpative procedure.

Despite careful attention to detail, revision of the fold is often necessary at the second operation. Unfortunately, folds created by external fixation techniques not only may appear unnatural, but when followed over a period of years, can lose their definition. Internal fixation of the fold can also lose definition over time (Fig. 6-11).

There are several methods of creating the inframammary fold with permanent sutures placed internally. In the case of total submuscular placement, it may be necessary to plicate the lower capsule and muscle to give the fold more definition. One method is to incise the anterior capsule several centimeters cephalad to the proposed fold area and suture the lower margin of capsule to the chest wall. Alternatively the upper margin can be pulled back to the chest wall and secured.

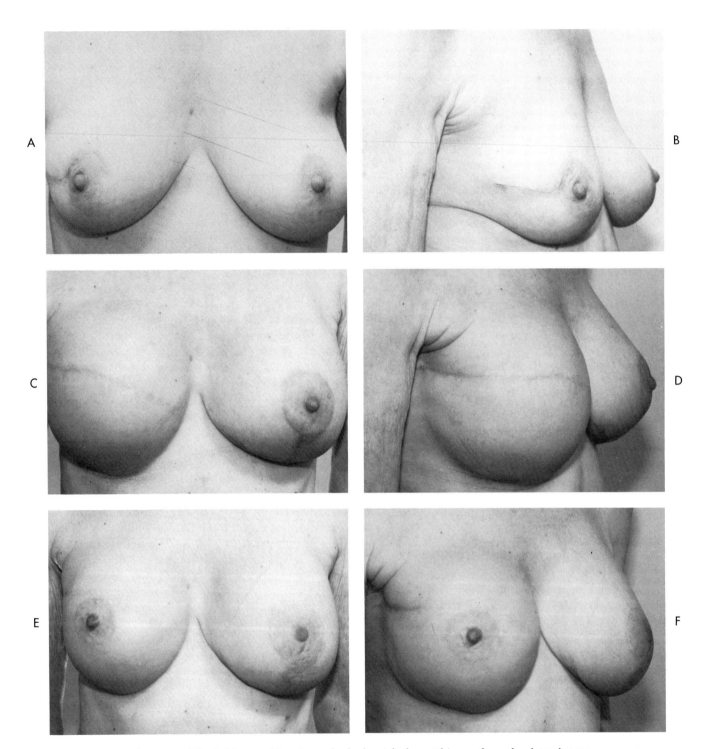

Fig. 6-9 **A** and **B** A 53-year-old patient who had a right breast biopsy through a lateral transverse incision. **C** and **D,** Immediate reconstruction was begun by placement of a right submuscular expander. A mastopexy with augmentation of the left side was performed at the time of the initial operation. The patient was seen 4 months later at completion of the expansion. In patients with ptotic contralateral breasts the expander should be placed slightly below the true horizontal plane of the remaining inframammary fold to improve the illusion of symmetry. **E** and **F,** The reconstruction has been completed by replacement of the expander with a polyurethane implant on the right side. The inframammary fold was created with the expander and is actually 2 cm below the patient's left inframammary fold. In patients with ptosis even after a mastopexy, a certain degree of ptosis will recur. Placing the right reconstructed mound slightly lower than the mastopexy side gives the appearance of reasonable symmetry.

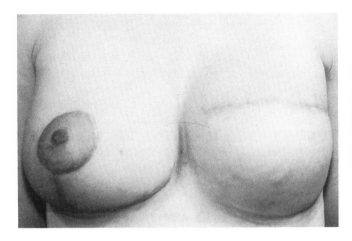

Fig. 6-10 A 42-year-old patient after placement of a tissue expander in a secondary reconstruction procedure. The patient had a mastopexy on the right side at the time the expander was placed on the left. Unlike the patient in Figure 6-9, this mastopexy created a nonptotic breast, and the expander on the left was placed at the same level as the inframammary fold on the right.

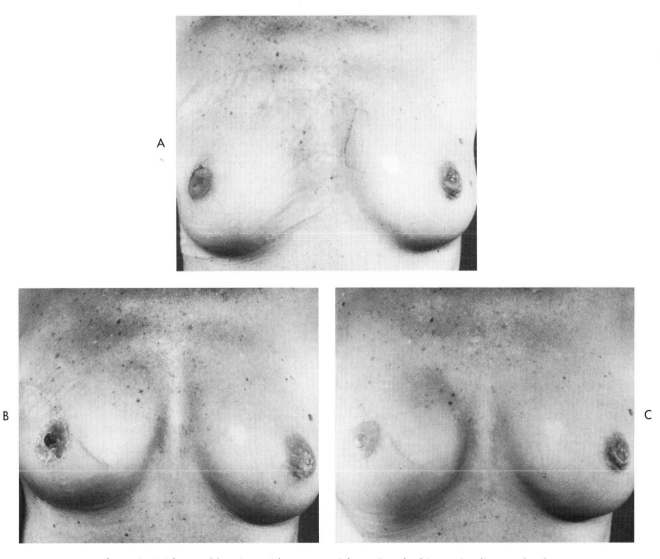

Fig. 6-11 **A,** A 36-year-old patient with a recent right periareolar biopsy site diagnosed as breast cancer. **B,** The patient had reconstruction, including creation of an inframammary fold by the internal suture fixation technique. **C,** The recreated fold looked good for approximately 8 months and then began to lose its definition as seen 1 year after the picture in Fig. 6-11, **B.**

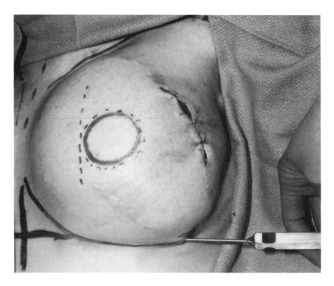

Fig. 6-12 The expander has been replaced with a permanent implant, and a small liposuction cannula is used to highlight the inframammary fold.

With either approach the depth of the sutures is altered depending on the amount of subcutaneous fat. It may be necessary to divide or remove muscle in the area to place the suture in a more subcutaneous layer for better definition of the fold. Liposuction with a small cannula along the line of the inframammary fold can add extra definition to the fold, especially in the patient with a fair amount of subcutaneous fat in the area. Turning the cannula opening toward the skin surface is especially effective in creating a crease in this area (Fig. 6-12).

OVEREXPANSION

In the early years of tissue expansion there was a tendency to underexpand, which was soon replaced by a tendency to significantly overexpand under the impression that this would create a more natural ptotic breast. Currently I agree with overexpansion but to a limited degree.

In the thin patient, when creating a relatively small breast, conservative expansion (i.e., expanding only to the intended final volume) may be adequate. However, expansion is not a static phenomena and that which can be created, can be lost. This is most evident in cases of unexpected expander deflation. Several days after deflation the chest can appear perfectly flat as if no expansion had occurred. Therefore expanding only to the final planned breast size may be inadequate, since contraction can occur, distorting the final appearance of the breast.

Gross overexpansion is an attractive strategy to counteract rebound contraction of the skin. However, a grossly overexpanded device replaced by a much smaller implant can create a floppy, unattractive mound. The expanded tissue will contract over time to the implant surface area, but it is unpredictable and does not necessarily give the optimal result.

One current approach is to moderately overexpand by approximately 10% to 20% greater than the final volume. The key factor is to initially create the right shape, contour, width, and projection with the expander. The final volume is then slightly reduced with the replacement implant or, in the case of long-term expanders, to soften the breast and create a more natural appearance.

USING POLYURETHANE IMPLANTS AFTER EXPANDER REMOVAL AND POLYURETHANE IMPLANTS WITH STACKING: "THE SECOND OPERATION"

Capsule formation has advantages and disadvantages in breast reconstruction with tissue expansion. Formation of a capsule around the expander, which is advantageous, helps create the inframammary fold and determines to a great degree the overall final shape and contour of the reconstructed breast. However, the lack of control over capsule formation during expansion is problematic, especially if the capsule is thick and rigid.

The real issue is not necessarily prevention of a capsule but rather controlling or limiting its formation. In the first phase of reconstruction with the expander, many patients do well with smooth-surface tissue expanders. However, there are a significant number of patients who develop such severe capsules that expansion is unsuccessful in creating an adequate breast mound.

Textured expanders modify the capsular response by reducing linear contraction. This facilitates expansion, making the overlying skin envelope, rather than the capsule, the limiting factor to expansion.

A major issue in breast reconstruction with expansion relates to capsular contracture associated with the final implant. Once the forces of the expander are removed, contracture or volume loss can occur, and although many patients do well with smooth-walled implants, there remains a significant incidence of capsular contracture.

Polyurethane implants have been of great benefit in these cases.[6]* Not only is the incidence of capsular contracture after replacement of the expander reduced, but intraoperative implant customization can be performed because of the ability to stack the implants in the same expanded pocket. Stacking allows intraoperative manipulation of the final breast shape to enhance projection and contour (Fig. 6-13). This is advantageous, since the breast mound often exhibits a significant lack of projection after expansion. Hester[13]

*Surgitek, Plastic Surgery Division, Paso Robles, Calif.

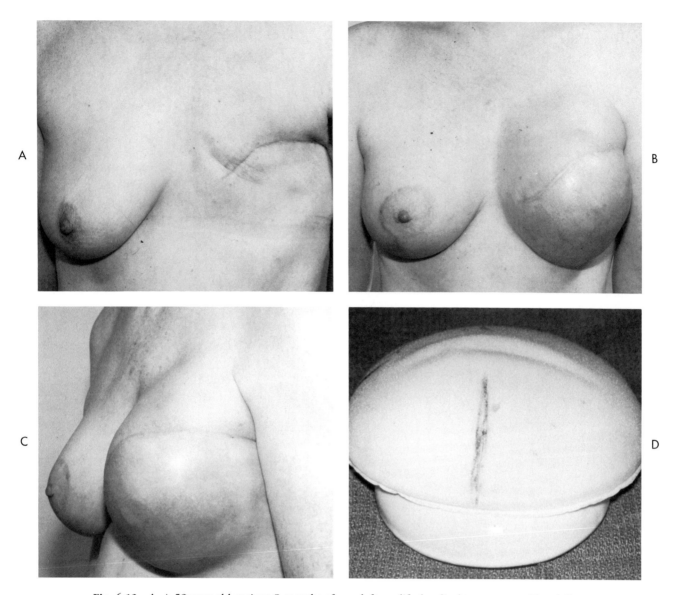

Fig. 6-13   A, A 52-year-old patient 8 months after a left-modified radical mastectomy. **B** and **C,** Three months after initial placement of a stacked, double-chamber expander (total volume 700 ml saline). **D,** The stacked expander was replaced with stacked polyurethane implants. Using temporary sizers the larger implant was a 385 g Replicon of correct base diameter. Next, a smaller group of sizers were inserted with the patient in the upright position and a 115 g Replicon was placed posterior to the larger implant.

described the concept of stacking polyurethane implants, which has become a common strategy of many surgeons. Stacking is an easy process that enhances the final result and can be summarized in a series of steps.

Step one

Determine the width of the breast mound in the final result, and compare this with the implant. For example, if a 14.0-cm-wide breast mound is required, the only replicon implants that will provide this are the 385-to-445 g devices.

Step two

Determine the final volume of fluid on completion of the expansion. I tend to overexpand approximately 20%. Therefore if a 700 ml expansion has provided a reasonable contour, I will plan on a 500-to-550 ml final implant volume.

Step three

Mark the patient preoperatively in the upright position. This confirms the location of the inframammary

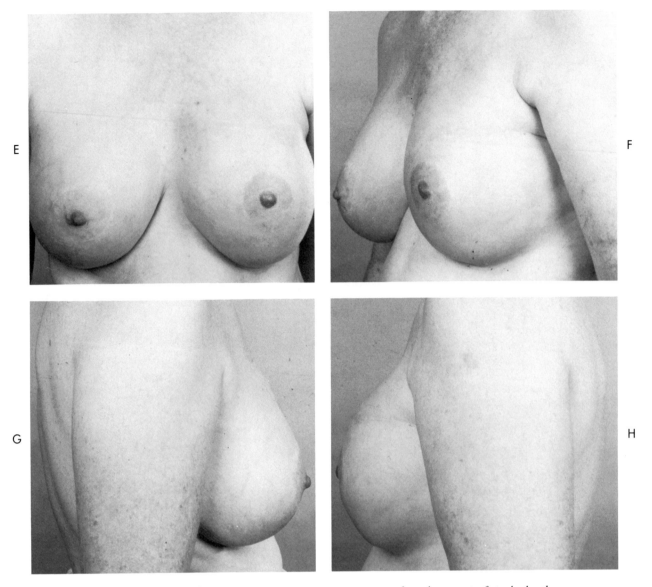

Fig. 6-13, cont'd **E** and **F**, The patients' appearance one year after placement of stacked polyurethane implants beneath expanded tissue on the left and a mastopexy/augmentation on the right. **G**, A lateral view of the mastopexy—augmentation side. **H**, A lateral view of the stacked polyurethane implant—reconstructed side, demonstrating a similar projection.

fold and identifies any modifications that need to be made in either the fold or mound contour.

Step four

A 445 g Replicon temporary sizer is placed in the pocket, the wound closed temporarily, and the patient placed in the upright position. Adjustment in size and base diameter can then be made according to the appearance of the reconstructed mound in this position. For example, if the 445 g implant is too wide, and is folded on itself, a 385 g permanent implant would be chosen.

Step five

Projection is then obtained by placing a smaller sizer in the 80-to-120-g range on top of the main implant. A custom implant has now been created with a total volume equal to that of the two implants added together. In this case, with the 115 g adjustment implant, the final volume would be 500 ml. This is more advantageous than simply inserting a 500 g implant because the larger implant has too wide a base diameter and will probably wrinkle and give less projection. Stacking implants allows volume adjustment within the confines of a specific base diameter, thereby giving ad-

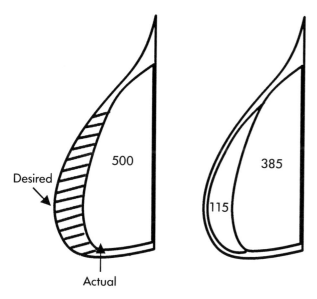

Fig. 6-14   Diagram showing concept of stacking. Total volume of 500 g Replicon may be too wide with inadequate projection. Placing a 385-g Replicon with a 115-g Replicon limits width while maintaining projection and volume.

equate projection (Fig. 6-14). The second smaller implant can be placed either anterior or posterior to the main implant.

Many patients get excellent results with a single implant replacing the expander and do not need stacked implants. However, in some patients, stacking can significantly enhance the final result. Care is advised, however, in choosing the size of the second implant. A too large device can displace the first implant superiorly and result in a fullness in the superior breast mound (Fig. 6-15).

My experience with stacking over the last 3 years has been good. These multiple implants in one pocket (I have used up to three in one breast reconstruction) remain in position. On three occasions I have gone back to modify stacked polyurethane implants and found that the devices had maintained their positions. It would be advantageous if these implants were adjustable, which would allow for secondary change without replacing the device. Implants of this type may become available in the future.

Polyurethane implants in contact with the capsule of the expander usually become adherent. If the expanded pocket is soft and of the correct shape and location, then the capsule should be left alone. If areas of the capsule need to be adjusted, then partial capsulectomies and adjustments should be made before inserting the polyurethane implants. Most important, do not destroy the shape and location of the inframammary fold created by the expander. One criticism of this

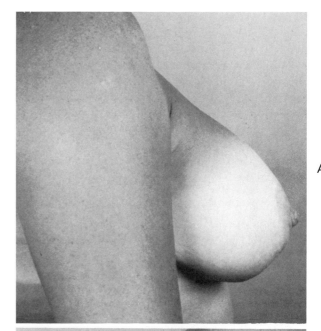

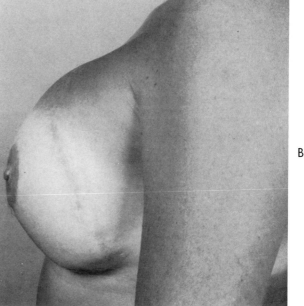

Fig. 6-15   A, The patient's normal breast. **B,** Reconstruction with stacked polyurethane implants. The smaller of the two implants was too large and displaced the larger implant superiorly, creating the superior fullness. Care must be taken when stacking implants to avoid this problem, which is usually caused by using too large of a second implant.

method is that polyurethane implants need to be in contact with virgin tissue to reduce capsular contracture. However, if the pocket created by expansion has a thin capsule, placing a polyurethane implant in contact with this capsule appears to be effective and has not led to problems with capsular contracture. This situation should not be confused with severe capsular contracture, where total capsulectomy is indicated before placement of polyurethane implants to prevent recurrence of the contracture.

I use textured expanders in most cases in attempt to reduce capsular contracture and facilitate contour control of the final result. I then use polyurethane implants to further reduce capsular contracture and increase projection of the breast mound. The ability to place multiple implants in the same pocket also allows for the creation of an intraoperative custom breast reconstruction.

INTRAOPERATIVE EXPANSION

Occasionally, because of secondary capsular contracture, expansion fails to give the correct contour and volume required. One adjunctive procedure is to remove the expander and capsule and intraoperatively overinflate with a temporary expander. This may give the extra volume needed to complete the reconstruction. It can also be used to correct abnormalities of contour intraoperatively. Another group of patients who may benefit from intraoperative expansion are those with previous reconstructions that lack the necessary volume. Here the implant is removed and the appropriate area of capsule excised. This may require a total capsulectomy. The temporary expander is then inserted and inflated to maximum capacity, stretching the tissue. The final implant is then inserted. This has been useful in cases where the surgeon wishes to avoid repeating the whole course of expansion and only moderate gains are necessary to get an acceptable result.

PROBLEMS AND COMPLICATIONS

In my preoperative discussion with patients, I now tell them that I have a 10% complication rate with tissue expansion breast reconstruction. This includes infection, valve or expander problems, inadequate expansion, or the need to use other reconstructive alternatives. I find this rate acceptable, and I doubt I could significantly lower it. There are reports in the literature of much higher complication rates with tissue expansion for breast reconstruction.[18] However, this technique has a significant learning curve in both patient selection and surgical technique.

Tissue expansion remains the most common technique for breast reconstruction. Excellent results are obtained with the majority of patients. Experience and attention to detail are critical. Complications and un-satisfactory results can occur, and it is imperative to learn to deal with these problems logically. No matter how careful or experienced the surgeon, there will be failures that will require alternate techniques of reconstruction. There will continue to be refinements in expanders that will enhance reconstruction surgery, but none of these developments will supercede surgical skill.

Three common problems encountered in breast reconstruction and the surgical solutions to employ in each case follow.

Inadequate Expansion with Severe Capsular Contracture

History
The patient is a 47-year-old woman who underwent secondary breast reconstruction with a smooth-wall-tissue expander with a self-contained valve. The patient developed a tight capsular contracture that prevented adequate expansion (Figs. 6-16, *A* and *B*).

Solution
Three months after insertion of the expander, a second operation was performed. The expander was removed and a total capsulectomy performed. A temporary expander was inserted and inflated with 1100 ml of saline over three cycles (Fig. 6-16, *C*). After obtaining appropriate hemostasis, stacked polyurethane implants were inserted. First, after considering base diameter, a 600 g sizer was inserted, and the patient was raised to the sitting position. The sizer was replaced with a 600 ml Replicon implant. Next, smaller temporary implants were inserted, and an 80 g Replicon was chosen for placement posterior to the larger implant along its inferior margin (Fig. 6-16, *D*). Again, the table was raised to properly evaluate the implant position and size. The appearance of the reconstruction 18 months later (Fig. 6-16, *F*) showed maintenance of projection compared with the normal side (Fig. 6-16, *E*).

Discussion
Intraoperative expansion can significantly improve what would have been a mediocre result. The extra expansion at the time of implant placement gives enough increase in volume to give a satisfactory outcome to difficult cases.

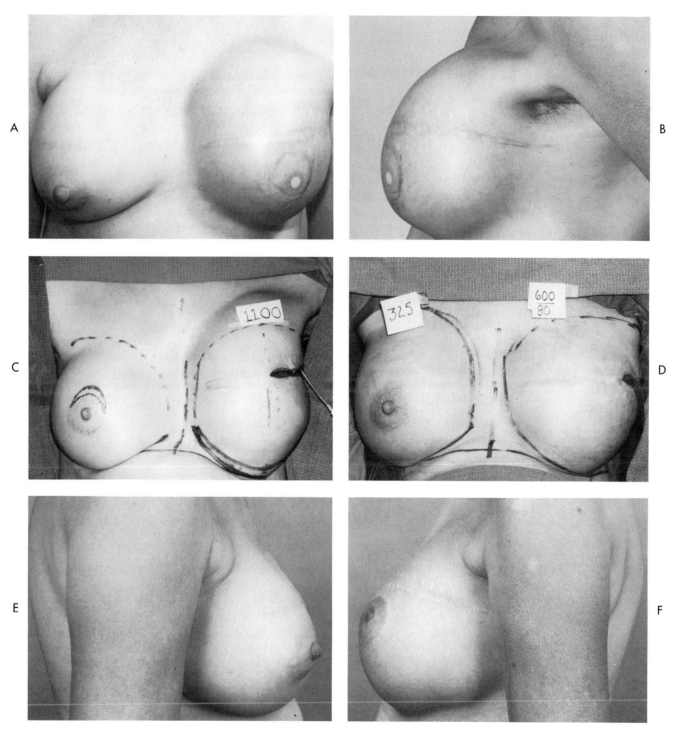

Fig. 6-16   A to **F,** Problem case no. 1.

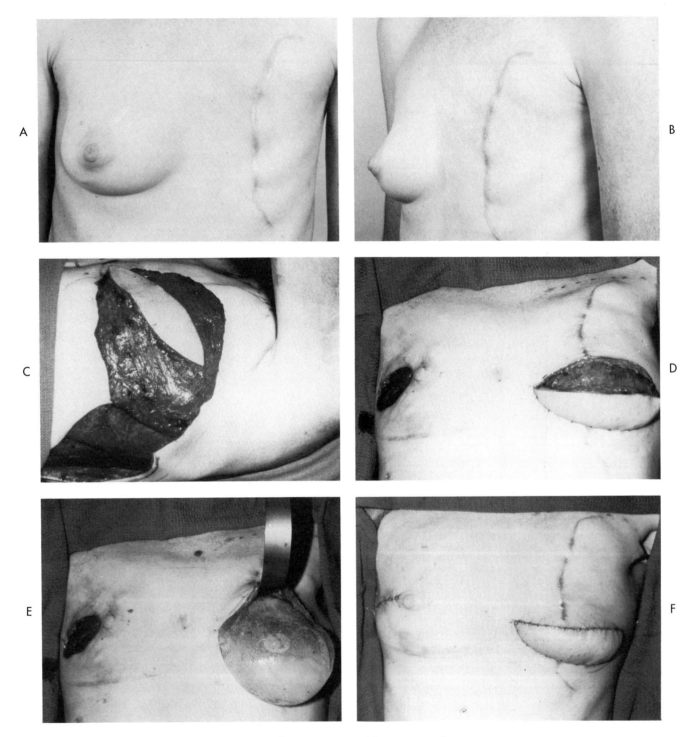

Fig. 6-17   **A** to **F**, Problem case no. 2.

G 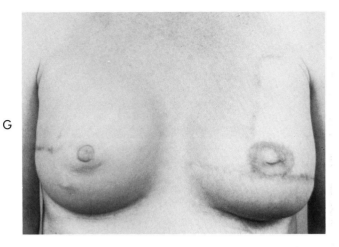 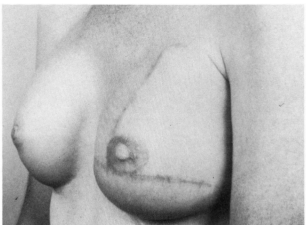 H

Fig. 6-17 cont'd **G** to **H**

Inadequate Local Tissue

History

A 39-year-old woman 2 years after a mastectomy with a long vertical scar and an atrophic pectoralis major muscle. The patient weighted 96 pounds, had no subcutaneous fat, and had a perfectly flat abdomen (Figs. 6-17, *A* and *B*).

Solution

During the first operation the surgeon placed a latissimus dorsi myocutaneous flap transversely at a right angle to the mastectomy scar. The flap was inset along the proposed inframammary fold (Figs. 6-17, *C* and *D*). A textured Biospan expander (400 ml) was placed beneath the latissimus dorsi muscle (Figs. 6-17, *E* and *F*). A subcutaneous mastectomy was simultaneously performed on the right side and also reconstructed with a 400 ml Biospan expander. After completion of the expansion 4 months later, the expanders were removed and replaced with a

385 g Replicon implant on the right side and a 325 g implant on the left (Figs. 6-17, *G* and *H*).

Discussion

Certainly there are alternative methods of reconstructing this patient. A TRAM flap could have been performed, but this patient had a perfectly flat and tight abdomen with no fat. An implant or expander would still have been necessary with the TRAM. A latissimus dorsi myocutaneous flap used with a tissue expander gives excellent results, and I frequently use this flap with tissue expansion. However, in this case it would have been important to ignore the mastectomy scar and to have inset the flap along the proposed inframammary fold. Placing the flap in a vertical plane would have severely limited the expansion, as well as compromised the creation of the inframammary fold.

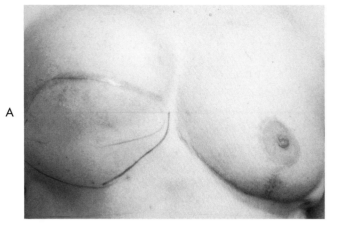

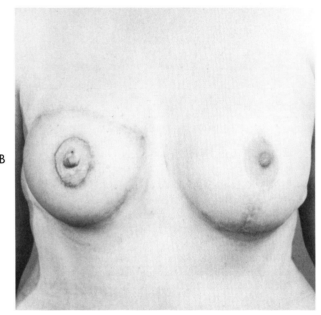

Fig. 6-18   A and **B,** Problem case no. 3.

Unsuccessful Expansion

History

Within 1 year this patient underwent two operations for tissue expansion. Expansion was inadequate, particularly in the inferior area. The patient was first seen after the second expander had been placed in conjunction with an open capsulectomy (Fig. 6-18, *A*). After initial consultation, expansion was continued for several more weeks but with little improvement.

Solution

This patient had an excellent abdomen for a TRAM reconstruction. The expander was removed and the flap oriented along the plane of the inframammary fold (Fig. 6-18, *B*). No implant was required.

Discussion

All surgeons have had patients with whom tissue expansion was unsuccessful. It is difficult to regroup after considerable effort has been invested in one method of reconstruction, but with some patients it is in their best interest to totally change the surgical plan. In this case, after a thorough discussion with the patient, it was elected to remove the expander and reconstruct the breast with a TRAM flap. The flap was inset transversely along the proposed inframammary fold, ignoring the previous area of limited expansion. Another alternative that I have used after unsuccessful expansion is a latissimus dorsi flap, with placement of an expander beneath the flap. This is another excellent option when it is necessary to regroup and start over.

REFERENCES

1. Argenta LC, Marks MW, and Grabb WC: Selective use of serial expansion in breast reconstruction, Ann Plast Surg 11:188, 1983.

2. Argenta LC: Reconstruction of the breast by tissue expansion, Clin Plast Surg 11:257, 1984.

3. Bailey MH et al: Immediate breast reconstruction: reducing the risks, Plast Reconstr Surg 83(5):845-51, 1989.

4. Becker H: The expandable mammary implant, Plast Reconstr Surg 79(4):631-7, 1987.

5. Becker H: The permanent tissue expander, Clin Plast Surg 14(3):519-27, 1987.

6. Brand KG: Foam-covered mammary implants, Clin Plast Surg 15(4):533, 1988.

7. Dickson MG and Sharpe DT: The complications of tissue expansion in breast reconstruction: a review of 75 cases, Br J Plast Surg 40(6):629-35, 1987.

8. Fisher J, Maxwell GP, Woods J: Surgical alternatives in subcutaneous mastectomy reconstruction, Clin Plast Surg 15(4):667-76, 1988.

9. Fodor PB and Swistel AJ: Chest wall deformity following expansion of irradiated soft tissue for breast reconstruction, NY State J Med 89(7):419-20, 1989.

10. Gibbons WP: Caution in expanding radiated tissue, Plast Reconstr Surg 80(6):871, 1987.

11. Gibney J: Use of a permanent tissue expander for breast reconstruction, Plast Reconstr Surg 84(4):607-17, 1989.

12. Gold A: Elliptical tissue expansion for breast reconstruction, Ann Plast Reconstr Surg (in press).

13. Hester TR et al: A 5-year experience with polyurethane-covered mammary prostheses for treatment of capsular contracture, primary augmentation mammoplasty, and breast reconstructions, Clin Plast Surg 15(4):569, 1988.

14. Maxwell GP and Fisher J: One hundred consecutive breast reconstructions in 68 patients using a textured silicone tissue expander. Proceedings of the sixty-ninth annual meeting of the American Association of Plastic Surgeons, Hot Springs, Va, 1990.

15. Radovan C: Tissue expansion in soft-tissue reconstruction, Plast Reconstr Surg 74:482, 1984.

16. Russell IS et al: The use of tissue expansion for immediate breast reconstruction after mastectomy, Med J Aust 152(12):632-635, 1989.

17. Seckel BR and Hyland WT: Soft-tissue expander for delayed and immediate breast reconstruction, Surg Clin North Am 65:383, 1985.

18. Slavin SA and Colen SR: Sixty consecutive breast reconstructions with the inflatable expander: a critical appraisal, Plast Reconstr Surg 86(5):910, 1990.

19. Versaci AD: Reconstruction of a pendulous breast utilizing a shaped expander, Ann Plast Surg 23(6):469-78, 1989.

CHAPTER 7

Prevention and Management of Complications in TRAM Flap Surgery

Carl R. Hartrampf, Jr,
Joseph R. Barnthouse,
G. Kristine Bennett

Autogenous breast reconstruction using the transverse abdominal island flap has many advantages over synthetic materials, however, complications can still occur. This chapter deals with these complications as they have occurred in practice and our experience with the complications of other surgeons doing TRAM flap surgery. Over the past 10 years, a total of 628 breast reconstructions in 534 patients using the TRAM island flap have been performed. The patients ranged in age from 17 to 90, with a mean age of 47 years. Fifty-six percent of the defects resulted from modified radical mastectomies, 26% from subcutaneous total or simple mastectomies, 12% from radical mastectomies, and the remaining 6% from a variety of causes, including congenital defects.

This chapter analyzes the results of these patients and discusses the occurrence, management, and prevention of various complications. Subjective assessment of results in the first 300 patients surveyed is presented.

A complication is an untoward event occurring intraoperatively or postoperatively, including the following (see Table 7-1):
1. Total flap loss.
2. Partial full-thickness flap loss.
3. Fat necrosis.
4. Abdominal wall weakness.
5. Abdominal wall hernia.
6. Delayed abdominal wound healing.
7. Loss of the umbilicus.
8. Pulmonary problems.
9. Deep venous thrombosis.
10. Wound infection.
11. Hematoma.

Poor breast shape, lack of projection, and asymmetry are subjective assessments related to artistic skill, surgical technique, and experience with the procedure and are difficult to evaluate objectively. We attempt to address these aesthetic factors with the patient survey and discussion of procedures we have performed to revise the reconstructed breast so that it will more closely match the opposite breast.

INHERENT PROBLEMS
Scarring

The abdominal donor site scar can be significant in some patients, especially when tissue harvest is great and the abdominal skin closure is tight. The scar may be red and wide and, in some individuals, may extend far laterally or high on the abdomen, making it difficult to conceal. However, a low transverse abdominal scar, which is easily hidden, is most common.

The breast scar will be present on the reconstructed breast mound, and, in most cases, the exact location is dictated by the level and direction of the mastectomy scar. These scars, however, fade with time but can be obvious for several years after the procedure. Breast scarring can be minimized if a plastic surgeon helps plan the mastectomy. A major advance in breast reconstruction has been the evolution of the skin-sparing mastectomy.

Symptoms of prolonged abdominal healing

Abdominal discomfort and swelling are the most common complaints after this procedure. Most patients experience a temporary loss of definition at the waist and varying degrees of suprapubic swelling. Excess suprapubic adipose tissue and redundant tissue in the upper hips, lateral to the abdominal scar, can be removed at the time of nipple reconstruction, using suction-assisted lipectomy. General abdominal discomfort and tightness usually persist for 6 weeks and may last 3 to 6 months. Approximately 1% of our patients complain of abdominal pain lasting 1 year or more. A persistent finding in these few patients is postoperative weight gain. Patients often complain of abdominal paresthesias and pain in the mid-abdominal region and over the anterior thighs.

It is the surgeon's responsibility to be certain that the patient thoroughly understands these inherent problems before this procedure is performed.

MAJOR AND MINOR FLAP COMPLICATIONS
Total flap loss

Of the 628 flap reconstructions in our practice, two total flap failures (0.3%) have occurred in the past 10 years. In one case, a technical error resulted in division of the deep superior epigastric pedicle. The patient was overweight, had an inordinately wide rectus muscle, a 7-cm diastasis, and a barrel-shaped chest. Anatomically, the vascular pedicles were located much farther laterally than usual, and on one side, the pedicle was severed. Revascularization using microvascular technique failed. In a second patient, an abdominoplasty had been performed 20 years previously, and a higher-than-usual upper abdominal TRAM flap procedure was attempted. The patient was aware of the risk of flap failure. Interestingly, this flap appeared viable for 3 days before a sudden loss of vascularity. During a second procedure the pedicle had thrombosed because of excessive stretch over the rib margin. Unfortunately, this case does not answer the questions of whether the perforators reconstituted after a previous abdominoplasty. In both cases, poor patient selection was the main error.

Subtotal flap loss

Thirty-two patients (6.7%) experienced subtotal flap loss. A tissue loss greater than 50% occurred in 4 flaps (0.8% of patients), a 25% to 50% loss occurred in 7 flaps (1.5% of patients), and a loss of less than 25% occurred in 21 flaps (4.4% of patients). These complications all required major surgical revision, including the use of a silicone implant, a latissimus dorsi flap, a triceps flap, or a revision of the TRAM flap.

Fat necrosis

In the first 119 patients, approximately 15% had areas of hardness in the buried portion of the TRAM flap that represented areas of fat necrosis. The majority of these patients had undergone a radical mastectomy and required a large flap extending across both sides of the lower abdomen. It became clear that the high incidence of fat necrosis seen in the early developmental stages of this procedure could be attributed to the overdependence on a single pedicle to nourish the abdominal tissue on the opposite side of the midline. We now believe that a single pedicle will reliably nourish only 60% to 70% of the abdominal tissue in a healthy patient. We learned that the major fat compartment between the skin and Scarpa's fascia receives its blood supply from the subdermal plexus. Therefore trimming the flap is now accomplished by removing fat on the underside of the flap, thereby shaping it down to a well-vascularized, thin dermal edge.

Causes of major and minor flap complications

The main cause of flap loss was attributable to injudicious patient selection and use of the flap beyond its reliable limits. The other causes of flap loss in order of frequency were technical error, excessive tension on the vascular pedicle, and venous obstruction caused by a hematoma under the pedicle. Cigarette smoking and previous chest wall irradiation did not statistically increase the rate of flap loss. Our current perioperative routine and operative technique have been continually modified to avoid total flap loss, partial flap loss, and fat necrosis.

SALVAGE PROCEDURES

The following procedures have been used after total or partial flap loss to achieve a more satisfactory breast size and shape.

Silicone implants

If after subtotal flap loss there is only a breast volume deficiency, then a silicone implant can be placed under the pectoralis major muscle if present; if the muscle is absent, the implant can be placed under the flap, but often only small volume implants are needed. The manufacturers will provide implants in the 50- to 100-ml range on special request. We have used both smooth and polyurethane-coated implants with equal success.

Latissimus dorsi muscle or musculocutaneous flap

The latissimus dorsi muscle can be used as a muscle flap to provide additional breast volume. On the other hand, the latissimus musculocutaneous flap provides skin and breast volume in cases where partial TRAM flap loss has resulted in full-thickness skin and volume deficiency. This flap has become a useful aid in restoring minor defects in the upper and outer portions of the reconstructed breast.

Triceps musculocutaneous flap

A long head of the triceps musculocutaneous flap was used in five patients after subtotal TRAM flap loss. All of these patients had undergone reconstruction for radical mastectomy defects. Four patients had previous radiation therapy after extirpative surgery. In four cases the safe limit of a single pedicle TRAM flap was unknowingly exceeded. The long head of the triceps musculocutaneous island flap was therefore developed to provide additional tissue either in the upper anterior chest (*N, 4*) or in the lateral and lower inframammary crease area (*N, 1*). The only prerequisite for using this flap is redundant tissue of the upper arm, which is often present in middle-aged patients and in those patients with postmastectomy lymphedema.

TRAM flap sharing

In one patient who had undergone bilateral TRAM flap reconstructions with total loss of the left flap, a portion of the large surviving right TRAM flap was transposed to the opposite breast on the original pedicle. Total and partial TRAM flap loss is unfortunate for all concerned, however, through salvage procedures and revisions, all but 2 of the 32 patients had acceptable outcomes.

ABDOMINAL WALL COMPLICATIONS

In assessing abdominal wall strength, almost half of our mastectomy patients could not perform sit-ups before the procedure. Of the patients who could perform sit-ups before surgery, 83% with unilateral muscle harvest could perform sit-ups after the procedure. In patients who had undergone bilateral muscle harvest, however, only 36% retained the ability to perform sit-ups. Postoperative back pain was common immediately after surgery but was rapidly resolved. Long-term chronic back pain has not been a problem in our patients.

Abdominal herniation may occur infrequently if a conservative rectus muscle and sheath harvest and a multilayered direct closure are practiced. In bilateral and double pedicle cases, a competent direct closure will be possible in more than half of the cases, and a synthetic mesh as an overlay support will be required in the remaining cases.

Reasons that postoperative hernias develop include the following:
1. Overzealous harvest of the rectus muscle and sheath.
2. Overdependence on synthetic mesh.
3. Suture failure (e.g., use of absorbable material).
4. Repair failure (e.g., too small tissue bites cause the knots to fail.)

Hernia/abdominal wall weakness

Six patients (1.3%) developed a lower abdominal wall hernia after TRAM flap surgery. Two hernias occurred in the first 100 patients; there were no hernias in the next 175 patients, and four hernias occurred in

the next 30 patients. There were no hernias in the last 71 patients. The four hernias that occurred in patients numbered 375, 385, 399, and 404 were a direct result of a change in the abdominal closure routine from two layers of nylon to one layer of polyglycolic suture followed by one layer of nylon and the application of stainless steel fascial staples. When the hernia rate was recognized higher than usual, we reestablished our traditional technique of a two-layer closure with double stranded #0 nylon and have been satisfied with our results. All six hernias were successfully repaired.

Two patients developed small defects in the upper rectus sheath not requiring repair. In the early developmental phase of the TRAM flap procedure, a strip of anterior rectus was not included with muscle but was completely dissected off the muscle. In each of these cases a small rent was made in the anterior sheath at the location of the dense adherence to the upper transverse inscription. We now perform a composite dissection of the sheath and muscle.

Two patients demonstrated postoperative abdominal wall laxity after single pedicle TRAM flap reconstruction. This had not been a problem in the single pedicle reconstruction since 1983 when we began to plicate the anterior rectus sheath on the nonpedicle side.

Improvement in the abdominal appearance and a return of abdominal wall strength has been the rule in our series.

Delayed suprapubic abdominal wound healing

Necrosis of an area of abdominal skin just below the reconstructed umbilicus, which healed without requiring a graft, occurred in 2% of the patients. All but one of these patients were former smokers. Former smokers were 58.5 times as likely to have skin loss as nonsmokers (*P* = .001). One patient required a skin graft to the suprapubic area after granulation tissue had covered exposed prolene mesh.

Loss of the umbilicus

In less than 1% of our patients (all bilateral muscle harvest) the umbilicus became devascularized and was lost. After spontaneous healing, most have a residual skin dimple with an acceptable appearance. We now retain some fat with its blood supply on the umbilical stalk to prevent this occurrence.

OTHER COMPLICATIONS
Pulmonary complications

A tight abdominal closure will stress pulmonary function. Basilar atelectasis and small pleural effusions are a frequent radiographic finding. Four patients had pulmonary emboli after TRAM flap surgery and were treated with systemic anticoagulants.

Risk Factor Classification in Patient Selection for TRAM Operation

Class I	No risk factors and a score of 0 on the risk rating scale. Patients in this class are most likely to do well with surgery.
Class II	One risk factor with a score of 2 or less. Patients in this category are still good candidates for the TRAM flap procedure, but the surgeon should institute measures to minimize the risk.
Class III	Two risk factors or a combined score of less than 5. These patients are marginal candidates for the TRAM flap procedure.
Class IV	Three or more risk factors or a combined score of 5 or greater. Patients in this category are not good candidates for reconstruction with the TRAM flap.

Deep venous thrombosis

In our series, three patients developed calf or ileofemoral deep venous thrombosis and were treated with anticoagulants.

We have developed a regimen for patients who have a history of deep venous thrombosis or who are 15% to 25% over their ideal body weight. We now administer intravenous low-dose continuous heparin the night before surgery until the patients are mobile. This heparin dose should not act as an anticoagulant but instead should maintain normal coagulation studies.

Wound infection

Three patients (0.6%) developed breast flap wound infections. One patient developed an *Escherichia coli* infection in an unrecognized breast hematoma. The other two patients developed a *Staphylococcus aureus* wound infection along the ellipse chest wall skin suture line, which was successfully treated with drainage and oral antibiotics. All three of these patients were former smokers.

Six patients (1.2%) developed localized abdominal wound infections, which were treated with local wound care.

Hematoma/seroma

During the developmental stages of this procedure, 26% of our patients developed persistent abdominal seromas requiring aspiration or drainage. Abdominal seroma formation has occurred infrequently with the past 275 patients. We attribute this dramatic decrease to careful hemostasis and external drainage with four small (3 mm) nonirritative silicone tubes.

Eight patients (1.6%) developed hematomas under the abdominal flap. Two patients had hematomas that occurred in the epigastrium and could have been prevented by better hemostasis in the epigastric tunnel region. Several abdominal hematomas occurred in obese patients, and two went unrecognized because of the obese abdomens. One hematoma occurred in an obese patient within the repaired rectus sheath and was secondary to an uncontrolled deep inferior epigastric vessel. This patient later developed an abdominal hernia. The deep inferior epigastric vessels are now controlled by double vascular clips.

We believe that the combination of meticulous hemostasis and adequate drainage with external, closed-suctioned drainage systems, has contributed to our current low rate of breast and abdominal hematomas.

CONTRAINDICATIONS AND RISK FACTORS

The TRAM procedure takes 3 to 4 hours to perform with unilateral reconstruction and 4 to 6 hours with bilateral reconstruction. It requires invading tissue planes from the pubis to the upper chest, followed by a tight abdominal wall closure, which can compromise pulmonary function. The tissue insult and subsequent stress on body systems during and after this procedure are considerable. Therefore the prudent surgeon only will consider this procedure for the healthy patient. The absolute contraindications for this procedure include chronic pulmonary disease, severe cardiovascular disease, uncontrolled hypertension, and insulin-dependent diabetes mellitus. These contraindications are obvious. However, there are certain risk factors that may not be so apparent, and the compounding of these factors in one patient may insidiously increase the chances of a complication in that patient beyond the acceptable range.

Risk factors for the TRAM procedure and my estimate of the severity of that risk are listed in Table 7-1. These risk factors can be translated into a risk classification (see Box) that will help determine good candidates for this procedure.

PATIENT SELF-ASSESSMENT OF THE TRAM FLAP

The overall response rate to a patient questionnaire sent to our first 300 patients was 97.6%. Patients perceived their sense of well being and general appearance to be improved after surgery (94% in unilateral reconstruction and 90% in bilateral reconstructions). Ninety-eight percent of the patients believed that breast reconstruction using the TRAM flap was worth their time and effort. Ninety-eight and one half percent of the patients would recommend this method of breast reconstruction to other patients.

Patient assessment of preoperative abdominal wall strength was elicited by questioning whether the patients could perform sit-ups before and after surgery. Approximately half of the patients could not perform sit-ups before reconstruction (and this has been our objective finding). Of the patients who could perform sit-ups, 87% of the patients with unilateral muscle harvest and 36% of the patients with bilateral muscle harvest TRAM flaps were able to perform sit-ups after surgery. Abdominal appearance was improved in 78% of the patients with unilateral reconstructions and in 82% of the patients with bilateral reconstructions. Thirteen percent of the patients with unilateral reconstructions and 12% with bilateral reconstructions believed their abdominal appearance was worse. However, most of these patients were thin and objected to the noticeable abdominal scar. Approximately 50% of the patients in both unilateral and bilateral reconstructions believed that their posture had not changed after surgery, and approximately 41% in both groups believed it had improved. Ninety-four percent of the patients with unilateral reconstruction and 90% of the patients with bilateral reconstruction believed that their general appearance and emotional state had improved after TRAM flap surgery. Postoperative back pain was common immediately after this procedure but rapidly resolved so that no long-term problem with back pain occurred. Ability to participate in activities such as tennis, golf, jogging, and swimming was the same or improved in 92% of the patients.

SUMMARY

A continuing honest appraisal of complications that have occurred and the technical errors that have been made is critical to improving surgical performance and autogenous reconstructive results. Predictably, good results with few complications can be achieved with autogenous breast reconstruction by the TRAM flap method if strict patient selection guidelines are adhered to and the surgeon is mentally prepared and gains experience in a self-critical manner.

Table 7-1

Risk Factors of the TRAM Flap Procedure

Risk factor	Score (1 to 10)
OBESITY	
Moderate: <25% above IBW	1
Severe: >25% over IBW	5
SMALL VESSEL DISEASE	
Light to moderate smoking (1+ pack/day for 2 to 10 years)	1
Chronic heavy smoking (10-20 pack years)	2
Chronic heavy smoking (20-30 pack years)	5
Autoimmune disease (scleroderma, Raynaud's)	8
Non-insulin-dependent diabetes mellitus	5
Insulin-dependent diabetes mellitus	10
PSYCHOSOCIAL PROBLEMS	
Unstable emotional state (life crisis)	2
Personality disorder	3
Substance abuse	5
ABDOMINAL SCARS	
If "planned out" of flap design	0.5
Disruption of vascular perforators; transection of superior epigastric vessels (Chevron incision, abdominoplasty)	10
PATIENT'S ATTITUDE	
Patient unwilling or unable to invest time required for healing or objects to abdominal scar	10
SURGEON'S INEXPERIENCE	
Less than 10 TRAM flaps	1
A MAJOR SYSTEM DISEASE PROCESS	
Chronic lung disease	10
Severe cardiovascular disease	10

SUGGESTED READINGS

Hartrampf CR: Transverse abdominal island flap technique for breast reconstruction after mastectomy, Baltimore, 1984, University Park Press.

Hartrampf CR and Bennett GK: Autogenous tissue reconstruction in the mastectomy patient—a critical review of 300 patients, Ann Surg 205:508-519, 1987.

Hartrampf CR: Breast reconstruction with living tissue, Norfolk, Va, 1990, Hampton Press.

CHAPTER 8

Facial Sculpturing: Aesthetic Craniofacial Surgery

Kenneth E. Salyer

Today, improved results can be achieved in facial skeletal surgery by applying aesthetic craniofacial surgical principles and using osteotomy and/or augmentation materials. New and refined techniques offer improvement of the bony architecture by adjusting angulation and projection at desired points of the face, thus allowing for refinement of deformed, displaced, or aesthetically undesirable facial skeletal proportion. Aesthetic facial skeletal sculpturing provides the foundation for and makes the difference between good and excellent results in facial proportions. When shape or contour is abnormal, simply cutting and moving the bone does not yield optimal results. In infant surgery, for example, the shape of the bone must be totally altered and repositioned to achieve superior aesthetic results. After maxillary or mandibular repositioning, additional contouring is necessary to balance asymmetries that may lack projection of the malar contour, the chin, the mandible, the orbits, or forehead. This may be achieved by hard-tissue alteration or augmentation. A recent method using native bone, splits the lamella into two segments. This is called the lamellar split osteotomy technique. Autogenous or alloplastic materials, which may also be used, offer alternative choices to this native bone osteotomy.

Achieving balance and harmony are the surgeon's ultimate goals in facial hard-tissue sculpturing. Although many surgeons use implantation of materials, as well as osteotomies of the existing skeleton, the classic bilamellar shift of the bone is one of the main methods used to obtain a new contour of the face. When this contouring is related to the maxilla and/or mandible, ultimate positioning is frequently determined by dental occlusion. However, there are times when dental occlusion may not be the optimal guideline for achieving an aesthetically pleasing face. Planning for facial contouring should rely on the basic principles of aesthetic

proportions, not dental occlusion. Plastic surgical principles and techniques applied to the facial skeleton allow for optimal results and changes, which are referred to in this chapter as facial sculpturing (Fig. 8-1).

The techniques presented in this chapter have been successful in my practice of craniofacial surgery,

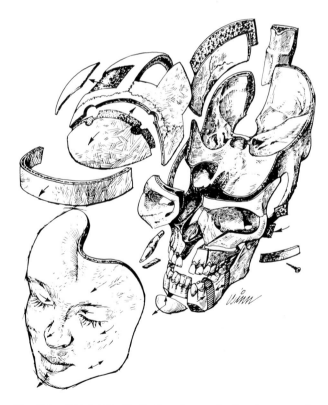

Fig. 8-1 Composite illustration demonstrating the present technology in craniomaxillofacial surgery. The use of split cranial bone and the split lamellar technique, as well as more classic osteotomies are depicted.

111

Donor Site vs. Recipient Site in Bone Grafting; Yes—good choice; No—poor choice

	MALAR	MAXILLA	MANDIBLE	CRANIAL VAULT	ORBITS	FOREHEAD	CHIN
Split cranial	Yes	Yes*	Yes*	Yes*	Yes*	Yes*	**
Split rib	Yes*	Yes*	No	No	Yes	No	No
Iliac cancellous	No	Yes	No	No	Yes	Yes	No
Split Iliac	No	Yes (rare)	No	No	Yes	Yes	No

*Preferred sources
†Alloplastic or osteotomy

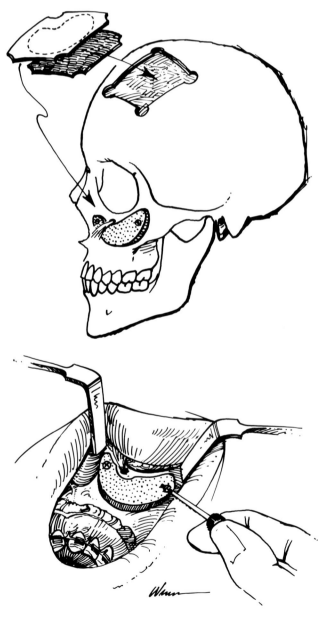

Fig. 8-2 Split cranial bone graft with screw fixation.

including techniques and methods others have found to be useful for changing the shape, form, and aesthetic balance of the facial skeleton. My new and proved technique of the lamellar split osteotomy will be featured as an example of one means to change and balance the facial skeleton by changing the contour. While the facelift—superficial or deep-plane rhytidectomy—has given us the ability to detail the soft tissues of the face, the lamellar split osteotomy allows for detailing of the facial skeleton and provides an alternative to alloplastic augmentation as a means of facial sculpturing.[9] Many of the ideas and techniques presented here are described in greater detail in *Techniques in Aesthetic Craniofacial Surgery.*[17]

BONE GRAFTS

The use of bone grafts is an intricate and important aspect of facial sculpturing. Grafts are essential in performing osteotomies that allow translocation of major segments of the face. The spaces created by maxillary, mandibular, and orbital cranial osteotomies are frequently filled with cancellous or cortical bone grafts. Bone from rib, hip, or cranium can be used. These grafts reshape and balance the face and cranium and enable the surgeon to refine his results. Although they undergo more resorption than inlay grafts, onlay grafts augmented by soft-tissue shifts of the galea and muscle, enable the surgeon to sculpt the face instead of simply moving the jaw or performing segmental osteotomies to move teeth. Bone grafts offer the surgeon one of the best materials for changing the aesthetic contour of the face.

THE CONCEPT OF SPLIT CRANIAL BONE GRAFTS

Cranial bone grafts are useful because they resorb less than rib or iliac crest grafts. Split cranial bone is readily available and offers a good, safe donor site for intracranial procedures. Obtaining cranial bone may risk intracranial damage in older patients because it is

A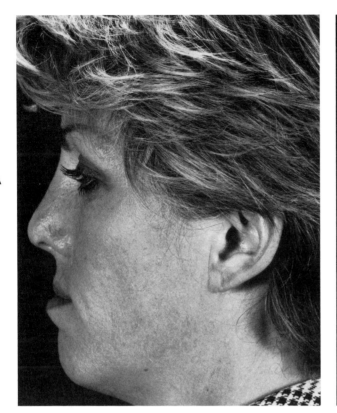   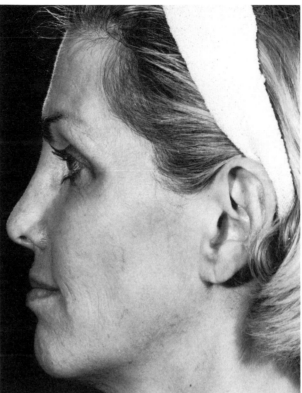B

Fig. 8-3   **A,** Preoperative lateral view showing straight profile with lip disproportion secondary to skeletal deficiency of the maxilla. **B,** Appearance 21 months after a Lefort I maxillary advancement and malar cheek augmentation with split cranial bone using the intraoral approach.

more brittle and cannot be contoured as well as rib grafts. Although we have used various techniques for harvesting cranial bone extracranially, no technique has proved ideal when large quantities of bone are needed. Split cranial bone is more predictably obtained through intracranial exposure provided by the neurosurgeon.[19] This allows harvesting of a large quantity of bone. It is also a safer procedure because direct visualization during harvesting is possible. After testing multiple techniques for in situ split cranial bone grafts, we have found that removal of an entire intracranial block of bone is the easiest, most straightforward, and potentially complication-free method (Fig. 8-2).

Cranial bone may be rather thin in younger patients, and this factor prevents its use when it is less than 4 to 5 mm thick. Although cranial bone is brittle, it is still excellent for maxillary, mandibular, cranial, malar, and nasal augmentation in the older patient. The graft is usually inserted through a coronal incision because this approach allows securing the grafts in a more superior location, particularly in malar augmentation, as a result of the inferior undisturbed soft tissue. An element of resorption and remodeling is invariably present, but the graft material is structurally sound (Fig. 8-3).

Forehead remodeling

In craniofacial surgery the bandeau has come to mean the area located at the base of the frontocranial region and includes the supraorbital rims. It is frequently treated as a separate unit in frontocranial reconstruction (Fig. 8-4).

Anatomy and aesthetics

The bandeau or supraorbital bar typically includes the supraorbital rim, glabellar region, and the nasofrontal angle, which together form the lower portion of the forehead. The normal supraorbital bar is obliquely and anteriorly directed, forming an angle of 90 to 120 degrees with the nose. The forehead begins to curve approximately 1 cm above the orbital rim and passes vertically and gently backward toward the vertex.[2,10] The inclination, width, height, relative prominence of the supraorbital rims, and the relationship of these measurements to the face are all important considerations in the correction of the upper craniofacial skeleton. Normal values have been obtained from the anthropometric analysis of a normal population and help to distinguish the dysmorphic from the orthomorphic facial skeleton.[3,4]

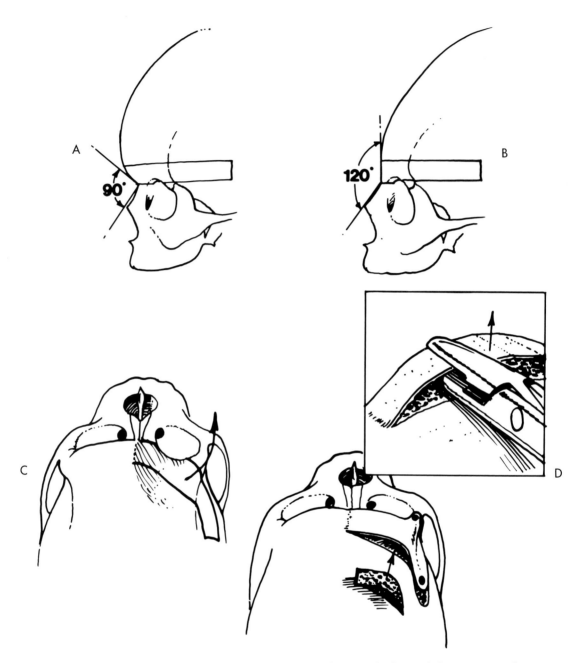

Fig. 8-4   A and B, The normal bandeau is obliquely and anteriorly directed, forming an angle between 90 degrees and 120 degrees with the nose. **C and D,** Unilateral advancement of bandeau using lamellar split technique. Frontal bone may be split along the diploic space with a reciprocating saw to provide additional graft as needed. *Inset,* The unilateral split lamellar bandeau is left attached at the midline, and contouring is performed in situ with Tessier bone forceps.

The explosive cerebral growth of the healthy infant results in predictable changes with development. Early in life, the infant has a high anterior protruding forehead relative to the face.[2] The supraorbital ridges are flat and blend into the forehead. The healthy infant appears proptotic relative to the adult, with one half to one third of the eye protruding beyond the bony orbit. These proportions change as the rapid cerebral and orbital growth of the infant ceases, near 6 years of age, and the midface and mandible continue to grow. The forehead then becomes relatively smaller, eventually achieving a slight posterior inclination, with increasing prominence of the supraorbital rims. In contrast to the infant, the adult eye is encased almost entirely within the bony orbit. The average adult forehead inclination varies from -10 degrees in the male to -6.6 degrees in the female. The average adult nasofrontal angle varies from 130.5 degrees in the male to 134.0 degrees in the female. The cornea lies 8 to 10 mm behind the supraorbital rim.[3] The prominence of the supraorbital region relative to the forehead and lower face is important in determining the "maleness" or "femaleness" of a given forehead and is greater in the male than the female.[13] If the supraorbital region is excessively prominent in the male, it can lead to a "simian" appearance.[1]

It is important not only to understand the normal distribution of facial measurements as they vary with race, sex, and age, but also to be cognizant of the proportions that make a given person attractive in a specific culture. An understanding of that which is deemed beautiful may be a useful guide in achieving harmony and proportion when the abnormal or unaesthetic is reconstructed. Again, anthropometric examination of subjects judged to be especially attractive can help us understand what is necessary to achieve the best possible aesthetic result.[16,22] Although the average adult woman's forehead is tipped backward at an angle of approximately 6 degrees from the vertical, the measurements of a group of especially attractive female faces studied by Farkas and Kolar had a slightly more vertical inclination of minus 2.4 degrees.[4,5,16] This demonstrates that seemingly slight differences in positioning are important.

Surgical techniques

We prefer a bilateral craniotomy with an advancement that allows a one-piece forehead and avoids a visible seam down the midline. Since 1986 we have also used a lamellar split technique where the bone is split in situ along the diploic space with a reciprocating saw. This is performed in selected patients over 3 years of age if we are not interested in increasing the intracranial volume, and the bone is of sufficient thickness to split. Remodeling of the outer table in this way allows us to achieve a subtle correction in patients with mild-to-moderate asymmetry or other deformity of contour, shape, and position.[21]

Fixation

Since the popular use of miniplate fixation, it is possible to achieve stable fixation easily without specifically using such osteotomy designs as the tongue-in-groove or lateral Z-plasty. Rigid fixation has prevented relapse at the osteotomy sites through the traction of soft tissues at the time of closure. In our experience, rigid fixation may theoretically decrease the rate of bony resorption of the bandeau and frontal reconstruction just as it has been proved to decrease resorption in onlay bone grafts.

With our current understanding, however, we believe that it is important to remove plates and screws in the growing infant after a short period (3 to 6 months) to use fully the reshaping forces of the rapidly growing brain. In older patients we do not remove the plates unless they are causing specific problems or are conveniently removed at the time of a secondary procedure.

Manipulation of the bandeau

Once the bandeau has been cut it can be manipulated in various ways. This can be removed and done on the back table, or in situ, as when it is green-sticked forward and left attached at the midline in the unilateral technique. After remodeling, the bandeau is examined in many different orientations before advancement. It is not always replaced in its original orientation. It may need to be tilted slightly or rotated to one side or another. Occasionally it is possible to obtain the proper nasofrontal angle by flipping the bandeau 180 degrees.

Replacement of the bandeau

At times the original frontal bone is unsuitable for remodeling (Fig. 8-5). Therefore when harvesting cranial bone for the bandeau, we are also careful to preserve a suitable portion to reconstruct the forehead. We prefer to use on piece if possible, to avoid seams under the forehead skin. Although not as thin as nasal skin, forehead skin also tends to show every underlying irregularity once postoperative edema has resolved. It is helpful to wet the forehead skin with water to check the contour as we redrape the bicoronal flap, much as one would do with a rhinoplasty. The inclination of the replaced forehead is carefully checked from the side before final fixation to the bandeau.

We have, in selected cases, discarded a grossly malformed bandeau, or placed it in the occiput, and if the frontal bone was of an appropriate shape, lowered it in

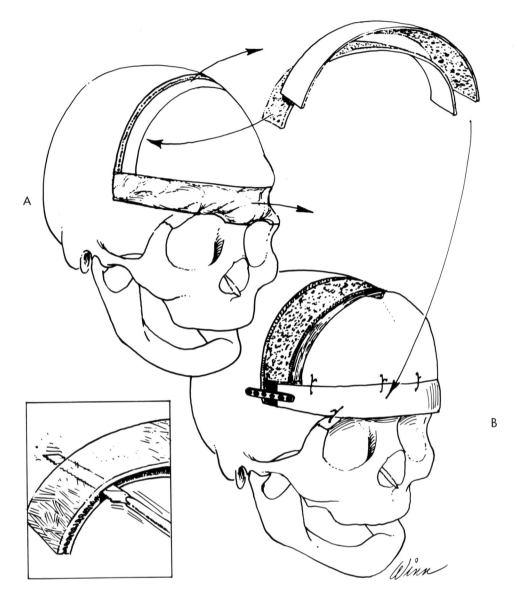

Fig. 8-5 A, Full thickness calvarium is harvested by the pediatric neurosurgeon and split with a
reciprocating saw using the inner table to reconstruct the donor defect. **B** The outer table is
used to reconstruct the bandeau. It is advanced and held in position with miniplate fixation
along with the temporal region. The inner table is returned to reconstruct the donor site, where
it is wired into position. If frontal advancement is to be performed, the parietal strip is taken
wider than the width of the required bandeau, and the remaining portion of the outer table is
returned to reconstruct the advancement gap. *Inset,* Detail showing the calvarium being split
with a reciprocating saw.

one piece to form both a bandeau and forehead. Split
cranial bone can also be used when the frontal bone is
unsuitable for remodeling (Fig. 8-6). It is more often
the case that the bandeau and frontal bone need to be
treated separately to achieve the proper shape and orientation. Since 1980, 215 cases have required a bandeau remodeling or advancement, and we have used
this technique 28 times. It has been especially useful in
secondary reconstruction where it would have been

quite difficult, if not impossible, to achieve a good result with other methods.

Orbital contour

   Aesthetically desirable orbits are best achieved by
performing osteotomies of the native bone, allowing
change of shape if necessary, moving the orbit into a
new position, and filling the gaps with grafts. Cranial,
iliac, or rib bone are all equally satisfactory as inlay ma-

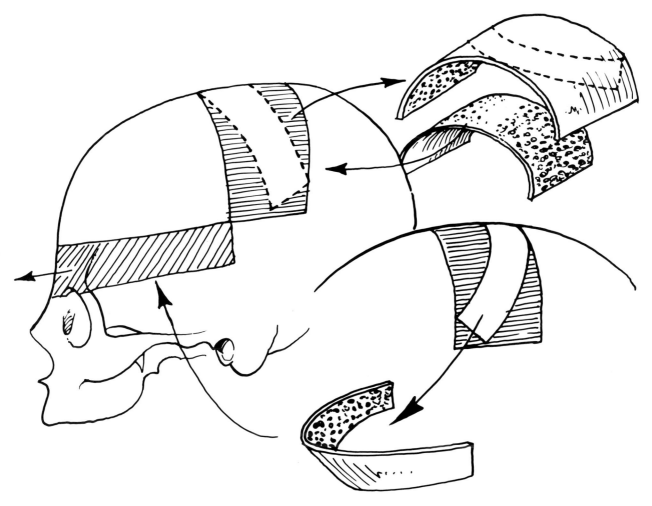

Fig. 8-6 The bandeau template is adjusted on the parietal graft to give the appropriate shape. A large portion of cranium can be taken by the neurosurgeon, leaving an ample portion of intact split cranial bone for reconstruction after returning the inner table to the donor site.

terial. Native bone is preferred for the orbits using the split lamellar technique. The newly created spaces are fitted with grafts of split cranium.

Correction of any disproportion of eye and orbit leading to proptosis is corrected by orbital osteotomy. The only exception is in hyperthyroid exophthalmus where there is hypertrophy of the periorbital tissue. In these cases, the best results are now achieved by removal of the lateral inferior orbit and malar bone using a modified osteotomy.[11]

Maxilla

In specific areas of maxillary deficiency it is best to elevate the periosteum only in the area to be grafted so that the periosteum can hold the graft or implant. For major deficiencies, the entire periosteum is elevated in a wide plane, and the augmentation and/or osteotomy is performed.

Mandible

Contour grafting of the mandible is much more difficult because of the greater propensity for resorption of bone grafts. Cranial bone is the material of choice. For the chin, osteotomy of the native bone with chin advancement and a cranial bone graft as an inlay instead of an onlay reduces resorption. Using the split lamellar technique is helpful here. Grafts placed between split bone segments, as in a sagittal split, do better than grafts placed on the surface of the mandible. Native bone seems to demonstrate less resorption and remodeling than bone from a distance, regardless of the source.

In mandibular lengthening procedures where the temporal mandibular joint (TMJ) or condyle is absent, the treatment of choice is a rib costochondral graft. Rib cartilage obtained from the contralateral side gives superior angulation and contour reconstruction to the ascending ramus and body of the mandible to the chin point. Inlay grafts from the hip or cranial bone give inferior results to rib in congenital cases repairing replacement of the TMJ. The anatomical fusion of cartilage to bone makes this a unique specialized source to use in TMJ reconstruction. Rib is the only graft offering growth potential, although it is unpredictable in any given case.

Genioplasties

Surgical alteration of the chin's shape, position, or relative proportion can make a significant contribution to aesthetic facial balance. Many patients who require orthognathic surgery and/or rhinoplasty are improved by alteration of their chin profile to achieve optimal balance to their face. Most patients are unaware of the chin's importance in facial profile. Chin augmentation, however, is one of the more frequently performed surgical procedures by surgeons who deal with facial balance. The surgeon's orientation and training usually dictate the preferred procedure. Most plastic surgeons today prefer an alloplastic implant for augmentation of the chin. Implants are easy to insert under local anesthesia with minimal complications. Most surgeons trained in maxillofacial and craniofacial techniques prefer chin osteotomy.

Wolford[24] uses porous hydroxyapatite with screw fixation for chin augmentation. The implant is usually in two pieces and extends around the chin as much as possible. After assessing both procedures I prefer the horizontal mandibular osteotomy. Chin advancement performed as an osteotomy can effectively influence the soft tissue and the bony contour, giving a more natural appearance.

CHIN AUGMENTATION

The most frequently used augmentation materials for the chin are porous firm or soft sponge silicone rubber, polypropylene, proplast, or porous hydroxyapatite. The softer sponge material is particularly popular. The harder materials such as proplast, hydroxyapatite, and other carbon teflon combinations have been used to a lesser extent.

An extraoral approach using a submental skin crease incision or an intraoral approach using a labial sulcus incision is used. However, the intraoral approach is preferred. The dissection is performed just above the periosteal plane, making a small pocket the size of the implant that is large enough for insertion and stabilization.

The main controversy is the placement of the implant. When used under the periosteum there is long-term erosion of the underlying bone, which subsequently defeats the original purpose of the augmenta-

tion. Placing the implant above the periosteum seems to prevent resorption, but fixation by a periosteal pocket is sacrificed. In our experience, the main disadvantage of an implant is the risk of extrusion. With minor augmentation of 3 to 5 mm, one may obtain a good result with minimal risk. When greater augmentation is indicated, an osteotomy generally produces a more aesthetically pleasing result. Many chin implants do not look natural and appear to be pasted on. The sliding horizontal mandibular osteotomy produces a more consistent aesthetic result in my experience.

Chin advancement

With chin advancement the procedure of choice is a single-tiered horizontal mandibular osteotomy that can give an 8 to 12 mm advancement depending on the thickness of the bone and the general craniofacial skeletal contour. We have used this procedure alone or in combination with rhinoplasty, maxillary, and/or mandibular osteotomies and in other skeletal surgery to improve the facial balance. General anesthesia is preferred because it offers consistent conditions for surgery (Fig. 8-7).

Technique

Under general anesthesia, the inferior labial sulcus, the chin, and the mental foramen along the border of the mandible are infiltrated with 1:1,000,000 epinephrine in 1% Xylocaine before prepping the patient. I currently use a new dissection needle called the boulder needle attached to the Valley lab electrode, which eliminates bleeding and is used to perform the soft tissue dissection. The initial incision is made in the labial sulcus on the lip mucosa side from one canine tooth to another. After the initial mucosal incision, the dissection is carried through the musculature at an inferior angle, preserving muscle attachment on the bone above the line of the osteotomy, which aids soft tissue closure. The dissection is then carried to bone through the periosteum 0.5 cm above the osteotomy level. Using a subperiosteal dissection, the anterior chin is degloved. This is done using the following technique:

1. The submental foramen with the infraorbital nerve are identified. This can be found at a variable vertical level on the mandible depending on the patient.
2. The osteotomy is performed 1 to 2 mm below the level of the nerve.
3. Lateral and inferior to the foramen, the periosteum is elevated from the lower border of the mandible toward the angle of the mandible.

Good, wide subperiosteal reflection facilitates exposure and the ease with which the osteotomy is performed.

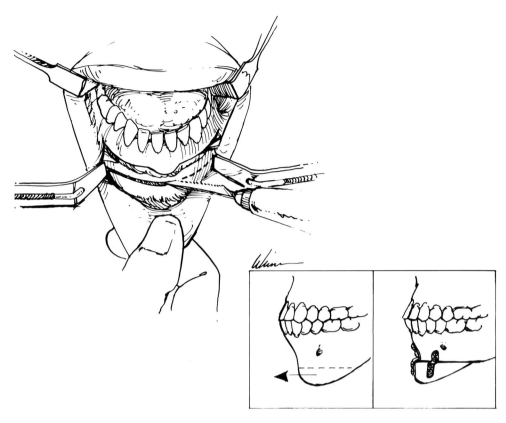

Fig. 8-7   Sliding horizontal mandibular genioplasty.

One of the keys to achieving an optimal result is angling the malleable saw blade in the horizontal plane. We prefer a reciprocating saw with a thin blade such as the air-driven Zimmer Hall. We also like the new Stryker and the electric Aesculap, both with self-irrigation. The currently available Aesculap saw blade is thicker than the Zimmer Hall blade, which is quite thin and malleable, but either one is excellent. We use two medium, lighted retractors of our own design to protect the nerve as it exits through the mental foramen.

The surgeon may stand on the right side of the patient, operating from below with nasal intubation, although it may also be done from the top of the head with nasal or oral intubation. The cut is usually initiated on the left side of the patient, cutting from left to right for a right-handed surgeon. It is important to first make a horizontal cut the full length of the blade through the anterior table of the mandible on one side and then turn the blade perpendicular to the plane of the cut mandible, cutting through the posterior table and completing the left side to the midline. This provides a level osteotomy. The incision is then repeated on the right side, bringing it up the border of the mandible an equal distance from the midline on both sides. It is important to taper the edge through the thickness of the mandible posteriorly, carrying it as far as possi-

ble to achieve optimal contour and to prevent a lateral step off after advancement of the chin.

With completion of the osteotomy the segment is readily freed with the fingertips and does not require an osteotome or other instrument for mobilization. We strongly prefer leaving the attachment of the soft tissues to the cut segment of the chin in as broad a base as possible. This provides better adaptation of the soft tissues without prolapse and improves vascularization of the chin segment by the attached soft tissues. The cut segment is then advanced the desired predetermined length. The last few millimeters of placement is decided by looking at the facial profile with the chin in various degrees of advancement and draped with the soft tissue. In a single-tiered advancement, up to 12 mm may be possible. The average advancement is 5 to 6 mm, depending on the degree of deformity.

Osteosynthesis is achieved by holding the chin with a grooved bone clamp in the midline. A drill hole is placed in the midline from the inner table of the advanced segment through the outer table of the proximal segment of the mandible. This aids in maintaining the chin in the advanced position. Two additional drill holes are placed lateral to the mental foramen when possible to give three-point fixation of the advanced chin segment. Soft stainless steel #26 prestretched

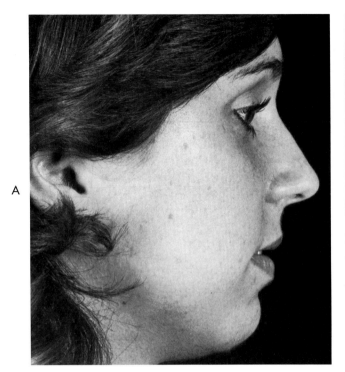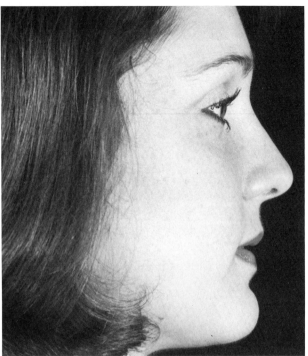

Fig. 8-8 A, Preoperative view of a patient with a retrognathic chin and excessive fat on the lower chin. **B,** Postoperative view following sliding advancement genioplasty and liposuction of the neck.

wire is used to secure the chin. The wires are twisted down into position, holding the chin segment in an advanced position with the bone-holding clamp or with the fingers. The wound is irrigated with one quarter strength betadine and saline and closed in two or three layers using 3-0 chromic sutures on the periosteum and muscle layers. The final layer of closure on the mucosa is achieved with 3-0 polydioxanone suture (PDS) running suture.

A compression dressing using a prefabricated elastic chin dressing with velcro straps is left in place for 3 to 5 days after surgery. If noncraniofacial surgeons were familiar with this technique, I believe that most would choose this procedure for patients requiring augmentation. When advancement greater than 12 mm is required, a two-level osteotomy may be used.

Combined procedures

The sliding genioplasty is often performed in combination with other orthomorphic surgery such as a sagittal split advancement of the mandible for a retrognathic microgenic deformity. The final adjustments of the facial proportions are made with the chin osteotomy for a minor, moderate, or extreme chin advancement, depending on the extent of the deformity.

One of the major advantages of the mandibular osteotomy procedure is that it produces an improvement in the soft tissue mandibular plane angle. Improvement

in the neckline can be achieved not only by removal of fat and skin and the posterior pull on the superficial musculoaponeurotic tissue as in a rhytidectomy, but also by an anterior pull of the muscles attached to the lower symphaseal fragment by a sliding genioplasty. Combining mandibular osteotomy and submental dissection with tightening of the skin and/or superficial musculoaponeurotic system improves the submental neckline, giving improvement in the obtuse neckline not achieved with chin augmentation.

Suction lipectomy can also be used as an adjunctive procedure in combination with a horizontal mandibular osteotomy with advancement. Again, this is a method that allows changing the obtuse angle and removing fat without making skin incisions or dissecting facial rhytidectomy. We have seen good results by using this adjunctive measure in selected genioplasty patients (Fig. 8-8).

THE CONCEPT OF THE LAMELLAR SPLIT OSTEOTOMY

The lamellar split osteotomy offers many advantages to aesthetic facial contour surgery.[20] This technique can be applied to surgery of the frontal bone, the orbits, malar region, maxilla, and mandible. The use of the in situ lamellar technique was introduced in 1987 and has been continuously refined.

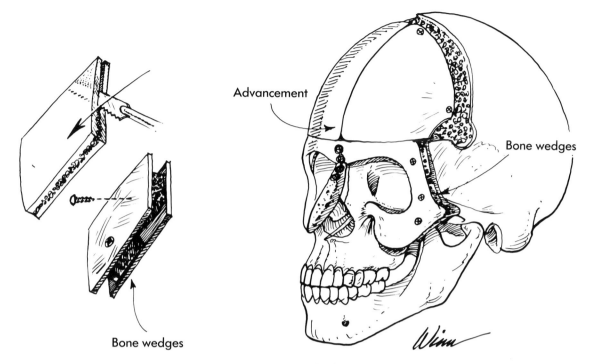

Fig. 8-9 The lamellar split procedure is shown in the frontal orbital malar region as a composite procedure. The inserts on the left demonstrate splitting the inner and outer tables in two portions, changing the shape and contour and repositioning these using lag screw fixation where interpositional bone grafting can be used.

This osteotomy is a new technique in which the facial skeleton is split between the internal and external bony lamella. The osteotomy allows a quantifiable translocation of the external table against the native position of the internal bony table. This interlamellar osteotomy has led to improved aesthetic results in the orthomorphic reconstruction of congenital deformities and can now be applied to all types of cases, including aesthetic surgery.

We developed the split orbitofacial osteotomy after performing over 400 orbitofacial osteotomies. Technical improvements in surgical equipment now allows an interlamellar splitting of bone. The split orbitofacial osteotomy appears to be safe. The interlamellar nature of this osteotomy also offers greater osseous stability, since rapid, rigid, precise fixation of the mobile external lamella to the stationary internal lamella is achieved. More important, this osteotomy allows better quantitative shifts of the desired new contour of bone, which improves the aesthetic results. Increased surface area for bone grafts, screw fixation, and/or miniplates is another important advantage. Postoperative comparison of anthropomorphic data and predictive drawings reveals that most of the patients have realized 90% of their idealized norms. Because infant surgery requires translocation of the entire bone to allow space for growth and development, this technique is recommended only for patients 3 years of age and older (Fig. 8-9).

Surgical techniques and approaches
Extracranial approach

The craniofacial skeleton is exposed through an extracranial approach using the classic bicoronal approach. This allows access to the entire zygomatic arch down to the maxilla and the infraorbital nerve from above and down to the pyriform apperature from above. In addition, the canthal ligaments along the medial orbital wall are exposed, and there is a higher exposure of the frontal bone. An extracranial approach requires a slower, more careful split, although anatomic limitations exist in the area where intracranial dura is present on the inside of the bone. When performing a major intracranial procedure, or when using an intracranial approach for whatever reason, the safe protection of the intracranial contents allows a rapid lamellar split of any of the frontal, temporal, parietal, orbital, or zygomatic regions.

Intracranial approach

A standard intracranial approach through a bifrontal craniotomy with protection of the frontal lobes is

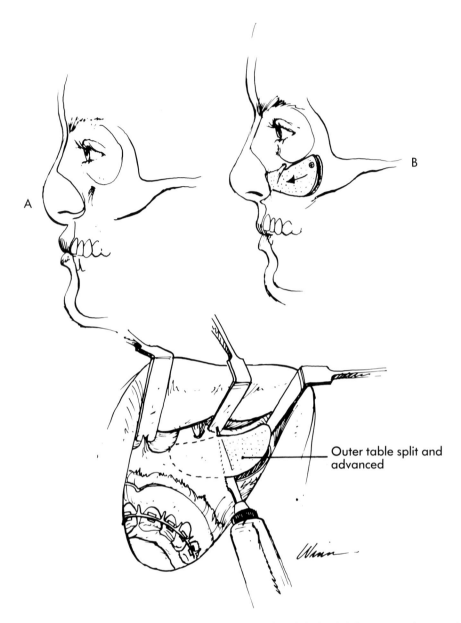

Fig. 8-10 **A,** Shows a preoperative lateral view of a midfacial skeletal deficiency with normal occlusion. **B,** Postoperative view after the advancement using split lamellar technique changing shape, contour, and position using lag screw fixation. The ossilating saw is used for the split lamellar technique in situ through a transoral approach.

used. A bilamellar bandeau or an in situ lamellar split may be performed. The bilamellar split can be continued through the lateral orbit and the zygoma down through the front of the maxilla into the pyriform aperature below the infraorbital nerve. The hemifacial bony mask developed on either side can then be moved or shifted in a three dimensional plane and fixed with lag screws and/or interpositional bone grafting. When the zygoma is split from above, it is not necessary to take down the inferior muscle attachment. The split bone can be advanced with the muscle attached, producing a smooth contour.

Extracranial/intraoral approach

The standard extracranial approach is through an intraoral transvestibular incision that exposes the entire front of the maxilla. The nasal mucosa is freed from the pyriform apperature, as well as from the vomer, to allow retraction and protection of the mucosa. The dissection is carried to the maxillary buttress, then up and over the zygomatic arch where the muscular attachment to the zygoma is taken down when performed from below. Using special instrumentation developed for this technique, the dissection is carried from below

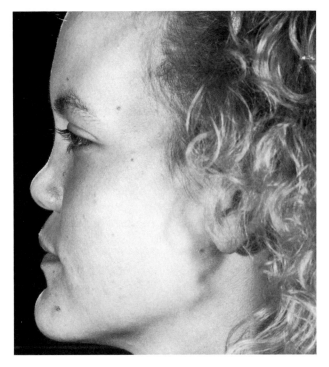
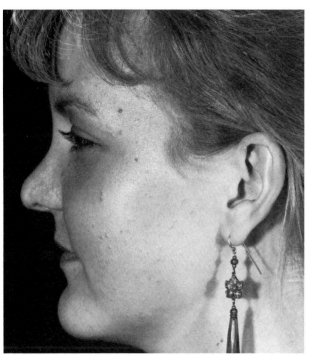

A   B

Fig. 8-11   A, Preoperative lateral view showing midface deficiency with foreshortened nose as a result of lack of skeletal development. **B,** Postoperative view following lamellar split as described in the text. In addition to cranial bone grafting to the nose, this shows the dramatic change in the balance and harmony of the face as a result of the techniques and methods discussed in this text.

to the orbit and the periosteum of the inferior orbital floor. Retraction of the orbital floor from below protects the globe from the oscillating saw, which is used to transect the front of the maxilla from the zygomatic arch. A small right angle saw allows the lateral upper perimeter of the cut to be made over the zygoma from below. The zygomatic arch is split from below with a feathered edge, tapering into the arch. The arch is then advanced, and interpositional bone grafts are placed and secured with lag screw fixation using 1 to 1.5 mm screws with low profile heads. We prefer either resorpable screws made of polyglycolic acid or removable screw heads (Figs. 8-10 and 8-11).

The technical aspects of performing this procedure are much more extensive and demanding than using a prefabricated insert or implant of any kind. Once an optimum result is achieved with this technique, however, the surgeon has little worry of future loss of the implant, migration, infection, or even growth disturbances. I have found this technique to be advantageous in major and in some minor congenital craniomaxillofacial orthomorphic surgical corrections. The extension of this technique to pure aesthetic contouring of the face offers change in the skeleton, which is not possible with alloplastic implants. This technique offers

many possibilities for future surgical exploration and development. The use of this contouring technique in combination with maxillary LeFort I, II, and III and mandibular sagittal splits, Inverted L, and sliding genioplasty permits adjustment of the middle and lower face. The use of the bilamellar cranial vault shift and forehead reconstruction, combined with the lamellar split adjustment, gives one the ability to change three dimensionally the contour of the cranial vault and face. This can also be done on individual segments of the craniofacial skeleton.

SOFT TISSUE GRAFTS AND FLAPS
Dermal fat grafts

The use of dermal fat grafts has remained controversial because of major resorption. I have used dermal fat grafts for many years as an adjunctive contouring material in craniofacial surgery. In more than 100 cases I have found a variable amount of fat resorption and liquification with approximately a 50% graft survival. Most of the surviving elements are dermal with some fat cells, although this has not been documented by quantative measurements. There seems to be a difference in dermal fat grafts obtained from different donor sites. Obwegeser[12] believes that dermal fat from the buttocks is different from and superior to other donor areas. He used this as his chosen donor site when large segments were needed for contouring the face. We have used this same donor site in a number of cases and have indeed found this to be satisfactory. Other donor sites from the abdomen, the groin, and the thigh, have also been used with success. The amount of resorption of these grafts varies from 40% to 60%. This technique is beneficial, and we recommend it as an adjunctive measure in facial contouring.

Contouring procedures—liposuction

Liposuction has been used for the last 7 years as an adjunctive measure in patients with craniofacial deformity where optimal aesthetic change is desired. It offers definite contour improvement in and around the neck, particularly in the submental region. Liposuction is performed as an adjunctive measure after the skeletal correction. There is a tendency for the submandibular fat to be excessive in patients who have had a mandibular setback. The use of submental lypolysis has been beneficial in improving this residual defect that results from posterior skeletal shifts. It is also helpful as a secondary procedure for contour restoration after free flap reconstruction and is performed 6 months after the first procedure.

Buccal fat pad

Aesthetic and craniofacial soft tissue refinements can be achieved by excision and/or transfer of the buccal fat pad for facial contouring. The buccal fat pad may be removed for slight aesthetic contour improvement of the malar cheek region. This can be done under local anesthesia in the office or in the operating room under general anesthesia in combination with other procedures. The buccal fat pad is best found in the retromolar area of the maxilla. This is freed, dissected, and teased out. The pedicle is cross clamped, electrocoagulated, and the fat is removed.

ALLOPLASTIC MATERIALS

Autogenous onlay bone grafts have long been the mainstay of maxillofacial reconstruction, allowing for augmentation of deficient areas and recontouring of deformities. The disadvantages of autogenous bone grafting are donor-site morbidity, unpredictable resorption and remodeling, and donor availability for staged reconstructions. Although a bone-graft substitute would eliminate the problems of donor-site morbidity and availability, the substitute must be stable, nonreactive, highly permeable, and of uniform pore diameter to facilitate ingrowth and eventual replacement by contiguous bone. Since the early 1970s, bone substitution materials have been studied. I have studied porous hy-droxyapatite in both laboratory animals and humans and evaluated this material as an onlay substitute for autogenous bone grafts in maxillofacial surgery.[8]

Porous hydroxyapatite*

Calcium Carbonate is harvested in the South Seas as coral, genus parietes. This coral has a uniform porosity of 180 to 200 microns. The coral is transformed by the replamineform process into porous hydroxyapatite, calcium triphosphate, which maintains the physical structure of the original coral. The uniform porosity enables bone regeneration and metabolism to occur throughout the implant. Research studies using this material have resulted in its development commercially as Interpore 200*. The first clinical trials as onlay grafts were performed between 1984 and 1985 using 45 hydroxyapatite implants compared with 23 bone grafts.[18] The complications were minimal. One patient had extrusion because granules, rather than block material, were used. There were no other cases where the material was a problem in this series of patients. This material is difficult to handle because it is easily fractured. However, it can be contoured with a diamond bur or carefully carved with a knife blade. To eliminate small particles and fragments, the wound should be thoroughly washed before implantation. Carving or contouring should be done on the back table away from the surgical wound because of potential contamination by the particles. Very careful contouring should be performed on this material before implantation because sharp edges or ridges will not remodel, and resorption of this material is minimal (Fig. 8-12).

Our series of patients has done well and has been followed for 5 years. We have observed thinning of soft tissue coverage over time and show-through of the hydroxyapatite edges in a few cases. This occurrence required the surgical removal of the hydroxyapatite graft and replacement with split cranial bone.

This material has been used as inlay material in combination with osteotomes.[14,24] We used hydroxyapatite in the early 1980s but continue to prefer bone.

Proplast I and II

Proplast was initially marketed by Vitek Inc. Proplast I is black and composes porous carbon as an added teflon molecule. Proplast II is a white material combining teflon and alumina and has received favorable reports from Whitaker et al.[23] The complication rate has been minimal when used as a maxillary onlay, but there have been an increased number of complications when used for mandible augmentation.

---

*Interpore 200, Interpore International, Irvine, Calif.

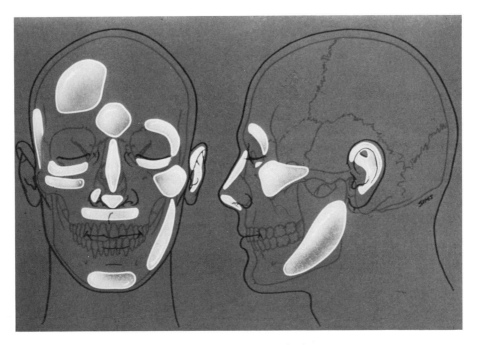

Fig. 8-12 Hydroxyapatite graft placement.

This material is available for implantation in a number of shapes and forms. It has high porosity and is soft, with a low modulous of elasticity, and has easy wetability. Ingrowth with vascularized fibrous tissue helps Proplast II rapidly adhere to adjacent structures. Proplast is porous in volume by 70% to 90%, with a pore size ranging from 50 to 400 microns. It is resilient, autoclavable, and easily carved. Extensive experience has shown this material to be chemically inert, biocompatible, and nonallergic.

Impregnating Proplast with antibiotic solution before implantation has minimized secondary infection. Proplast is available for chin, periorbital rim, nasal dorsum, zygomatic malar, and zygomatic orbital rim implants. Custom implants are also available. The advantage of this material is its ease of insertion when wet and pliable. Thousands of these implants have been used with low complication rates, particularly in malar or maxillary augmentation. They eliminate the problem of resorption seen with bone grafts.

Proplast hydroxyapatite

This new material combines porous hydroxyapatite and Proplast II. It looks, feels, and adapts very much like Proplast II. Both substances contain an ultraporous polymer base with 70% to 90% porous volume and are lightweight with a low modulus and a softness similar to tissue. Like Proplast II, it is wetable and may be impregnated with antibiotics. Its pliability allows it to be shaped with a sharp scalpel.

Adding the hydroxyapatite theoretically creates an osteoconductive material, whereas Proplast alone allows only fibrous tissue ingrowth. This material is available in block and sheeting, in preformed implant shapes for the chin and malar areas, in custom implants, and as a TMJ. Time and further experience are needed to confirm the advantages and disadvantages of this new material; it deserves further evaluation as an onlay material.

Solid hydroxyapatite calcitite*

This material contains a solid form of hydroxyapatite, but in my opinion has less appeal than the porous hydroxyapatite. It acts primarily as a spacer without bone ingrowth.

Methyl methacrylate†

Methyl methacrylate has been used by most neurosurgeons performing cranioplasties. This material is an acceptable space filler with no resorption. In craniofacial surgery it has been our experience that this material is not readily resistant to infection and/or trauma and may become exposed and/or infected or cause erosion. Although easily used because it can be shaped at the table, it is thermic and generates a considerable amount of heat at the time of hardening. The use of methyl methacrylate in major craniofacial surgery of the growing face is not the material of choice in my opinion. We have seen patients who required implant

*Calcitek, Inc, San Diego, Calif.

†Cranioplast, Codman, and Shuntleff, Inc., Randolph, Mass.

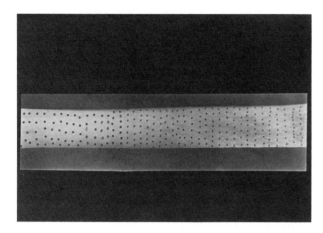

Fig. 8-13   Perforated bone used for preparation of perforated decalcified bone matrix.

removal, which was technically very difficult. The potential for infection is high in major craniofacial cases where the cranial vault is opened to the mouth or sinuses.

Lyophilized cartilage

This material reacts differently than the material used by Sailer because of processing currently unavailable in the United States. Its use was popularized in Europe more than 20 years ago. Sailer[15] published a monograph on lyophilized cartilage, scientifically documenting the advantages and disadvantages of this material. It may be used as an inlay or an onlay grafting material in craniomaxillofacial surgery. It is a good material for contouring and can be cut with the dermatome or knife blade. It is used for soft tissue augmentation, particularly for asymmetries of the face. The material does not have a memory and is not distorted by cutting or carving. This material has proved effective in contour reconstruction of the face.

Radiated homograft cartilage

This material has been extensively used in Europe. I have used irradiated homograft cartilage on a number of occasions as a bone filler when bone was resorbed or in an infected bed where there was potential for repeated loss. In a number of cases, this material acted as a good salvage material for permanent contour and filling of craniofacial defects. The material demonstrates minimal problems of rejection when used for contouring and can be recommended as a space filler.

Allograft bone (cadaver bone)

We have had no experience with cadaver bone. This non-living bone is treated by various methods and may act as a lattice or space filler for new bone formation. We recently operated on a patient who had lyophilized banked bone implanted in his mandible fol-

lowing repair of a traumatic deformity. At the time of surgery it bled very little from the surface. Because of poor positioning we did a split of the mandible and secured it with lag screws. It gave a marked aesthetic improvement and the patient continues to do well.

Demineralized bone paste

Demineralized bone paste has been developed by Glowacki and others[7] and offers new possibilities. This material comprises living osteoblasts derived from treated homograft materials, which provide osteogenic cells that are capable of regenerating bone. This material has not yet received Federal Drug Administration (FDA) approval. However, clinical trials are still in process. Theoretically, demineralized bone paste could be used alone or with a material such as porous hydroxyapatite, which offers support as the basic porous structure of bone. This combination may offer advantages as a graft that provides a structural supporting matrix combined with cells that have osteogenic capabilities. When implanted in the shark, a non-bone forming mammal, the material has proved to be osteogenic, producing bone.

PERFORATED DEMINERALIZED BONE MATRIX

Gendler[6] has reported the use of perforated decalcified bone matrix (PDBM) as a new form of osteoinductive material. Samples of perforated bone matrix were implanted subcutaneously in the sternal region of 30-day-old Long-Evans rats. Ninety Days after implantation the bone matrix had undergone considerable resorption and was replaced by new bone and bone marrow. Gendler concluded that the mechanism of action of PDBM appears to be similar to that previously described for other forms of decalcified bone matrix such as nonperforated matrix and powdered bone matrix. The advantages of PDBM over powdered preparations include highly localized centers of osteogenesis, the creation of endochondral osteogenesis that allow easy assessment of morphology and the option to form the PDBM to fit inside the bone defect, thereby stimulating bone regrowth and fracture healing (Fig. 8-13).

This material, unlike demineralized bone paste, is readily available from the Pacific Bone Bank in Los Angeles and is promising in craniofacial surgery. We have begun to use this material and will report our results in the future. The preliminary results are encouraging.

Silastic

Prefabricated silastic, or silastic 382, which is cured at the time of the surgical procedure, gives an immediately available form to the material and has been used extensively as an implant in the face. A recent long-term follow-up of these patients has shown this material to migrate. It is nonreactive to the adjacent tissues, it is not adherent, and it is prone to loss secondary to trauma with potential development for infection and extrusion. At this time, I do not recommend this material for use as a bone replacement material in the craniofacial region. However, a number of surgeons continue to use it in the face.

Polyethylene or polypropylene

This material is readily contoured, cut, and adapted and has been used for augmentation in and around the face. It is relatively pliable and soft and has a low extrusion rate. This material should be considered in certain select places for those who need a soft, pliable, easily cut material. There would seem to be better biologic materials on the market, but it is superior to some of the nonporous materials available today. However, I have no clinical experience with this material.

Polyetherurethane and polyethylene terephthalate cloth mesh

Polyetherurethane and polyethylene terephthalate cloth mesh have been used as a space filler with autogenous bone grafts. In noninfection-prone areas, when large segments of bone replacement are needed, the results have been very favorable.

TEMPOROMANDIBULAR JOINT REPLACEMENT

We advocate the use of costocondral rib replacement when there is congenital absence or other reason to replace the temporomandibular joint. Our preference remains autogenous tissue replacement. A discussion of joint replacement would not be complete without mentioning the prosthetic joint. Vitek has been working on and marketing such a joint. Their most recent version involves the use of high molecular polyethylene that fits into the glenoid fossa, articulating against a metabolic condylar implant of cobalt chrome. Although this implant has been used successfully, I believe that ultimately most of these implants must be removed.

SUMMARY

Orthomorphic techniques improve craniofacial surgical results by altering the shape, contour, projection, and angulation of the underlying displaced and deformed skeleton. These aesthetic refinements are achieved through a combination of reshaping, osteotomy, and addition of onlay and inlay augmentation materials for providing a new skeletal framework. The soft tissue facial mask is redraped and altered as necessary to effect an optimum aesthetic craniofacial change. Simply moving bone is not enough.

Lamellar splitting is a new technique that allows a three dimensional contour change of the outer lamella while maintaining the reference points of the inner lamellar bone. The use of additional split cranial bone is called for when the native in situ bone is too thin, hypoplastic, or inadequate to achieve a lamellar split. Our preference is for an in situ lamellar split with interpositional bone grafting. When this is possible, detrimental remodeling or resorption is minimized or nonexistent. No late contour surface defects have been observed when using in situ split lamellar reconstruction. These advantages determine our choice for using the split cranial bone and the lamellar split technique to achieve balance, harmony, and long-term, consistent results that are not at risk for early or late rejection, infection, mobility, or resorption of the reconstructed face. An additional advantage of these two techniques is that they can be used after the age of 3 years without the potential adverse problems of adding foreign body or alloplastic materials. This is especially important in the young, growing face. Therefore our primary choice for malar, orbital, and maxillary augmentation, nondependent on tooth positioning, is split lamellar bone.

Facial contouring removes the "stereotyped" look that may result from dental dependent surgery. This look is frequently seen in patients when surgical planning was based on dental proportions oriented toward jaw movement. Aesthetic contouring or "sculpturing" allows for individualization and creation of a more interesting face. Projection of the malar region, nose, and chin result in a light reflex from these surfaces that adds angulation and is perceived as an aesthetically pleasing facial feature.

The surgeon's choice of alloplastic or autogenous implants, osteotomy, or combinations of these techniques is dependent on many factors. Plastic surgery in the future will continue to use more hard tissue techniques for reconstruction as a means of sculpting the face in purely aesthetic cases. Having the full spectrum of surgical modalities available allows for optimum flexibility by the surgeon while striving for aesthetic balance and harmony in facial surgery.

REFERENCES

1. Edgerton MT: Discussion, Plast Reconstr Surg 79:712, 1987.
2. Enlow DH: Handbook of facial growth, Philadelphia, 1975, WB Saunders Co.
3. Farkas LG: Anthropometry of the head and face in medicine, New York, 1981, Elsevier Science Publishing Co Inc.
4. Farkas LG and Kolar JC: Anthropometric guidelines in cranio-orbital surgery, Clin Plast Surg 14:1, 1978.
5. Farkas LG and Kolar JC: Anthropometrics and art in the aesthetics of women's faces, Clin Plast Surg 14:599, 1987.
6. Gendler E: Perforated demineralized bone matrix: a new form of osteoinductive biomaterial, J Biomed Mater Res 20:687, 1986.
7. Glowacki J et al: Application of the biological principle of induced osteogenesis for craniofacial defects, Lancet 1:959, 1981.
8. Holmes RE and Salyer KE: Bone regeneration in a coraline hy-

droxyapatite implant, Surg Forum 24:611, 1978.

9. Joganic EF and Salyer KE: Analysis of facial proportions: what do I have, what do I want, and how do I get there? In Vistnes L: How they do it—procedures in plastic and reconstructive surgery, Boston, 1991, Little, Brown & Co Inc.

10. Marchac D and Renier D: Basic surgical principles in the treatment of craniosynostosis. In Craniofacial Surgery for Craniosynostosis, Boston, 1982, Little, Brown & Co Inc.

11. Matton G: Surgical decompression of the orbit in dysthyroid exopthalmos. Waldon Lecture presented to the American Society of Maxillofacial Surgeons, Toronto, Ontario, 1988.

12. Obwegeser H: Personal Communication, September 14, 1988.

13. Ousterhout DK: Feminization of the forehead: contour changing to improve female aesthetics, Plast Reconstr Surg 79:701, 1987.

14. Rosen HM: Porous hydroxyapatite as an interpositional bone graft substitute in orthognathic surgery, Plast Reconstr Surg 83:985, 1989.

15. Sailer HF: Transplantation of lyophilized cartilage in maxillofacial surgery: experimental foundations and clinical success, New York, 1983, Karger.

16. Salyer KE, Vasconez H, and Genecov J: Analysis of facial proportions in twenty beautiful faces, Plast Surg Forum 10:129, 1987.

17. Salyer KE: Techniques in aesthetic craniofacial surgery, New York, 1989, Gower Medical Publishing Ltd.

18. Salyer KE and Hall CD: Porous hydroxyapatite as an onlay bone graft substitute for maxillofacial surgery, Plast Reconstr Surg 84(2):236-244, 1989.

19. Salyer KE et al: Reconstruction using split cranial bone. Paper presented at the Sixth International Congress on Cleft Palate and Related Craniofacial Anomalies, Jerusalem, Israel, June 18-22, 1989.

20. Salyer KE et al: Lamellar split osteotomy: a new craniofacial technique, Plast Reconstr Surg 86:5, 1990.

21. Salyer KE and Hall JD: Bandeau—the focal point of frontocranial remodeling, J Craniofac Surg 1:18, 1990.

22. Whitaker LA et al: Aesthetic surgery of the supraorbital ridge and forehead structures, Plast Reconstr Surg 8:23, 1986.

23. Whitaker LA et al: Anesthetic Augmentation of the malar—mid-face structures, Plast Reconstr Surg 80:337, 1987.

24. Wolford LM et al: Coraline, porous hydroxyapatite in orthognathic surgery, J Oral Maxillofac Surg 45:1034, 1987.

CHAPTER 9

Cleft Orthognathic Surgery

Jeffrey C. Posnick

MANAGEMENT OF CLEFT LIP AND PALATE

The satisfactory management of patients with cleft lip and palate presents challenging clinical problems for the maxillofacial surgeon and orthodontist.[36] Orthognathic surgery is often the final procedure to consider in the patient's rehabilitation. It is also a procedure likely to be labeled "too risky" or "too big an operation" for a patient who already "has come a long way."

Adding further difficulty is a lack of information about the exact surgical technique required for each of the cleft types: unilateral cleft lip and palate (UCLP), bilateral cleft lip and palate (BCLP), and isolated cleft palate (ICP). With each type come a different set of residual cleft problems for the adolescent patient. Thus different surgical techniques are required if safe orthognathic surgery is to be provided for each patient's final reconstruction.

The surgeon and orthodontist must agree on the goals and methods of surgery, since they are key members of a multidisciplinary team designed to provide effective orthognathic surgery.[10]

Integrated team approach

The care of a patient with cleft palate is best delivered by a cleft lip and palate team that meets regularly to discuss cleft protocols in general, as well as the nature and quality of the care of specific patients. It is no longer adequate for individual practitioners, whether surgeons, orthodontists, or speech pathologists, to carry out extensive treatment plans without considering the views of the other team members.

The plastic surgeon plays a primary role in coordinating the patient's care, which must transcend his own area of expertise and facilitate effective, coordinated care throughout adolescence. The orthodontist may provide preoperative orthopedics in infancy and interceptive orthodontic treatment in childhood, identify early abnormal growth patterns of the facial skele-

ton,* and carry out final orthodontic treatment in conjunction with orthognathic surgery when required.

The speech pathologist plays a critical role in speech assessment, which involves a clinical examination, nasendoscopy, and videofluoroscopy. Before orthognathic surgery is even contemplated[46,60], these procedures are necessary to characterize both velopharyngeal function and anterior articulation problems resulting in sibilant distortion. Such evaluation is important because velopharyngeal function tends to deteriorate after maxillary Le Fort I osteotomy with advancement.[61] Closure that was adequate before surgery may become borderline afterward, and closure that was borderline may become inadequate. Articulatory distortions because of malocclusion also are identified and cause-and-effect relationships determined. Intraoperative correction of crossbite, open bite, cleft-dental gaps, and residual oronasal fistulas can also correct sibilant distortions.[62]

Other team members make significant contributions to the care of cleft patients. The otolaryngologist and audiologist help prevent and manage middle ear problems, and the otolaryngologist also assists with potential airway problems; the geneticist helps with the interpretation of additional birth deformities and syndrome analysis, as well as with family planning, both for the parents and the teenager with a cleft palate; the social worker assists with family and community-related issues.

Historical perspective of the Le Fort I osteotomy

In general, the main problem for a patient with a cleft skeletal dysplasia and malocclusion is maxillary hypoplasia resulting from the original birth defect and previous surgical interventions.[17,43] The usual surgical procedure to consider is the Le Fort I maxillary osteot-

*References 4, 5, 12, 29, 43-45, 50.

TABLE 9-1

Le Fort I in Unilateral Cleft Patients: Horizontal Advancement and Relapse

Time after Operation	Effective Advancement (mm)				Mean Relapse from Previous Position (mm)
	Mean	SD	Min	Max	
1 week	6.7	2.6	1.7	12.2	Unknown
6 weeks	5.7	2.5			1.0
1 year	4.9	2.6			0.8
2 years	4.8	2.6	1.0	10.7	0.1

From Posnick JC and Ewing MP: Plast Reconstr Surg 85:706, 1990.

TABLE 9-2

Le Fort I in Unilateral Cleft Patients: Vertical Displacement and Relapse

Time after Operation	Downward Displacement (mm)				Mean Relapse from Previous Position (mm)
	Mean	SD	Min	Max	
1 week	2.6	3.0	−3.4	8.6	Unknown
6 weeks	1.4	2.7			1.2
1 year	1.2	2.5			0.2
2 years	1.2	2.5	−2.9	7.0	0.0

From Posnick JC and Ewing MP: Plast Reconst Surg 85:706, 1990.

omy in one or more segments. This procedure originated in Europe. In 1867 Cheever performed a unilateral Le Fort I osteotomy to remove a nasopharyngeal tumor.[28] Later, Wassmund[56] performed an osteotomy of the maxilla according to the fracture line described by LeFort[26] in a patient with an open bite deformity. Schuchardt[47] was the first to separate the Le Fort I osteotomy at the pterygoid plates. Obwegeser[30,31] showed that the down-fractured maxilla could be moved in any direction, either as one unit or in segments. Bell et al,[2] in an experiment with dogs, documented the flap blood supply, revascularization, and bone healing that occurred with this procedure when a horizontal-maxillary-circovestibular incision was used for exposure, extending from one zygomatic buttress to the other.

Generally, applying this information about the Le Fort I osteotomy to the cleft patient has resulted in inadequate flap circulation to the clefted maxillary segments, with reported cases of aseptic necrosis and tooth loss.[8,14,59] These problems have given cleft orthognathic surgery a bad name and led surgeons and orthodontists to take an overly conservative approach (see historical perspective of surgical technique).

Patient protocol

Patients referred for possible orthognathic surgery are seen by the orthodontist, surgeon, and speech pathologist. Additional consultations are held with the prosthodontist, pediatric dentist, and periodontist as indicated. Discussion with the medical and dental consultants, family, and patients results in a decision for or against surgery. If orthognathic surgery is planned, the patient is registered in a prospective database.

Preoperative records and tests include medical photographs with views of the face and occlusion, cephalometric and dental radiographs, speech assessment, including nasendoscopy, anthropometric surface measurements of the face, facial sensibility testing, and nasal airflow studies. Within 2 weeks of surgery, dental records are obtained, including algenate impressions,

bite registration, and a face-bow transfer. The articulated dental models are then jointly reviewed. After surgery, cephalometric and dental radiographs are obtained at the following standard intervals: immediately, within 5 days, at 6 to 8 weeks, at 1 year, and at 2 years. Speech is reassessed 1 year after surgery through clinical examination and nasendoscopy. Facial sensibility testing, anthropometric facial measurements, and nasal airflow studies are also completed at this time.

Timing of orthognathic surgery

Correction of jaw deformity should usually be planned when the skeleton is mature. Maxillofacial growth is generally complete between the ages of 14 and 16 in girls and between 16 and 18 in boys. However, skeletal growth is variable, and assessment of each patient must be based on either epiphyseal plate closure, documented on hand radiographs, or cessation of maxillofacial growth, documented on sequential cephalometric radiographs taken at 6-month intervals.

Only rarely will psychosocial considerations take precedence and require early jaw surgery in a cleft patient. Wolford, Cooper, and El Deeb[63] have shown that if early jaw surgery is undertaken in cleft patients, revision surgery will be required once skeletal maturity is reached. If mandibular hypoplasia is severe and documented peripheral sleep apnea results, such as with Pierre Robin syndrome, then either tracheostomy or a mandibular advancement procedure must be performed at an early age and revision osteotomy planned for the time of skeletal maturation.[42]

Skeletal stability and relapse patterns

Soft tissue changes associated with Le Fort I osteotomy and the skeletal stability achieved by the procedure have been reported.* In general, published studies of long-term skeletal stability tend to group populations that should be considered separately, have an in-

---

*References 1, 11, 13, 15, 19, 22, 32, 53, 57.

TABLE 9-3

Le Fort I in Unilateral Cleft Patients: Effect of Pharyngoplasty on Horizontal Advancement and Relapse

Pharyngoplasty in Place	Time after Operation	Effective Advancement (mm)		Mean Relapse from Previous Position (mm)
		Mean	SD	
No (N = 24)	1 week	7.4	2.5	
				2.2 mm
	1 year	5.2	2.6	
Yes (N = 6)	1 week	5.5	3.0	
				1.9 mm
	1 year	3.6	2.5	

From Posnick JC and Ewing MP: Plast Reconstr Surg 85:706, 1990.

TABLE 9-4

Le Fort I in Unilateral Cleft Patients: Comparison of Horizontal Advancement and Relapse Between Patients with Direct-Wire and Miniplate Fixation

Fixation	Time after Operation	Effective Advancement (mm)		Mean Relapse from Previous Position (mm)
		Mean	SD	
Direct wire (N = 25)	1 week	6.5	2.7	
				1.9 mm
	1 year	4.6	2.7	
Miniplate (N = 5)	1 week	8.0	1.7	
				1.6 mm
	1 year	6.4	2.2	

From Posnick JC and Ewing MP: Plast Reconstr Surg 85: 706, 1990.

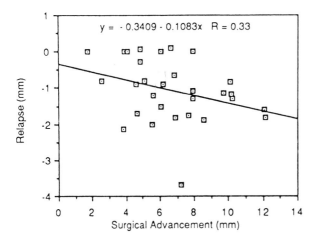

Fig. 9-1 Relationship between horizontal surgical advancement and relapse after 1 year. (From Posnick JC and Ewing MP: Plast Reconstr Surg 85:706, 1990.)

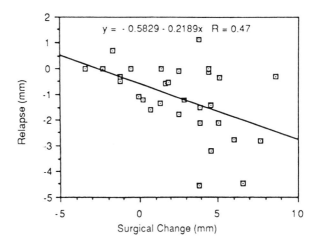

Fig. 9-2 Relationship between vertical surgical displacement and relapse after 1 year. (From Posnick JC and Ewing MP: Plast Reconstr Surg 85:706, 1990.)

adequate follow-up period, or fail to include a large enough sample to ensure statistically significant results. It was therefore decided to carry out a retrospective institutional review of long-term skeletal stability after Le Fort I maxillary advancement in patients with UCLP at The Hospital for Sick Children in Toronto, Ontario.[37]

A review of medical records and cephalometric radiographs identified 30 UCLP patients who underwent a Le Fort I maxillary advancement between 1973 and 1984.[37] The records were investigated to determine amount and timing of relapse, correlation between advancement and relapse, effect of performing multiple jaw procedures, effect of different types of bone grafts, effective pharyngoplasty in place at the time of osteotomy, and effectiveness of various methods of internal fixation. Tracings of preoperative and serial postoperative lateral cephalometrograms were digitized to calcu-

late horizontal and vertical maxillary changes (Tables 9-1 and 9-2).

No significant difference in outcome was seen between patients who had maxillary surgery alone and those who had operations on both jaws nor did the outcome vary significantly with the type of autogenous bone graft used or the segmentalization of the Le Fort I osteotomy. Mean "effective" advancement was greater immediately and 2 years after surgery in patients who did not have a pharyngoplasty in place before the operation (Table 9-3). Advancement also was greater immediately and after 2 years in the miniplate fixation group than in patients with direct-wire fixation (Table 9-4). Mean downward (vertical) displacement was 2.6 mm with a relapse of 1.4 mm after 2 years (Table 9-2). Amounts of relapse and advancement or displacement did not correlate significantly (Figs. 9-1 and 9-2).

UNILATERAL CLEFT LIP AND PALATE

Correction of the residual skeletal deformities of the UCLP adolescent challenges the ingenuity and skill of the maxillofacial surgeon. The central pathology in this type of patient is of maxillary hypoplasia combined with residual oronasal fistula, bony defects, and soft tissue scarring. In addition, the maxillary lateral incisor tooth at the cleft site is usually congenitally absent, resulting in a cleft-dental gap.

Residual deformities

The prevalence of residual clefting deformities in adolescents with UCLP varies widely, depending on the center's policy in regard to the staging of reconstruction and its available surgical expertise. In addition, despite a center's preferred method of management in infancy, childhood, and early adolescence, a subgroup of UCLP patients' presenting multiple residual clefting problems include the following:[40]

1. Maxillary hypoplasia. The maxilla is often vertically short, resulting in an edentulous look, and the occlusal plane is often canted. Arch width deficiency resulting in crossbite may be present in the transverse plane. The maxillary dental midline may be shifted off the facial midline, usually toward the clefted side. The hypoplastic maxilla is retruded in the horizontal plane, resulting in a concave midface profile, Class III malocclusion, and negative overjet. Greater and lesser maxillary segments vary in degree of dysplasia, making it difficult to achieve a satisfactory appearance by repositioning the maxilla in one unit rather than with segmental osteotomies.

2. Residual oronasal fistula. Despite the general preference for fistula closure in the mixed dentition, the UCLP candidate for orthognathic surgery will often have residual labial and palatal fistulas. Previous attempts at closure may have failed. Furthermore, buccal mucosa may have been placed over the cleft site, resulting in a lack of attached gingiva in the tooth-bearing surface region.

3. Residual bony defects. With cleft deformity there are significant bony defects, not just at the alveolus but throughout the palate and floor of the nose along the cleft site. This results in an inferiorly displaced floor of the nose and nasal seal.

4. Cleft-dental gap. The lateral incisor is frequently congenitally absent at the cleft site. A hypoplastic tooth may be present but with inadequate root development or with bony impaction in the cleft. Orthodontic closure of this gap with the movement of the canine tooth into the lateral incisor location is only occasionally accomplished, often with mesial angulation of the canine tooth. The result is often a dental gap at the cleft site between the central incisor and canine teeth.

5. Chin dysplasia. The UCLP patient will frequently be a mouthbreather with the resulting open-mouth posture.[18,48] The addition of a pharyngeal flap in childhood may increase this tendency. The result is a vertically long and retrognathic chin.

6. Mandibular dysplasia. True mandibular prognathism is uncommon in the UCLP patient. The need for mandibular osteotomy should be limited to facial asymmetries, occlusal plane canting, and true anteroposterior discrepancy.

Historical perspective of surgical technique

The literature warns of the possible complications of maxillary osteotomy in the UCLP patient but provides only limited descriptions of technique to guide the orthognathic surgeon in the performance of safe, reliable osteotomy to solve these problems. In 1974 Willmar reported on the complications of 17 UCLP patients undergoing a Le Fort I osteotomy.[59] One patient had aseptic necrosis and partial loss of the lesser segment of the maxilla. In 1974 Georgiade[16] suggested that a camouflage approach with mandibular osteotomy and setback was often preferred to direct maxillary surgery. Kiehn, Des Prez, and Brown[25] and Des Prez and Kiehn[7] warned of blood supply problems that might occur with maxillary surgery in cleft patients. In 1975 Henderson and Jackson[20] reported combining lip-scar revision, anterior fistula closure, and maxillary osteotomy in a one-stage procedure. Their concept was innovative, but they did not specify the details of the technique. In 1978 Jackson[23] further described the Le Fort I procedure as it applied to the cleft patient, stating that if a large fistula was present that required extensive flap mobilization for closure, the maxillary blood supply might be in danger. In such cases, he preferred a staged approach with fistula closure and bone grafting later followed by osteotomy. In general, surgeons have been leary about flap necrosis with loss of maxillary bone and teeth.

In 1980 Tideman, Stoelinga, and Gallia[54] further defined the maxillary Le Fort I osteotomy in cleft patients with a segmental palatal osteotomy. His incision placement, with significant subperiosteal degloving, risks flap circulation but without allowing direct exposure. In 1980 Sinn also reported on the simultaneous maxillary advancement, oronasal fistula repair, and bone grafting of the alveolar cleft.[49] He stressed the importance of preserving a vertical soft-tissue pedicle similar to that described by Tideman. He then completed bony osteotomies through tunnels rather than under direct vision and used a cheek rotation flap for oral-side closure of the labial and palatal oronasal fistulas. With his technique, nonkeritonized buccal mucosa, rather than attached gingiva, is brought into the cleft tooth-bearing region. In 1984 Ward-Booth, Bhatia, and Moos[55] analyzed the Le Fort II osteotomy used at his institution in 13 cleft patients for managing midface hypoplasia. They believed that the Le Fort II osteotomy was preferable to the Le Fort I osteotomy in providing an improved blood supply to the alveolar segments. The residual fistulas were not simultaneously closed, and fixation was with direct wires, intermaxillary fixation (IMF), and craniomaxillary external appliances. In 1985 James and Brook[24] described a variation for the correction of maxillary hypoplasia in patients with cleft lip and palate by transection of the hard palate. He raised an extensive palatal flap and used three vertical stab incisions for exposure on the labial aspects of the maxilla. Access was then achieved through subperiosteal tunneling without direct exposure. Fixation was with IMF and a "halo" head frame, which was maintained for 10 weeks. The second procedure was required for further bone grafting and palatal fistula closure. James expressed concern that a more direct down-fracture of the maxilla would risk vascular compromise to the segments. In 1985 Poole[33] proposed an additional modification of the Le Fort I osteotomy to be used in patients with cleft palate. With his technique, a partial-thickness palatal flap was elevated, leaving the greater palatine vessels in situ and allowing the maxilla to be repositioned anteriorly without displacement of the soft palate. Poole believed this approach would limit interference with the velopharyngeal function. He again used small vertical incisions on the labial aspect, requiring tunneling and lacking direct exposure for osteotomies, disimpaction, fistula closure, bone-graft placement, or plate-and-screw fixation. Fixation was with IMF, direct wires, and halo craniomaxillofacial fixation in this series.

Posnick[34,35,36,40] described modifications of the Le Fort I osteotomy for the UCLP deformity, placing the soft-tissue incision to permit direct exposure for dissection, osteotomies, disimpaction, fistula closure, bone grafting and application of plate-and-screw fixation but without risk of circulation injury to the dento-osseous-musculo-mucosal flaps. The increased visibility provided by these incisions make possible the incorporation of the routine surgical closure of the cleft-dental gap through differential maxillary segmental repositioning. This method of approximating the gap in the maxillary segments also closes the cleft dead space and brings together the labial and palatal flaps to permit closure of recalcitrant oronasal fistulas without tension.

Preferred surgical technique

A maxillary vestibular incision is made from one zygomatic buttress to the other without requiring maintenance of labial pedicles. Parallel incisions are then made in the region of the residual labial oronasal fistula, separating the oral and nasal mucosa on each side of the cleft. These incisions are perpendicular to the first incision and follow the line angles of the teeth adjacent to the cleft, generally along the mesial line angle of the canine tooth and the distal line angle of the central incisor. The nasal and palatal mucosa are also sharply incised along the palatal aspect of the residual oronasal fistula to complete the separation of mucosal layers and facilitate fistula closure (Fig. 9-3).

The anterior maxilla on each side is directly exposed by soft tissue subperiosteal dissection. After retractors have been put in place, horizontal osteotomies are carried out through the lateral, anterior, and medial maxillary walls with a reciprocating saw, as is customary for a Le Fort I osteotomy. The deviated nasal septum is separated from the maxilla with an anterior nasal spine chisel, and the pterygo-maxillary sutures are also separated with a chisel in the standard fashion. The maxilla is down-fractured with finger pressure and disimpacted with Tessier hooks, but no direct pressure is applied to the palatal mucosa, since doing so would compromise the flap's vascular supply.

Vomer flaps are elevated, and a submucosal resection of the inferior aspect of the vomer and cartilagenous septum is completed. The enlarged, bulbous, inferior turbinates are reduced, then the nasal mucosa is sutured along the palatal and labial aspects for a watertight nasal-side closure of the fistula tract.

The down-fractured maxilla is generally in two segments as a result of the original bony cleft. If this is not the case, and surgical closure of the cleft-dental gap is required, the segments are separated with a rotary drill. Bony spurs are shaved from the alveolar region along the distal aspect of the central incisor and mesial aspect of the canine tooth to allow good approximation of the segments. Care is taken to avoid penetrating the lamina dura or exposing the dental roots. Any impacted supernumerary teeth in the cleft site are removed at this stage. The maxillary segments are then ligated into the prefabricated acrylic occlusal splint. This procedure closes the cleft-dental gap and the dead space associated with the cleft, and approximates the labial and palatal mucosal flaps for adequate oral-site fistula closure. The maxilla and splint are then advanced onto the mandible and the IMF applied. The ideal vertical dimension, determined before the procedure, is achieved at the maxillary osteotomy site, and titanium bone miniplates are applied at each zygomatic buttress and piriform aperture.[6,9,21,27] An additional micro-bone plate is frequently applied across the cleft site to stabilize closure of the cleft-dental gap. The IMF is released and the occlusion checked. A few selected sutures may be placed in the palatal mucosa for oral-side

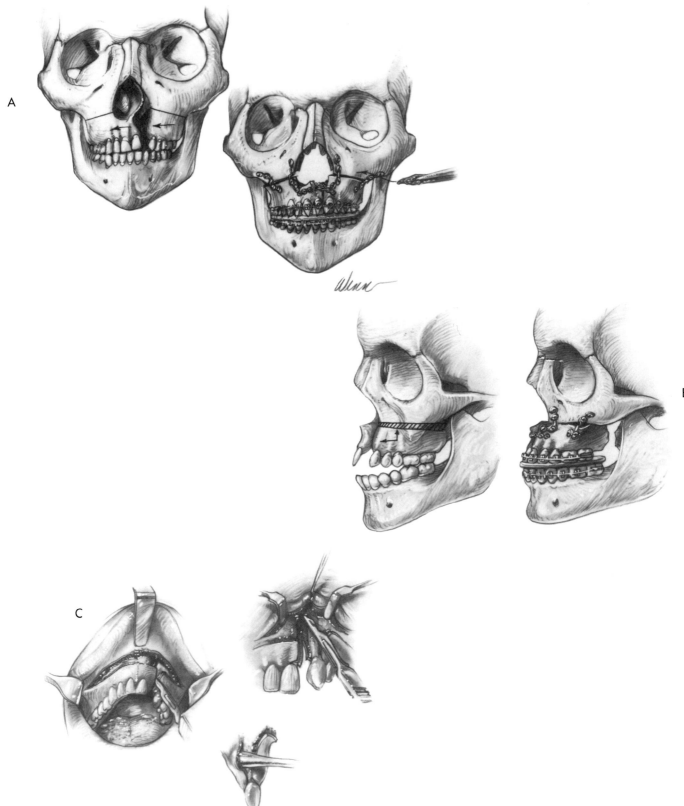

Fig. 9-3 Illustrations of modified Le Fort I osteotomy in two segments. **A,** Frontal view of bony skeleton before and just after fixation of Le Fort I osteotomy in two segments. The inferior tur-binates have been reduced, and a submucous resection of the deviated nasal septum has been performed. Iliac cancellous bone graft has been placed along the nasal floor. **B,** Lateral view of maxillofacial skeleton before and just after fixation of modified Le Fort I osteotomy. **C,** Illustration of direct incisions for completion of osteotomies and fistula closure.

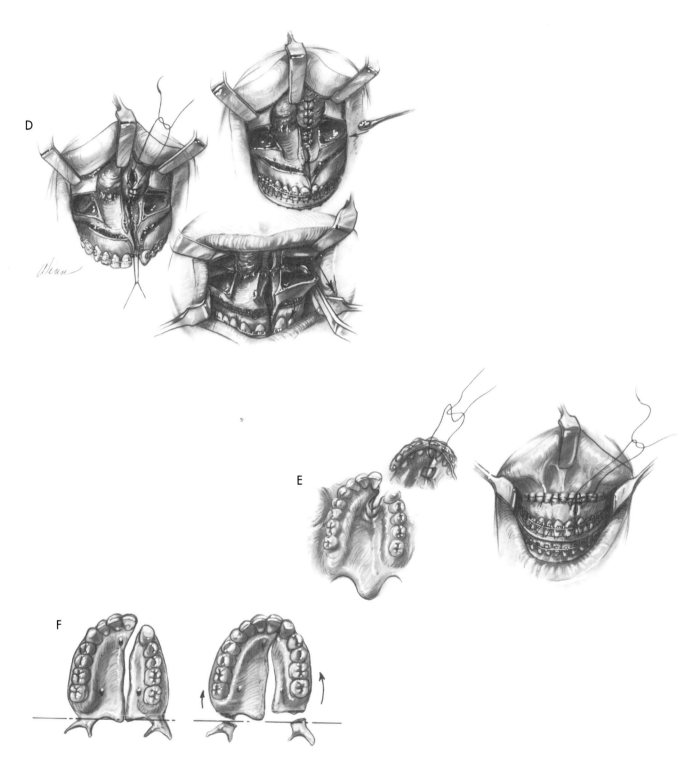

Fig. 9-3, cont'd. **D,** Illustration of down-fractured Le Fort I in two segments after submucous resection of the septum, reduction of inferior turbinate through the nasal mucosa opening, followed by watertight nasal-side closure. **E,** Illustration indicating oral-side wound closure on both labial and palatal aspects after differential segmental repositioning. **F,** Palatal view of bony segments before and after repositioning. (From Posnick JC: Secondary skeletal deformities in cleft patients. In Cohen and Mimis, eds: Mastery of surgery, Boston, Little, Brown and Co [in press]).

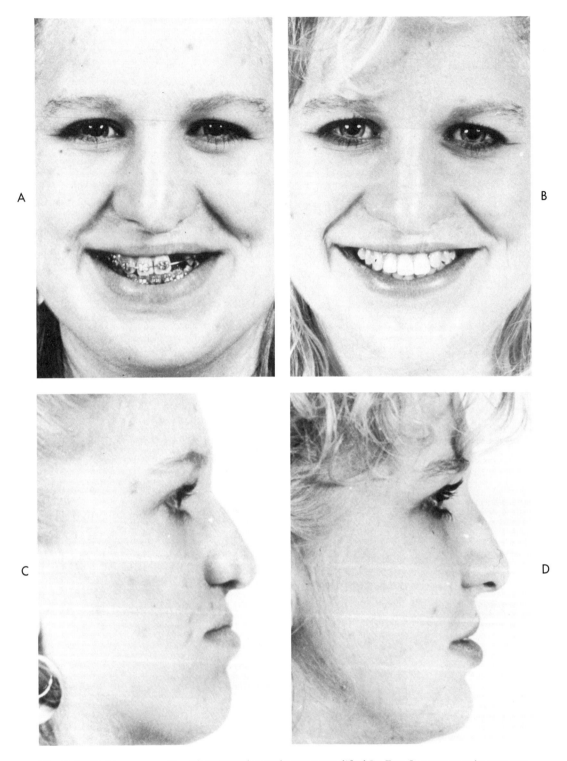

Fig. 9-4 Eighteen-year-old with UCLP who underwent modified Le Fort I osteotomy in two segments is shown before surgery and 2 years later. **A,** Preoperative frontal view. **B,** Postoperative frontal view. **C,** Preoperative profile view. **D,** Postoperative profile view.

fistula closure; however, they are not generally required, since the differential segmental repositioning nicely approximates the freshened mucosal edges along the palate.

An iliac cancellous bone graft is packed along the floor of the nose and into the cleft palate, beginning posteriorly and eventually filling the nasal sill.[52] The

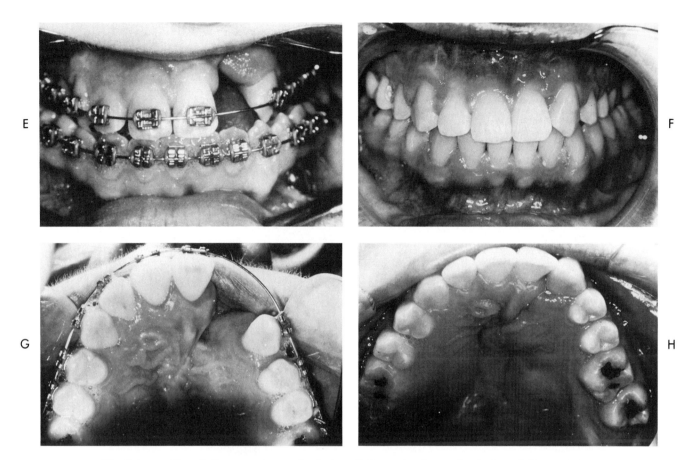

Fig. 9-4, cont'd. E, Preoperative occlusal view. **F,** Postoperative occlusal view. **G,** Preoperative palatal view. **H,** Postoperative palatal view. (From Posnick JC: Secondary skeletal deformities in cleft patients. In Cohen and Mimis, eds: Mastery of surgery, Boston, Little, Brown and Co [in press]).

dead space associated with the alveolar cleft has already been closed by the differential segmental repositioning. With the cleft-dental gap surgically closed, the gingival mucosal flaps on the labial aspects are approximated and directly sutured without the need for buccal mucosal rotation flaps.

The jaws are rewired, either at the end of the procedure or during the first few days, depending on perioperative airway needs, giving increased stability. IMF is generally released at 6 weeks, but the prefabricated acrylic splint remains ligated to the maxillary teeth for an additional 2 weeks. The segmental surgical arch wires are then replaced by one continuous wire, and orthodontic treatment is resumed.

Case examples
Case 1

This patient (Fig. 9-4), born with a complete cleft of the left lip and palate, underwent lip repair at 3 months of age, cleft palate repair with modified von Langenbeck flaps at 18 months, a pharyngoplasty at 6 years, and a cleft lip rhinoplasty at 15 years. Orthodontic brackets were placed at age 15 ½ years to align the

maxillary and mandibular teeth on each jaw. Although vertical and horizontal projection of the maxilla was generally adequate, at age 18 she was referred for surgical consideration of her multiple residual clefting problems.

Examination revealed transverse collapse of the greater and lesser maxillary segments with crossbite, a residual perialveolar oronasal fistula, a congenitally missing lateral incisor with a cleft-dental gap, poor alveolar bony support to the teeth adjacent to the cleft, and a shift of the maxillary dental midline of the facial midline with a poor overjet and overbite relationship at the incisors. A modified maxillary Le Fort I osteotomy was performed in two segments with differential repositioning to close the gap and residual oronasal fistulas. The maxillary dental midline was repositioned to match the facial midline, the posterior crossbites were corrected, a positive overjet and overbite were created, and periodontal support to the adjacent teeth was improved. The patient also underwent a vertical reduction and advancement genioplasty. She is shown 2 years after surgery and has an attractive smile. She did not need prosthetic rehabilitation.

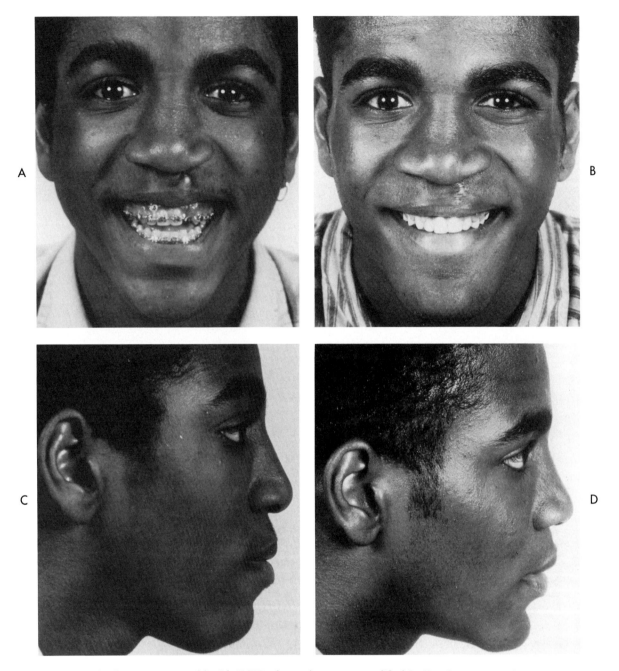

Fig. 9-5 Seventeen-year-old with UCLP who underwent a modified Le Fort I osteotomy in two segments is seen before surgery and 1 year after surgery. **A,** Preoperative frontal view. **B,** Postoperative frontal view. **C,** Preoperative profile view. **D,** Postoperative profile view.

Case 2

This patient (Fig. 9-5) was born with a complete cleft of the left lip and palate. He had undergone lip closure at 4 years of age, followed by a cleft palate repair with push-back flaps at age 6. Cleft lip revision and a pharyngoplasty were performed at age 15.

His residual problems included a cleft-dental gap with a poorly formed, palatally displaced, rudimentary lateral incisor tooth at the cleft site, a perialveolar oronasal fistula, an anterior open bite, a Class III malocclusion, and a vertically long and retrognathic chin. At age 16, the patient received orthodontic brackets to level and align the teeth on each maxillary segment and the mandible in preparation for orthognathic surgery carried out 1 year later.

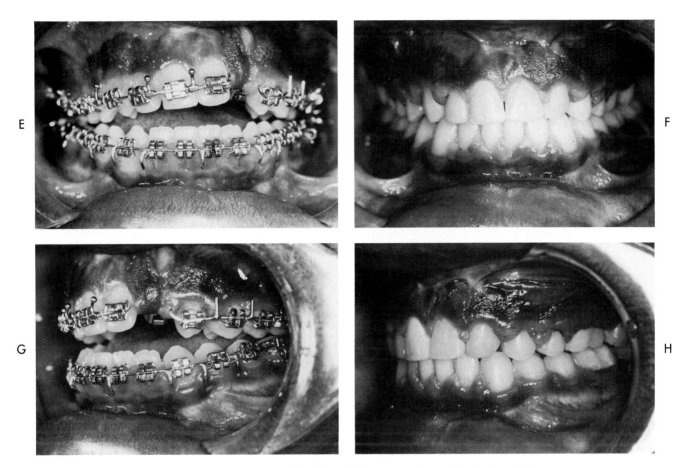

Fig. 9-5 cont'd. **E,** Preoperative occlusal view. **F,** Postoperative occlusal view. **G,** Preoperative lateral occlusal view. **H,** Postoperative lateral occlusal view.

He underwent a modified Le Fort I osteotomy in two segments with differential repositioning to close the gap and the oronasal fistula and to correct the anterior open bite and Class III malocclusion. A vertical reduction and advancement genioplasty was also performed.

He is shown 1 year after surgery with improved function and appearance and without the need for prosthetic rehabilitation.

Complications

I have used the modified Le Fort I osteotomy as previously described for the UCLP deformity in 45 patients over a 4-year period. There were no difficulties with aseptic necrosis or tooth loss, and 95% of the patients had successful oronasal fistula closure.

A variable degree of skeletal relapse occurs after surgery. Postoperative orthodontics are helpful in maintaining a positive or at least a neutral overjet for an overall satisfactory clinical result.

Some degree of velopharyngeal deterioration after a Le Fort I osteotomy with horizontal advancement in a cleft patient can be anticipated. I have not found it necessary to take down a pharyngeal flap at the time of Le Fort I osteotomy to achieve the desired intraoperative maxillary advancement. The scar tissue of the flap has not been a limiting factor in the advancement. To preserve adequate blood supply to the maxillary segments, it is best not to modify an existing pharyngeal flap to improve velopharyngeal function or set in a new one at the time of the osteotomy.

BILATERAL CLEFT LIP AND PALATE
Residual deformities

The (BCLP) adolescent seeking orthognathic surgery may have the following multiple residual clefting problems:[38]
1. Maxillary dysplasia. The premaxilla may be either vertically long, resulting in a gummy smile or horizontally short with an edentulous look. There may be a negative overjet, indicating horizontal deficiency. The arch width of the lateral segments is generally deficient in the transverse plane, with bilateral posterior crossbites and a degree of horizontal deficiency, with a Class III malocclusion.

2. Residual oronasal fistula. Despite the general preference for fistula closure and bone grafting in the mixed dentition, the BCLP candidate for orthognathic surgery will often have residual labial and palatal fistulas with loss of fluid through the nose while drinking and air leakage while speaking. Previous attempts at fistula closure may have failed because of inadequate available soft tissue for wound closure.

3. Cleft-dental gaps. Lateral incisors are most frequently absent at the cleft site. Rudimentary teeth may also be impacted within the cleft and, if so, are of no functional value. If hypoplastic lateral incisors do erupt in the lateral segment, they rarely have adequate root and bone support necessary for long-term functioning. The result is often a dental gap at the cleft site between the central incisor and canine teeth on each side.

4. Residual bony defects. Significant residual bony defects through the alveolus, floor of the nose, and palate are frequent, resulting in a mobile premaxilla secured only to the nasal septum.

5. Chin dysplasia. The BCLP patient will frequently be a mouthbreather with a resulting open-mouth posture.[18,48] The result is a vertically long and retrognathic chin.

6. Mandibular dysplasia. True mandibular prognathism in the BCLP patient is uncommon. The need for mandibular osteotomy should be limited to facial asymmetries, occlusal plane canting, and anteroposterior discrepancy.

Historical perspective of surgical technique

Surgical attempts to correct BCLP skeletal problems date back to Steinkamm's description in 1938 of a maxillary Le Fort I osteotomy in a bilateral cleft patient.[51] The literature since that time strongly warns of possible complications with maxillary osteotomy in this group but offers only an incomplete description of surgical technique to guide the surgeon in performing safe and reliable osteotomies. Henderson and Jackson[20] reported their classic one-stage procedure and Jackson[23] later discussed BCLP patients requiring jaw surgery, suggesting they first have fistula closure and bone grafting, then undergo either a standard Le Fort I or Le Fort II procedure. Ward-Booth, Bhatia, and Moos[55] described an approach with the Le Fort II osteotomy designed to protect circulation to the jaw segments.

In 1974, Willmar[59] reported on the complications associated with the Le Fort I osteotomy. Eight of his 106 patients who underwent surgery had BCLP, one of whom died afterward. However, details of the surgical technique were not mentioned. In 1980, Sinn[49] described modifications for bilateral maxillary alveolar cleft repair combined with the Le Fort I osteotomy. These entailed mobilization of the lateral segments and closure of the bilateral fistula with cheek flaps. Tideman[54] described at least one BCLP patient who underwent a Le Fort I advancement in which he used limited vertical incisions with subperiosteal tunneling for osteotomy exposure. Westbrook, West, and McNeil[58] described simultaneous maxillary advancement and closure of bilateral clefts and oronasal fistulas. He used limited incisions to maintain a safe blood supply to the lateral maxillary segments, which prevented direct exposure of the maxillary walls. He did not mention surgical dental-gap closure of the single BCLP patient described. James and Brook[24] and Poole, Robinson, and Nunn[33] also described cleft-orthognathic technique using indirect exposure with subperiosteal tunneling; they both believed that sequencing of the fistula closure and osteotomy were necessary to avoid flap necrosis.

I have described modifications of the maxillary Le Fort I osteotomy in patients with a BCLP deformity, which allow a routine, one-stage management of the multiple residual deformities of the BCLP adolescent.[34,35,38,40,41] The modifications are based on a rethinking of the circulatory needs after a Le Fort I osteotomy, which leads to the conclusion that flaps can be safely elevated to allow direct maxillary exposure. The surgical technique for the premaxillary osteotomy is based on a labial mucosal pedicle, first described by Wunderer[64] in 1962 and formerly used extensively in noncleft patients. Meticulous attention to detail is necessary to preserve the attachments of the soft-tissue-mucosal pedicle to the premaxilla. This ensures flap survival and safe repositioning of the segment. The technique of maintaining a blood supply to the posterior segments of the down-fractured maxilla after direct buccovestibular incision placement, described in this chapter, resembles that described by Bell and Levy,[3] which is used clinically in noncleft patients.

Preferred surgical technique

Precise incision placement is critical (Fig. 9-6). The buccal incisions are made in the depth of the vestibules and extend from the zygomatic buttress forward to the location of the residual labial oronasal fistula on each side, they are then taken down the mesial line angle of the canine teeth, or if these are missing, the most mesial tooth in each lateral segment. This incision separates the oral and nasal mucosa along each lateral segment. The premaxillary segment incisions

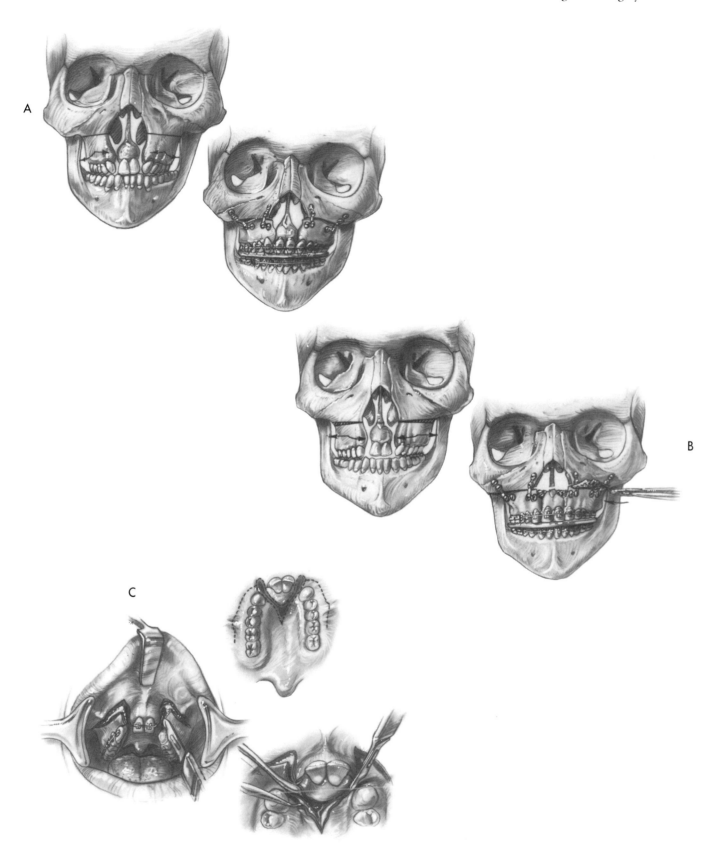

Fig. 9-6 Illustrations of modified Le Fort I osteotomy in two or three segments. **A,** Illustration of the BCLP patient before and after lateral segmental osteotomies and repositioning. **B,** Illustrations before and after three-part maxillary osteotomies with repositioning of the segments.

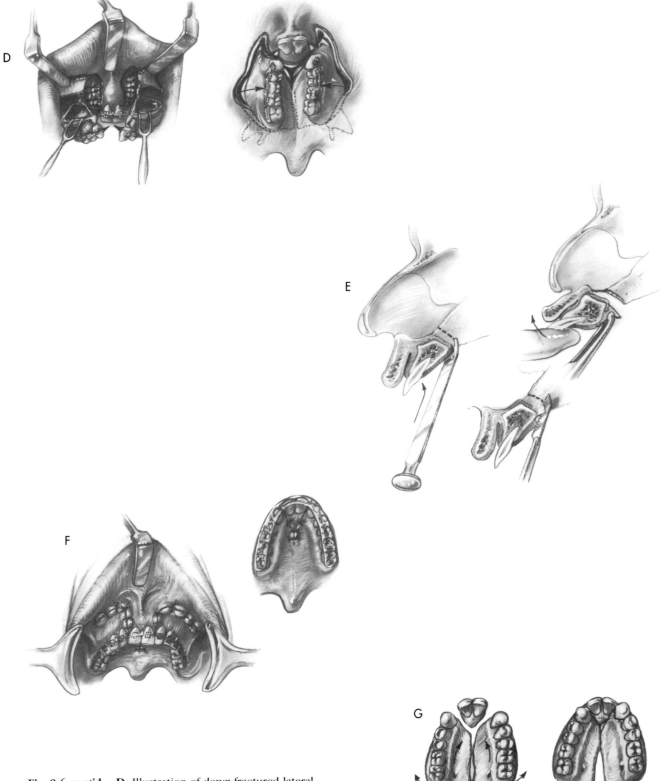

Fig. 9-6 cont'd.   D, Illustration of down-fractured lateral segments demonstrating exposure for nasal-side closure of oronasal fistula and additional view of oral mucosa incisions. **E,** Illustration of premaxillary osteotomy from palate side using either a chisel, rongeur, or reciprocating saw. **F,** Illustration demonstrating oral wounds sutured at the end of procedure. **G,** Palatal view of bony segments before and after repositioning for closure of cleft-dental gaps.

are placed adjacent to the distal line angle incisor on each side to separate the oral and nasal mucosa. Care is required to prevent any disruption of or incision into the mucosa on the labial vestibule of the premaxilla. The nasal and oral mucosa are also sharply incised and separated on the palatal aspect of the premaxilla and on each lateral segment.

A subperiosteal soft-tissue dissection provides direct exposure of the anterior maxilla on each side. Routine Le Fort I osteotomies are then performed through the lateral, anterior, and medial maxillary walls with a reciprocating saw. The pterygomaxillary sutures are separated with a mallet and chisel. The lateral segments are down-fractured with finger pressure, then disimpacted with Tessier hooks to release scar tissue for three dimensional repositioning. The vomer is rarely attached to the lateral segments, but if it is, an osteotomy is also required before the down-fracture.

The nasal mucosal flap is further dissected and separated from the palate side of the premaxilla, and an osteotomy is performed to free the premaxillary segment from the palate, avoiding separation of the labial vestibule mucosa from the premaxillary bone. This is done with the reciprocating saw, chisel and mallet, or rongeur. It is imperative that the labial vestibule mucosa to the premaxilla remain connected to its underlying periosteum and the bone, since blood flows through this pedicle into the premaxillary bone and teeth. The inferior turbinates, which are generally enlarged, are reduced with Mayo scissors to facilitate nasal-side fistula closure. If the nasal septum is deviated, then submucosal resection of the inferior aspect of the vomer and cartilage of the septum is completed. The nasal mucosal lining is sutured for a watertight nasal-side closure on both the left and right palatal and labial surfaces. The elevated vomer flaps assist in both submucosal septal resection and closure.

The lateral maxillary segments are advanced and ligated into the prefabricated acrylic occlusal splint, along with the premaxillary segment. Through this procedure, the cleft-dental gap on each side and the dead space associated with the bony clefts are closed. It may be necessary to shave a small amount of bone at the alveolar edges, using the rotary drill, to approximate the central incisor and canine tooth on each side. The differential segmental advancement approximates the labial and palatal mucosal flaps for adequate oral-side fistula closure. Intermaxillary fixation is applied through the splint. The ideal vertical dimension, determined before the procedure, is achieved at the maxillary osteotomy sites to improve the lip-to-tooth relationship and the appearance of the smile. Bone miniplates are applied across the osteotomy sites at the zygomatic but-

tresses and piriform apertures and secured with titanium screws.[6,9,21,27] The IMF is released and the occlusion checked. A few selected sutures may be placed in the palatal mucosa for oral-side fistula closure. These are not generally required, however, since the differential segmental repositioning has well approximated the freshened mucosal edges along the palate.

Iliac cancellous bone graft is packed along the floor of the nose and cleft palate on each side,[52] beginning in the posterior area and eventually filling the nasal sill. This step establishes an appropriate nasal floor level. The dead space associated with the alveolar cleft has already been closed by segmental repositioning. Iliac bone is also interposed along the bony gap in the anterior maxilla created when the lateral segments were advanced. Finally, with the cleft-dental gaps surgically closed, the gingival mucosal flaps on each side are directly approximated without the need for buccal mucosal rotation flaps.

The jaws are rewired, either at the end of the procedure or during the first few days, depending on perioperative airway needs, to provide increased stability. IMF is released at 6 weeks, but the splint remains ligated to the maxillary teeth for an additional 2 weeks. A continuous arch wire is then reapplied and active tooth movement reinitiated as required by the treating orthodontist.

Case examples
Case 3

A skeletally mature 17-year-old man, born with a complete bilateral cleft lip and palate, sought improvement in facial appearance (Fig. 9-7).[36] He was documented as having had a protruding, vertically long premaxilla during childhood. However, at skeletal maturity, his premaxilla proved to be hypoplastic. He had previously undergone a buccal flap in an unsuccessful attempt to close his oronasal fistula.

When first seen, he had maxillary hypoplasia, a mobile premaxilla, residual bilateral labial and palatal oronasal fistulas, residual bony clefts, bilateral cleft-dental gaps in the region of the congenitally absent lateral incisors, a vertically long and retrognathic chin, and a cleft-nasal deformity with a short columella.

When preoperative orthodontic treatment was complete, he underwent a maxillary Le Fort I osteotomy in three segments, simultaneous iliac bone grafting, closure of residual fistulas and cleft-dental gaps, and a vertical reduction and advancement genioplasty procedure. One year later, he had an open rhinoplasty, and when his postoperative orthodontic treatment was complete, he also had resin build-ups of his hypoplastic anterior teeth.

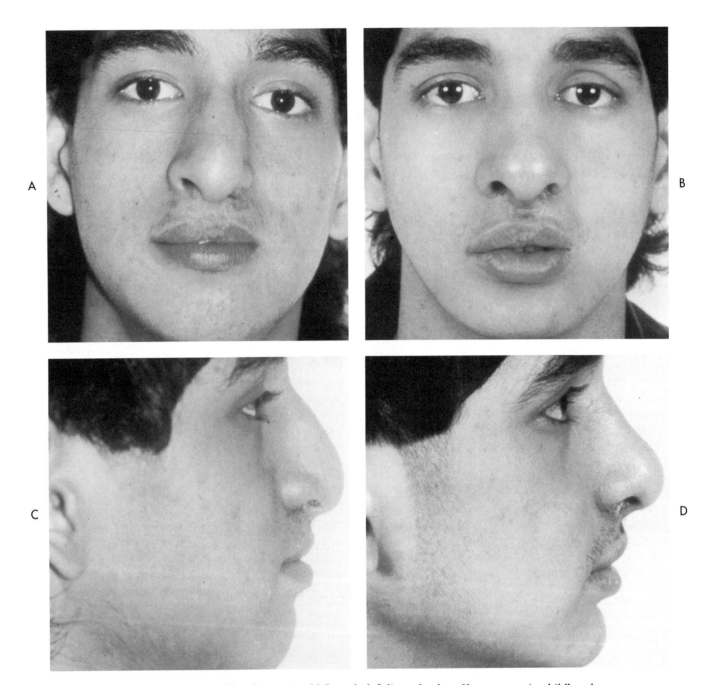

Fig. 9-7   A 17-year-old with a repaired bilateral cleft lip and palate. He was seen in childhood with an elongated hypoplastic premaxilla. By the time of skeletal maturity his premaxilla proved to be hypoplastic. His residual skeletal clefting problems were managed through a combined or-thognathic and orthodontic approach. One year later he underwent an open rhinoplasty. **A,** Preoperative frontal view. **B,** Postoperative frontal view. **C,** Preoperative lateral view. **D,** Postoperative lateral view. From Posnick JC et al: In Bardach J and Morris HL (eds): Multidisiplinary management of cleft lip and palate, Philadelphia, 1990, WB Saunders.

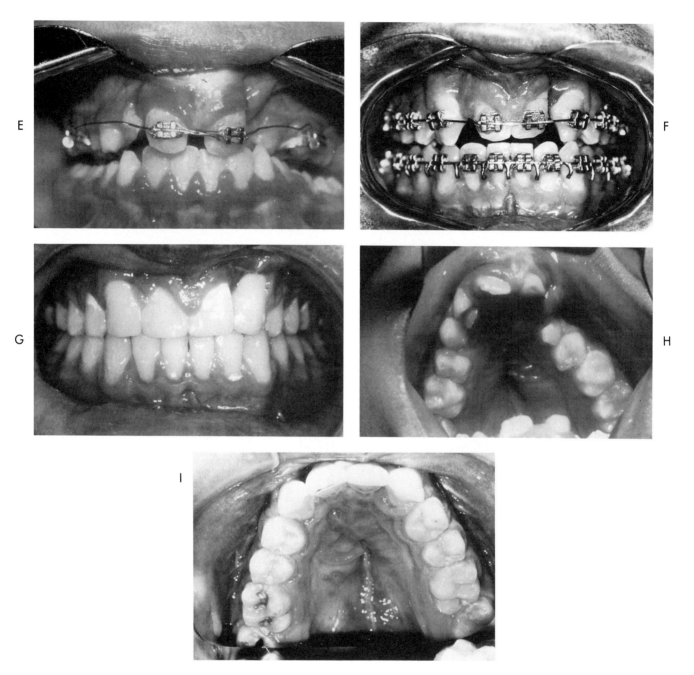

Fig. 9-7 cont'd. **E,** Preoperative occlusal view at 13 years of age. The premaxilla appears to be vertically long. **F,** After preoperative orthodontic treatment in preparation for jaw surgery at age 17. **G,** 18 months after surgery with completion of orthodontics and resin build-ups of the anterior teeth. **H,** Occlusal view in mixed dentition phase. The cheek rotation flap used for fistula closure has decreased the vestibular depths and placed nonkeritonized mucosa over the tooth-bearing surface. A sliding mucogingival rotation flap would have been preferable. **I,** Dental arch form after maxillary Le Fort I osteotomy with differential repositioning of segments to close fistulas and cleft-dental gaps in the regions of the congenitally absent lateral incisors.

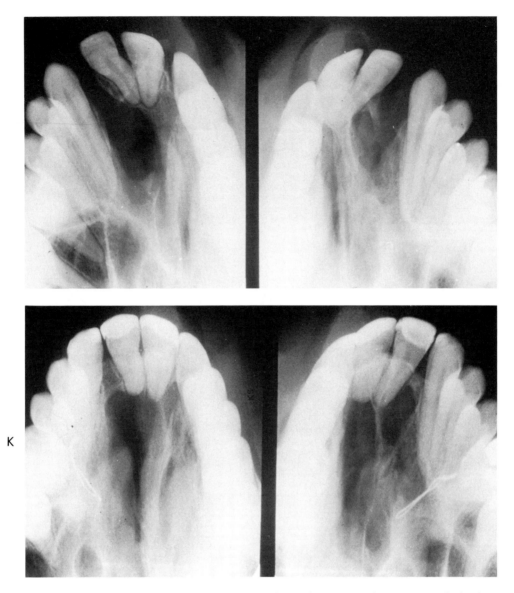

K

Fig. 9-7 cont'd.   J, Occlusal radiographs before orthognathic surgery demonstrating lack of continuity in the maxillary arch. **K,** Postoperative occlusal radiographs demonstrating bony bridges on both sides, stabilizing the maxilla.

Case 4

A skeletally mature 16-year-old girl, born with a bilateral cleft lip and palate, had correction surgery in infancy. She also had a pharyngoplasty and two cleft lip nasal revisions later in childhood (Fig. 9-8).

With the permanent dentition in place, she had orthodontic alignment of her maxillary and mandibular teeth. Her maxillary lateral incisors were present and aligned within the premaxillary segment. Unfortunately, there was limited alveolar bony support. Her canine teeth and three of four premolar teeth were maintained in the lesser segments but at the expense of se-

vere alveolar bone resorption along the mesial aspects of the canine tooth within each hypoplastic lateral maxillary segment. A marked residual oronasal fistula remained in the palate and along each alveolar cleft. There was residual mobility of the premaxilla and marked velopharyngeal incompetence with regurgitation of fluid while drinking and intake of air while speaking. She required a palatal prosthesis.

She was referred for surgical consideration of fistula closure. After discussion with her orthodontist and family, she underwent a modified maxillary Le Fort I osteotomy in three segments with differential reposi-

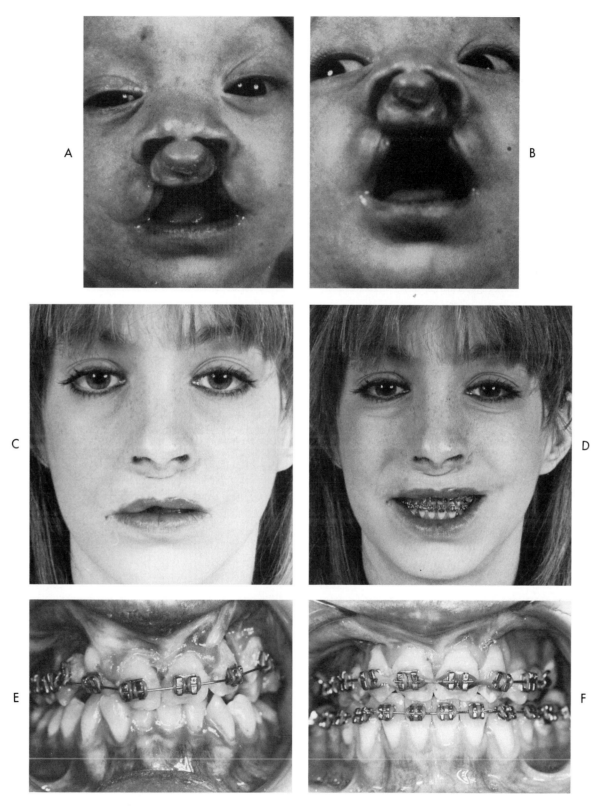

Fig. 9-8 A 16-year-old with repaired BCLP with a marked residual oronasal fistula and poor alveolar bone support to the teeth adjacent to each cleft. She underwent a combined orthognathic
and orthodontic approach. **A** and **B**, Initial cleft deformity at 8 weeks of age. **C**, Preoperative
frontal view. **D**, Six-month postoperative frontal view. **E**, Preoperative occlusal view. **F**, Six-
month postoperative occlusal view.

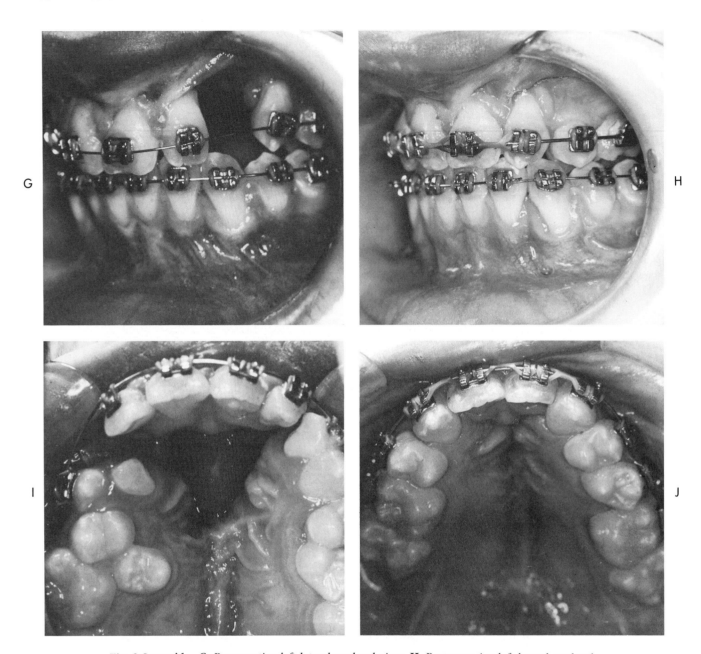

Fig. 9-8 cont'd.   G, Preoperative left lateral occlusal view. **H,** Postoperative left lateral occlusal view. **I,** Preoperative palatal view. **J,** Postoperative palatal view.

tioning. Through intraoperative extraction of the lateral incisors, it was possible to reposition the maxillary lateral segments and close the cleft-dental and alveolar gap at each cleft site. Closing this maxillary dead space also permitted effective oronasal fistula closure. Iliac bone graft, miniplate fixation, and a prefabricated

acrylic splint were used for osteotomy stabilization.

Six months later, her postoperative orthodontic treatment is near completion. There is marked improvement in velopharyngeal closure without the need for an obturator with the fistula closed, plus improved dental health and a more natural smile.

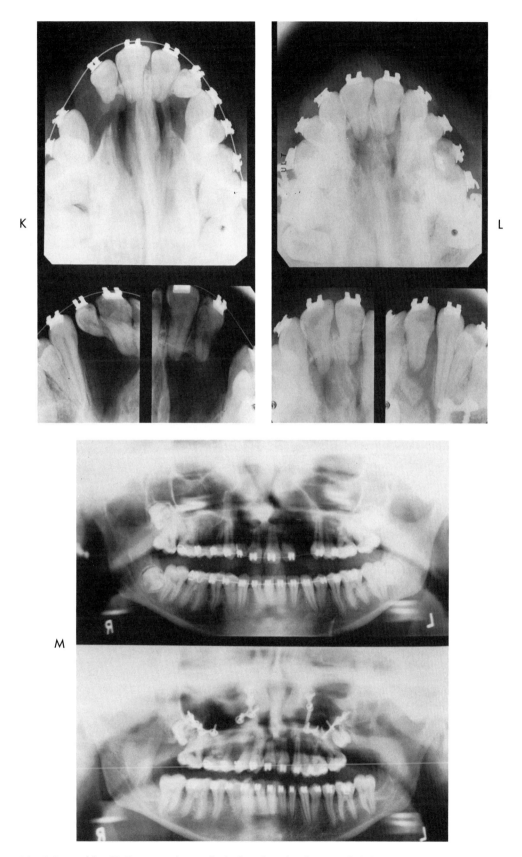

Fig. 9-8 cont'd.   K, Preoperative periapical and occlusal view of cleft. **L,** Postoperative periapical and occlusal view of cleft. **M,** Preoperative and postoperative panorex views.

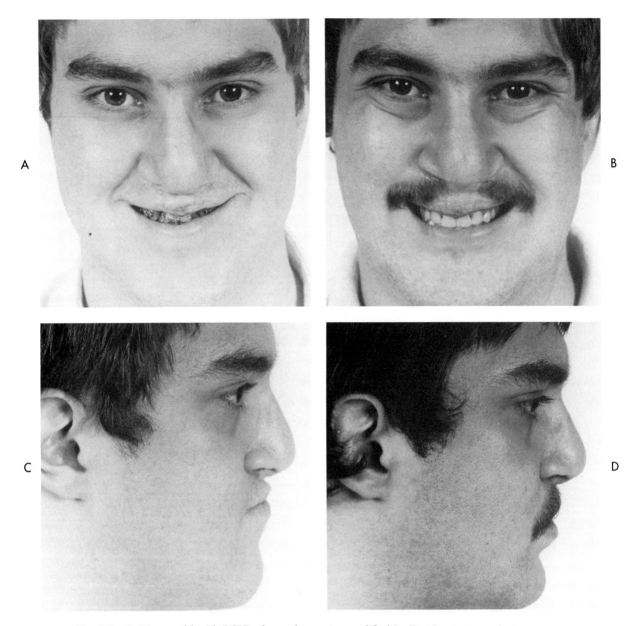

Fig. 9-9   A 17-year-old with BCLP who underwent a modified Le Fort I osteotomy in two segments with the premaxilla remaining intact. He is shown before surgery and 2 years later. **A,** Preoperative frontal view. **B,** Postoperative frontal view. **C,** Preoperative profile view. **D,** Postoperative profile view. From Posnick JC and Dagys AP: Orthognathic surgery in the bilateral cleft patient, Philadelphia, WB Saunders, 1991.

Case 5

This patient with BCLP underwent bilateral lip repair at 3 months of age, followed by cleft palate repair at 18 months with bilateral push-back flaps (Fig. 9-9).[41] He had lip-scar revision at age 2, followed by columella lengthening at age 4. At 13 years of age, brackets were placed for what was believed to be his final orthodontic treatment to align the teeth in each segment.

At age 16 the patient was referred for surgical correction of his mobile premaxilla and oronasal fistula closure in preparation for fixed bridgework to replace the missing lateral incisors. Examination revealed a mobile premaxilla, congenitally missing maxillary lateral incisors with cleft-dental gaps, labial and palatal residual oronasal fistulas, and a vertically long and retrognathic chin.

At age 17, he underwent a modified maxillary Le Fort I osteotomy to reposition the lateral segments differentially for closure of the cleft-dental gaps and oronasal fistulas, to stabilize the premaxillary segment, and to improve periodontal support for the teeth adjacent to each cleft. A vertical reduction and horizontal ad-

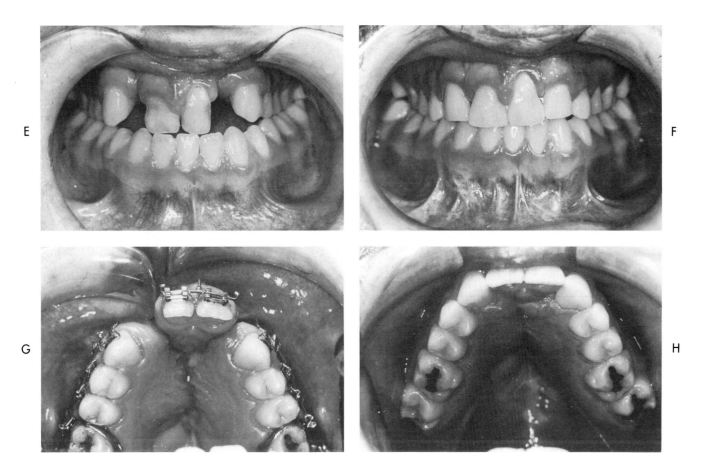

Fig. 9-9 cont'd.   **E,** Preoperative occlusal view. **F,** Postoperative occlusal view. **G,** Preoperative palatal view. **H,** Postoperative palatal view.

vancement genioplasty was also completed to improve his lip closure and appearance.

He is shown 2 years after surgery with successful management of these problems and a more attractive smile, without the need for prosthetic rehabilitation.

Complications

Since 1986, I have completed 22 modified maxillary Le Fort I osteotomies for correction of skeletal deformities in BCLP patients. There have been no postoperative difficulties with avascular necrosis or loss of teeth.

Approximately 20% of these patients retain small residual fistulas in the incisal foramen region with loss of some bone graft and a degree of residual mobility of the premaxilla. The orthognathic procedure has significantly reduced the size of the fistulas to the point where elevation of standard flaps for fistula closure with additional bone grafting from the same hip wound has successfully resolved these problems.

Postoperative velopharyngeal incompetence can be accurately predicted by speech assessment before surgery and is not considered a complication.[61] When velopharyngeal incompetence is either present before surgery or as a result of the Le Fort advancement, it is managed secondarily as described for the UCLP patient.

ISOLATED CLEFT PALATE
Residual deformities

1. Maxillary dysplasia. When maxillary dysplasia occurs, it generally follows one of two patterns. The first is horizontal maxillary retrusion, generally with a minor degree of vertical hypoplasia. The second is vertical maxillary excess with a minor degree of horizontal retrusion. The latter occurs more frequently in mouthbreathers. A pharyngeal flap was often placed in childhood.
2. Residual oronasal fistula. There may be a residual midline palatal fistula located in the region between the incisal foramen and the soft palate.
3. Residual bony defects. The alveolus is not clefted, but generally there are bony defects of the palate.
4. Chin dysplasia. The ICP patient will frequently be a

mouthbreather, with resulting open-mouth posture. The end result is a vertically long and retrognathic chin. If Pierre Robin syndrome is present, a retrognathic chin is also expected.

5. Mandibular dysplasia. True mandibular prognathism in the ICP patient is rare. Mandibular retrognathism may be part of a Pierre Robin syndrome. The need for mandibular osteotomy in addition to maxillary osteotomy is limited.

Preferred surgical technique

The surgical technique I prefer is a standard maxillary Le Fort I down-fracture osteotomy. The dissection may be complicated by residual palatal fistulas and the need to carefully separate the oral and nasal layers. Great care is taken to prevent subperiosteal dissection of the palatal mucosal flaps. If residual fistulas are present preoperatively in the ICP patient, they cannot be closed at the same time as the Le Fort I osteotomy.

Case examples
Case 6

A 19-year-old woman with an isolated cleft palate (Fig. 9-10) had undergone palate repair at 18 months of age.[36] No further revisions were required. On examination, she had marked maxillary hypoplasia with a Class III malocclusion and a vertically long and retrognathic chin.

Before surgery, nasendoscopy and videofluoroscopy indicated borderline velopharyngeal closure. There was a circular pattern of closure with occasional bubbling of mucosa through the velopharyngeal port. Resonance was normal, but nasal air emission was inconsistent. A sibilant distortion was attributed to abnormal tongue placement. The patient was considered a high risk for postoperative velopharyngeal incompetence.

Preoperative orthodontic therapy was carried out before performing a maxillary Le Fort I osteotomy with horizontal advancement and posterior vertical intrusion. The chin required vertical reduction and advancement. The maxilla was stabilized with titanium miniplates and screws and iliac bone graft. The chin was stabilized by direct transosseous wires.

Velopharyngeal incompetence and hypernasality were noted after the procedure despite evidence of a circular closure pattern with a Passavant's ridge. A superiorly based pharyngeal flap was carried out 6 months after surgery.

Case 7

A skeletally mature 16-year-old girl, born with an isolated cleft palate, was seen in consultation for or-

thognathic surgical correction of her facial appearance (Fig. 9-11). She had cleft palate repair at 1 year of age with a bilateral push-back procedure. She developed mouthbreathing because of a septal deviation requiring submucous resection when she was 8 years old. Her presenting problems included maxillary hypoplasia and a Class III malocclusion for which a combined orthognathic and orthodontic approach was planned.

Preoperative nasendoscopy indicated hyponasality and orthodontic treatment was carried out to correct dental alignment. Detailed surgical model planning indicated that her maxillary hypoplasia was associated with mandibular asymmetry and a vertically long chin.

Twelve months after orthodontic treatment, she had a maxillary Le Fort I osteotomy with vertical and horizontal lengthening, sagittal split mandibular osteotomies for a minor setback, correction of asymmetry, and a vertical reduction and advancement genioplasty. Stabilization was achieved with titanium miniplates and screws, using an autogenous iliac bone graft.

One year later, she has maintained a Class I occlusion, and her facial appearance is improved in both profile and frontal views. Her velopharyngeal closure remains adequate despite the maxillary advancement procedure.

Complications

Since 1986 I have completed 12 maxillary Le Fort I osteotomies for correction of skeletal deformities in ICP patients. No patient experienced postoperative necrosis, infection, or tooth loss.

SUMMARY

The cleft patient's care is best delivered by a dedicated cleft lip and palate team. There are multiple residual clefting problems in the adolescent patient that can be resolved by sequencing surgery and orthodontics. Each of the cleft types: UCLP, BCLP, and ICP present unique challenges requiring varied surgical techniques for safe orthognathic surgery. For the UCLP and BCLP patient, the modified Le Fort I osteotomy allows differential segmental repositioning followed by routine closure of cleft-dental gaps, dead space, and residual recalcitrant oronasal fistulas. Standard surgical technique is used when orthognathic surgery is required for patients with ICP.

Dental rehabilitation and improved function and appearance are achieved without the need for removable or fixed prosthetics. It is anticipated that these refinements will achieve an improved long-term quality of life in the care of patients with residual cleft deformities.

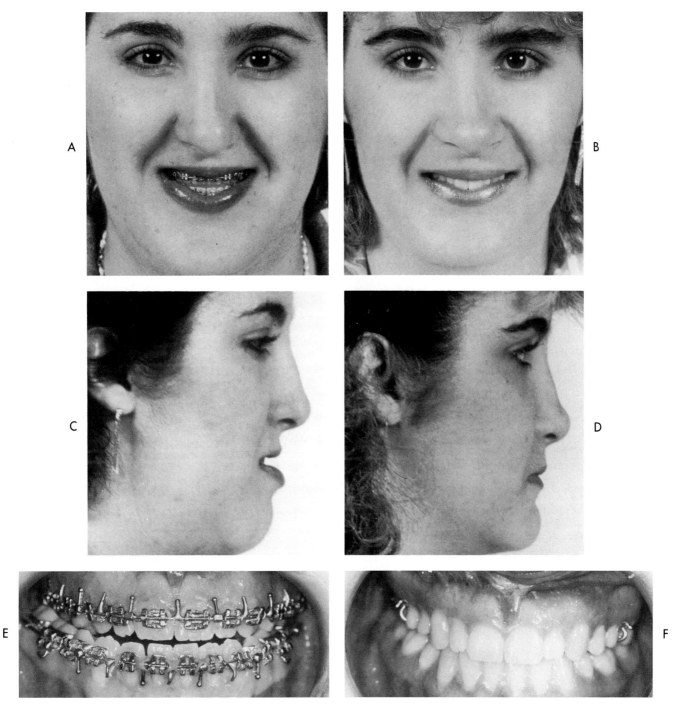

Fig. 9-10 A 19-year-old woman with isolated cleft palate. **A,** Frontal preoperative view. **B,** Frontal postoperative view. **C,** Lateral preoperative view. **D,** Lateral postoperative view. **E,** Occlusal view with orthodontic treatment under way. **F,** One year after surgery after removal of orthodontic bands. From Posnick JC et al: In Bardach J and Morris HL (eds): Multidisciplinary management of cleft lip and palate, Philadelphia, 1990, WB Saunders.

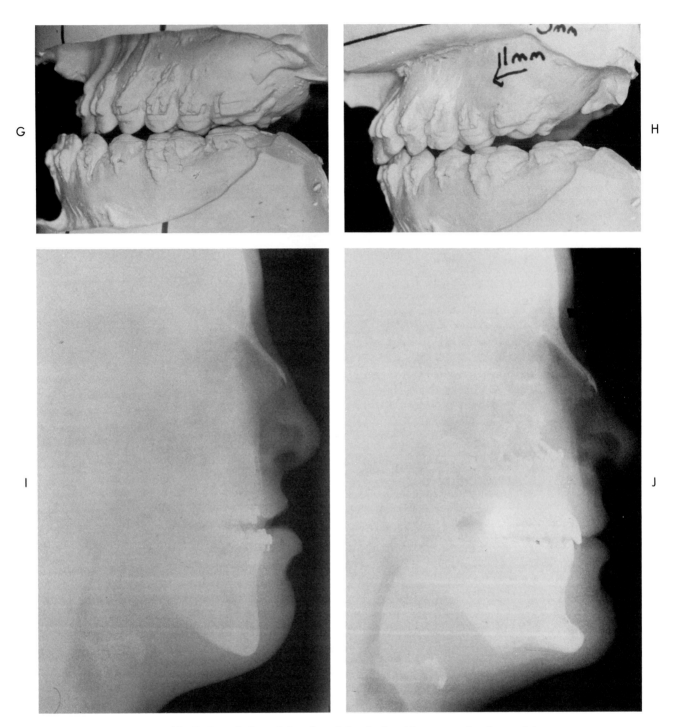

Fig. 9-10 cont'd   G, Lateral view of dental model articulated in preparation for model surgery.
H, Lateral view of articulated model repositioned through model surgery. **I,** Preoperative lateral
cephalometric radiograph. **J,** Postoperative lateral cephalometric radiograph.

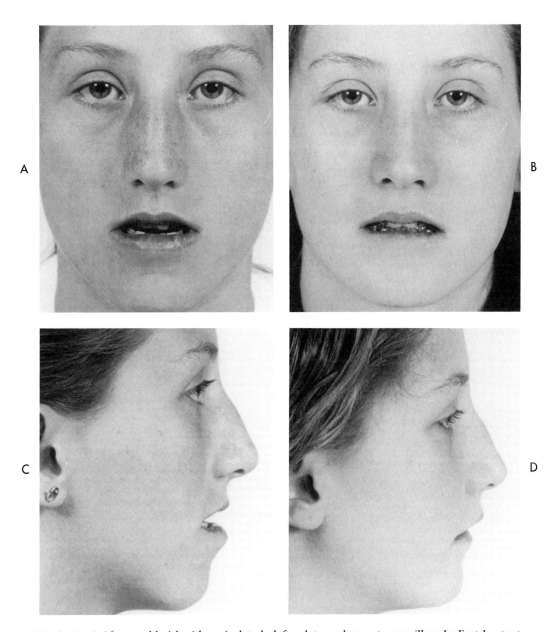

Fig. 9-11 A 16-year-old girl with an isolated cleft palate underwent a maxillary Le Fort I osteotomy with horizontal and vertical lengthening, bilateral sagittal split osteotomies of the mandible with correction of asymmetry and setback, and a vertical reduction and advancement genioplasty procedure. She is shown before surgery and 1 year later. **A,** Preoperative frontal view. **B,** Postoperative frontal view. **C,** Preoperative profile view. **D,** Postoperative profile view.

REFERENCES

1. Araujo A et al: Total maxillary advancement with and without bone grafting, J Oral Surg 36:849, 1978.
2. Bell WH et al: Bone Healing and revascularization after total maxillary osteotomy, J Oral Surg 33:253, 1975.
3. Bell WH and Levy BM: Revascularization and bone healing after posterior maxillary osteotomy, J Oral Surg 29:313, 1971.
4. Braun TW and Sotereanos GC: Orthognathic and secondary cleft reconstruction of adolescent patients with cleft palate: J Oral Surg 38(6):425-434, 1980.
5. Braun TW and Sotereanos GC: Orthognathic surgical reconstruction of adolescents with cleft palate deformities, J Oral Surg 39:255-263, 1981.
6. Champy M: Surgical treatment of midface deformities, Head Neck Surg 2 451-465, 1980.
7. DesPrez JD and Kiehn CL: Surgical positioning of the maxilla,

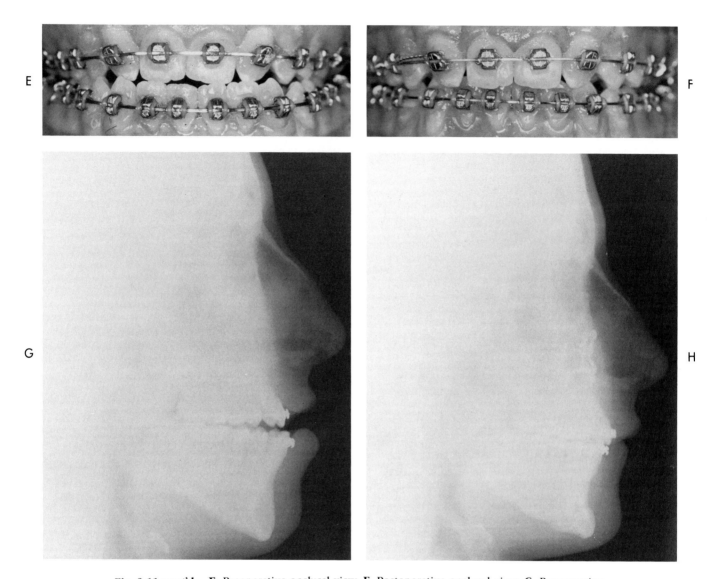

Fig. 9-11 cont'd. **E,** Preoperative occlusal view. **F,** Postoperative occlusal view. **G,** Preoperative soft-tissue cephalometric radiograph. **H,** Postoperative soft-tissue cephalometric radiograph.

Symp Man Cleft Lip Palate Assoc Deform 8:222-227, 1974.

8. Drommer R: Selecting angiographic studies prior to Le Fort I osteotomy in patients with cleft lip and palate, J Maxillofac Surg 7:264, 1979.

9. Drommer R and Luhr HG: The stabilization of osteotomized maxillary segments with Luhr mini-plates in secondary cleft surgery, J Maxillofac Surg 9:166, 1981.

10. Epker BN and Fish LC: Cleft lip-palate dentofacial deformity. In Dentofacial deformities: integrated orthodontic and surgical correction, St. Louis, 1986, The C V Mosby Co.

11. Fitzpatrick B: Mid-face osteotomy in the adolescent cleft patient, Aust Dent J 22(5):338-350, 1977.

12. Friede H and Pruzansky S: Longitudinal study of growth in bilateral cleft lip and palate from infancy to adolescence, Plast Reconstr Surg 49:392, 1972.

13. Freihofer HP Jr: Results of osteotomies of the facial skeleton in adolescence, J Maxillofac Surg 5:267, 1977.

14. Freihofer HPM and Brouns JA: Midfacial movements: a reappraisal, Oral Maxillofac Surg Clin N Am 2(4):761, 1990.

15. Garrison BT, Lapp TH, and Bussard DA: The stability of Le Fort I maxillary osteotomies in patients with simultaneous alveolar cleft bone grafts, J Oral Maxillofac Surg 45:761, 1987.

16. Georgiade NG: Mandibular osteotomy for the correction of facial disproportion in the cleft lip and palate patient, Am Plast Reconstr Surg 8:238-241, 1974.

17. Gillies HG and Rowe NL: L'osteotomie du maxillaire superieur envisagee essentiellement dans les cas de bec-de-lievre total, Rev Stomat 55, 545, 1954.

18. Hairfield WM, Warren DW, and Deaton DL: Prevalence of mouthbreathing in cleft lip and palate, Cleft Palate J 25:135, 1988.

19. Hedemark A and Freihofer HP Jr: The behavior of the maxillary vertical movements after Le Fort I osteotomy, J Maxillofac Surg 6:244, 1978.

20. Henderson D and Jackson IT: Combined cleft lip revision, anterior fistula closure, and maxillary osteotomy: a one-stage procedure, Br J Oral Surg 13:33, 1975.

21. Horster W: Experience with functionally stable plate osteosynthesis after forward displacement of the upper jaw, J Maxillofac Surg 8:176, 1980.
22. Houston WJ et al: Le Fort I maxillary osteotomies in cleft palate cases, J Craniomaxillofac Surg 17:9, 1989.
23. Jackson IT: Clefts and jaw deformities. Symp Reconstruct Jaw Deform 16:(11) 113-138, 1978.
24. James DR and Brook K: Maxillary hypoplasia in patients with cleft lip and palate deformity—the alternative surgical approach, Eur J Orthod 7:231, 1985.
25. Kiehn CL, Desprez JD, and Brown F: Maxillary osteotomy for late correction of occlusion and appearance in cleft lip and palate patients, Plast Reconstr Surg 42, 203, 1968.
26. Le Fort R: Experimental study of fractures of the upper jaw: parts I and II, Rev Chir de Paris 23:208-379, 1901.
27. Luhr HG: Aur stabilen osteosynthese bei unterkierferfrakturen durch mini-kompressionsplatten, Dtsch Zahnaerztl Z 23:754, 1968.
28. Maloney F and Worthington P: The origin of the Le Fort I maxillary osteotomy: cheever's operation, J Oral Surg 39:731, 1981.
29. Narula JK and Ross RB: Facial growth in children with complete bilateral cleft lip and palate, Cleft Palate J 7:239, 1970.
30. Obwegeser HL and Trauner R: Zur operationtechni bei der progenie und anderen unterkieferanomalien, Stsch Zach-, Mund-Keiferheilk 9:73, 1942.
31. Obwegeser HL: Surgical correction of maxillary deformities. In Grabb WC, Resenstein SW, and Brock KR: Cleft lip and palate, Boston, 1969, Little, Brown & Co Inc.
32. Obwegeser HL: Surgical correction of small or retrodisplaced maxillae: the "dish-face" deformity, Plast Reconstr Surg 43:351, 1969.
33. Poole MD, Robinson PP, and Nunn ME: Maxillary advancement in cleft lip and palate patients, J Maxillofac Surg 14:123-127, 1986.
34. Posnick JC and Dagys AP: Refinements in Orthognathic surgery in the cleft patient. Proceedings of the Sixth International Congress On Cleft Palate and Related Craniofoacial Anomalies, June, 1989.
35. Posnick JC: Refinements in cleft orthognathic surgery through modification of the maxillary Le Fort I: morbidity and long term results. Proceedings of the forty-fourth Annual Meeting of the Canadian Society of Plastic Surgeons, Monction, New Brunswick, June, 1990.
36. Posnick JC, Witzel MA, and Dagys AP: Management of jaw deformities in the cleft patient. In Bardach J and Morris HL (eds): Multidisciplinary management of cleft lip and palate, Philadelphia, 1990, WB Saunders Co.
37. Posnick JC and Ewing M: Skeletal stability after Le Fort I maxillary advancement in patients with unilateral cleft lip and palate, Plast Reconstr Surg 85:706, 1990.
38. Posnick JC: Discussion, orthognathic surgery in cleft patients treated by early bone grafting, Plast Reconstr Surg 87:840, 1991.
39. Reference deleted in proofs.
40. Posnick JC: Secondary skeletal deformities in cleft patients. In Cohen and Mimis, eds: Mastery of surgery, Boston, Little, Brown & Co (in press).
41. Posnick JC and Dagys AP: Orthognathic surgery in the bilateral cleft patient: an integrated surgical and orthodontic approach, Philadelphia, WB Saunders 1990.
42. Riley RW, Powell N, and Guilleminault C: Current surgical concepts for treating obstructive sleep apnea syndrome, J Oral Maxillofac Sur 45:149, 1987.
43. Ross RB: The Clinical implications of facial growth in cleft lip and palate, Cleft Palate J 7:37, 1970.
44. Ross RB and Johnston MC: Cleft lip and palate, Baltimore, 1972, Williams & Wilkins.
45. Ross RB: Treatment variables affecting facial growth in complete unilateral cleft lip and palate: an overview of treatment and facial growth, Cleft Palate J 24:75, 1987.
46. Sandor GKB, Witzel MA, and Posnick JC: The use of nesendoscopy in predicting velopharyngeal function after maxillary advancement. Proceedings of the forty-sixth Annual Meeting of the Cleft Palate-Craniofacial Association, April, 1989.
47. Schuchardt K: Ein Beitrag zur chirurgischen kieferorthopadie unter berucksichtigung ihrer bedeutung fur die behandlung angeborener und erworbener kieferdeformitaten bei soldaten, Deutsch Z M K-heilk 9, 73, 1942.
48. Seaton D et al: The posterior pharyngeal flap: effects on airway size and breathing, J Dent Res 67:259, 1988.
49. Sinn DP: Simultaneous maxillary expansion and advancement, repair of oronasal fistula, and bone grafting of the alveolar cleft. In Bell WH, Profit WR, and White RP (eds): Surgical correction dentofacial deformities, Philadelphia, 1980, WB Saunders Co.
50. Smahel Z: Craniofacial morphology in adults with bilateral complete cleft lip and palate, Cleft Palate J 21:159, 1984.
51. Steinkamm W: Die Pseudo-Progenie und ihre Behandlung, Inaug Diss, Berlin, 1938.
52. Tessier P and Tulanse JF: Secondary repair of cleft lip deformity, Clin Plast Surg 11(4):747-760, 1984.
53. Teuscher U and Sailer HF: Stability of Le Fort I osteotomy in Class III cases with retropositioned maxillae, J Maxillofac Surg 10:80, 1982.
54. Tideman H, Stoelinga P, and Gallia L: Le Fort I advancement with segmental palatal osteotomies in patients with cleft palates, J Oral Surg 38:196, 1980.
55. Ward-Booth RP, Bhatia SN, and Moos KF: A cephalometric analysis of the Le Fort II osteotomy in the adult cleft patient, J Maxillofac Surg 12:208, 1984.
56. Wassmund M: Praktischen chirurgie des mundes und der kiefer, Bd 1:260-282, Hermann Meusser, Leipzig, 1935.
57. West A: Orthognathic surgery, Oral Maxillofac Surg Clin North Am 2(4):761, 1990.
58. Westbrook MT Jr, West RA, and McNeil RW: Simultaneous maxillary advancement and closure of bilateral alveolar clefts and oronasal fistulas, J Oral Maxillofac Surg 41:257, 1983.
59. Willmar K: On Le Fort I osteotomy: a follow-up study of 106 operated patients with maxillo-facial deformity, Scand J Plast Reconstr Surg [Suppl 12], 1974.
60. Witzel MA and Posnick JC: Patterns and location of velopharyngeal valving problems: atypical findings on video nasopharyngoscopy, Cleft Palate J 26(1):63, 1989.
61. Witzel MA and Munro IR: Velopharyngeal insufficiency after maxillary advancement, Cleft Palate J 14:176, 1977.
62. Witzel MA, Ross RB, and Munro IR: Articulation skills before and after facial osteotomies, J Maxillofac Surg 8:195, 1980.
63. Wolford LM, Cooper RL, and El Deeb M: Orthognathic surgery in the young cleft patient and the effect on growth. Proceedings from the Forty-seventh Annual Meeting of the American Cleft Palate-Craniofacial Association, St. Louis, 1990.
64. Wunderer S: Die prognathieoperation mittels frontal gestielthem Maxillafragment, Oster Z Stomatol 59:98, 1962.

CHAPTER 10

Use of Hyperbaric Oxygen Therapy By Plastic Surgeons

Eric P. Kindwall
Lawrence J. Gottlieb

Since the early 1980s, the number of hospitals providing access to hyperbaric oxygenation facilities has increased steadily. More recently this growth has accelerated to over 30 new units each year. Some plastic surgeons have acquired their own chambers for adjunctive use with problem patients. For this reason, the American Society of Plastic and Reconstructive Surgeons (ASPRS) has included an instructional course on hyperbaric oxygen therapy at its annual meeting since 1989. In this chapter, hyperbaric oxygenation (HBO) refers to treatment in which the entire patient is placed in a chamber and breathes oxygen at increased atmospheric pressure. Treatment in which a limb is encased in a plastic bag or container with oxygen applied locally is sometimes confusingly referred to as hyperbaric therapy but is better termed *topical oxygen therapy* and has little physiological relation to HBO.

The hyperbaric oxygen chamber was first used for nondiving diseases in 1956 when Boerema, a Dutch cardiovascular surgeon, began using it intraoperatively in cardiac and vascular surgery. He and other investigators found that major vessels could be occluded for significantly longer periods and that certain cardiac repairs could be made if the procedures were performed in a large pressurized operating room.[6,57]

Boerema and his colleagues also carried out an experiment that graphically demonstrated the ability of HBO to deliver significant amounts of metabolic oxygen. They exsanguinated a pig that was breathing oxygen in the chamber at pressure and replaced the pig's blood with plasma. The oxygen physically dissolved in the plasma (6.4 volumes %) supported all of the pig's metabolic needs in the total absence of hemoglobin. The pig's own blood was subsequently retransfused, and the pig was decompressed without ill effect.[7] With the introduction of heart-lung machines, improved by-

pass techniques, and intraoperative hypothermia, however, the need to perform surgery in the chamber is rarely necessary. By the late 1960s, most of the surgical investigators had left the field, and many large operating room chambers were closed or dismantled.

For some years afterward relatively little good scientific research was carried out, and there were exaggerated claims by some hyperbaric enthusiasts that could not be substantiated. There was no regulation of hyperbaric chamber treatment, and no recognized medical specialty took responsibility for it. The usefulness of HBO therapy was touted far beyond what could be physiologically validated. Alarmed by these developments, the Undersea Medical Society (UMS), a 2000-member group of physicians and physiologists interested in the problems of deep sea diving, created a Committee on Hyperbaric Oxygenation in 1976. Its purpose was to investigate and define any valid indications for HBO therapy and to provide insurance companies with guidelines regarding diseases that should be legitimately reimbursed. This committee critically examined some 64 different disorders and found that many of them had no scientific basis for the application of HBO.[39] During its review, the committee consulted with the Health Care Finances Administration and the National Blue Cross/Blue Shield Association to determine their needs. They had received many claims for reimbursement for HBO therapy and had no criteria by which to judge their validity. The resulting committee report was adopted by the National Blue Cross/Blue Shield Association for use as a source document in determining reimbursement. Since that time the report has been updated approximately every 2 years. The current report lists only 11 disorders for which HBO therapy is approved for reimbursement (see box on p. 160).[45]

Disorders Currently Approved for HBO Therapy by the UHMS

1. Air or gas embolism
2. Carbon monoxide poisoning and smoke inhalation
3. Clostridial myonecrosis
4. Crush injury, compartment syndrome, and other acute traumatic ischemias
5. Decompression sickness
6. Enhancement of healing in selected problem wounds
7. Exceptional blood loss anemia
8. Necrotizing soft tissue infections
9. Osteomyelitis (refractory)
10. Radiation tissue damage
11. Skin grafts and flaps (compromised)
12. Thermal burns

When the report was first issued in 1977, there were only 37 clinical hyperbaric chambers operating in the United States. Today there are nearly 300.[19] As a reflection of this growth, in 1986 the UMS was renamed the Undersea and Hyperbaric Medical Society (UHMS).

Since 1977 an increasing number of articles have appeared in the peer-reviewed literature supporting the limited use of hyperbaric oxygen as an adjunctive tool for the plastic surgeon. This chapter will outline those uses of HBO of most interest to the plastic surgeon, as well as a description of the equipment used and the typical treatment protocols.

BASIC MECHANISMS OF ACTION

The therapeutic effects of hyperbaric oxygen are twofold: a purely mechanical effect and the effect of an elevated partial pressure of oxygen in the tissues. There is no other physiological basis for HBO treatment.

The mechanical effects are limited to the reduction in size of closed, gas containing spaces within the body. In this case, the therapeutic effect would be limited to the compression of gas bubbles within the body, primarily the vascular tree in cases of air embolism and decompression sickness, which obviously have important applications in diving but are also important to the surgeon dealing with air embolism. Iatrogenic air embolism stemming from the use of extracorporeal pump oxygenators, kidney dialysis, cardiac catheterization, lung biopsy, and detached central lines contribute most of the medically related etiologies. If the gas-containing cavity within the body is a normal structure, with its communication to the outside blocked, such as the sinuses or middle ear, increasing the pressure surrounding the patient causes barotrauma and may complicate HBO therapy. Clearing the middle ear is the most commonly encountered problem in treatment.

Boyle's law

Changes in gas volume are in accordance with Boyle's law, which states that the volume of a gas is inversely proportional to the pressure exerted on it. Doubling the absolute pressure halves the volume, while increasing the pressure by a factor of 4 reduces volume to one fourth of its original state. It is easily seen that the greatest reduction of volume occurs during the application of the first additional atmosphere of pressure (the volume is halved). Increasing pressure from 6 to 7 atmospheres further reduces volume from 16.7% to 14.3% of its original state. The practical point here is that the first few pounds of pressure produce the greatest change in volume and cause the patient the most trouble in equalizing pressure in the ears and sinuses.

Elevated oxygen pressure

The chamber's ability to raise oxygen tensions in tissue is most important to the plastic surgeon. Oxygen breathed at 2 atmospheres pressure results in an approximate 20% decrease in blood flow to forearm muscle,[5] as measured by plethysmography. However, this is more than compensated by the increased oxygen tension in that tissue, which may reach 250 to 300 mm of mercury when HBO is applied. Wounds heal as a function of the oxygen tension available in tissue, not the quantity. Gram for gram, a healing wound uses only about one tenth of the oxygen required by brain tissue.

Normal tissue pO_2's are 30 to 40 mm of mercury, but in ischemia caused by infection, trauma, or edema, oxygen levels fall much lower. Below 30 mm of mercury, fibroblast and leukocyte function are severely compromised. Although hypoxia (15 mm Hg) is optimal for stimulation of capillary budding, the increase in collagen formation afforded by HBO permits more rapid capillary growth and arcading by providing the necessary matrix for capillary support. The necessary hypoxia is present between HBO treatments. Lactate also serves as a strong stimulus to capillary growth, even in the presence of high oxygen tensions. HBO therapy enables fibroblast replication, collagen formation, and increased bacteriocidal function of leukocytes to take place while the patient is in the chamber. Concomitant stimulation of neovascularization is important in providing a long-term increase in tissue pO_2. These effects will be discussed in more detail as individual indications are considered.

CONTRAINDICATIONS

HBO as with any other modality, has contraindications and side effects. Untreated pneumothorax is an absolute contraindication as is concurrent therapy with doxorubicin (Adriamycin),[92] cis-platinum,[60], and disulfiram (Antabuse).[31] Topical Sulfamylon (mafenide) should also not be used in conjunction with HBO.

Doxorubicin has been shown to produce a high mortality when combined with HBO in animals and is probably secondary to cardiac toxicity. Cis-platinum given concomitantly with HBO decreases the strength of healing incisions while disulfiram blocks production of superoxide dismutase. SOD protects some tissues against damage from high partial pressures of oxygen. Sulfamylon is a carbonic anhydrase inhibitor, which causes a peripheral vasodilatation. When combined with the central vasoconstriction produced by HBO, the results are worse than when either is used alone. Relative contraindications include the following:

1. Upper respiratory infections, which make clearing the ears and sinuses difficult.
2. Low seizure threshold, which can be mitigated by anticonvulsants.
3. Emphysema with CO_2 retention where breathing is dependent on the stimulus for low arterial pO_2.
4. High fevers, which lower seizure threshold.
5. Congenital spherocytosis, which may provoke hemolysis.

Pregnancy does not appear to be a contraindication.

The Russians treated a large series of gravid females who had habitual spontaneous abortions because of congenital heart disease. Treatment was carried out during all three trimesters, with some babies delivered in the chamber. No retrolental fibroplasia or premature closure of the patent ductus was observed in the several hundred cases treated.

SIDE EFFECTS
Barotrauma

Barotrauma to the middle ear is the most common problem. It is similar to the discomfort experienced on a commercial aircraft when landing. It is eased with decongestants and slow pressurization. Pressure equalization tubes are often needed with intubated patients and patients who have postoperative edema of the pharynx. If the patient is only to be treated once, as with carbon monoxide (CO) poisoning, simple myringotomy will suffice if the patient has an absolute ear block.

Oxygen toxicity

Oxygen is toxic under pressure. The two organs most susceptible to toxicity are the brain and lungs. Nearly everyone will experience a grand mal seizure if allowed to continuously breath 100% oxygen for longer than 3 hours at 3 atmospheres absolute (ATA). For this reason, frequent air breathing periods are interposed when giving oxygen at the higher pressures. Two hours of continuous exposure at 2 ATA almost never provokes a seizure in a healthy person. In clinical practice, seizures are rare, resulting in about 1.3 seizures per 10,000 treatment exposures at 2.4 ATA.[16] However, seizures are usually benign, with no long-term sequelae.[21] Pulmonary oxygen toxicity will begin to become manifest after about 6 hours of breathing oxygen at 2 ATA. Since uninterrupted clinical exposures are limited to 2 hours, pulmonary oxygen toxicity has never been a clinical problem. If a patient requires an FIO_2 of greater than 40% when not in the chamber, particular care must be taken to monitor for early signs of pulmonary oxygen toxicity.

Temporary refractive changes

Some older patients receiving more than 20 HBO treatments will experience a temporary change in the refractive power of the lens, making focusing on distant objects difficult. Conversely, the ability to read without glasses improves. These effects usually disappear within 6 weeks after treatment cessation.[16]

Cataracts

Patients with cataracts may experience earlier maturation of the cataracts after many treatments. *De novo* production of cataracts, using the clinical regimens employed in the United States, has not been reported, although Swedish investigators have reported it in elderly patients receiving more than 500 treatments.

TYPES OF HYPERBARIC CHAMBERS

There are two general types of hyperbaric chambers available: Class A, or multiplace chambers, and Class B, monoplace chambers.

Multiplace chamber

Multiplace chambers can accommodate two or more persons, including an inside attendant (Fig. 10-1). They range from 4 to 12 feet in diameter and between 8 and 40 feet in length. Most clinical chambers have at least two locks or compartments so that personnel can be locked in or out while the patient is under treatment, without altering the treatment compartment pressure. Recompression chambers, traditionally used by divers, have been provided with circular doors, which are lighter and less expensive. For clinical

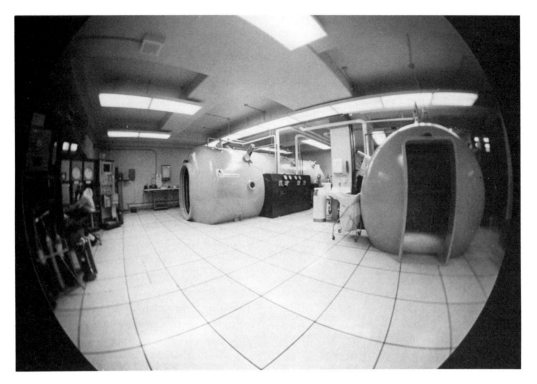

Fig. 10-1 Multiplace hyperbaric chambers are capable of 7 ATA. Note the rectangular door on the chamber to the right, allowing easy entry of gurneys. These are so-called double-lock chambers, each having two compartments so that personnel may enter and leave the inner compartment while the patient is at pressure. Courtesy St. Luke's Medical Center, Milwaukee.

work, however, most chambers are equipped with rectangular doors, which allow patients to be rolled in or out on gurneys or in wheel chairs. These chambers are pressurized with compressed air, but the patient breathes 100% oxygen from a mask, head tent, or endotracheal tube. Although rarely necessary, most multiplace chambers have a 6 ATA pressure capability, which is equal to a pressure of 165 feet of sea water. These chambers are usually equipped with small pass-through locks through which drugs, intravenous (IV) supplies, and similar equipment may be passed. Multiplace chambers require a separate room for air compressors, volume tanks, and fire suppression equipment. Some large chambers, which may hold 18 to 24 patients, are quite sophisticated with airconditioning and computerized atmosphere and depth control.

The primary advantage of the multiplace chamber is that patients with multiple IVs and monitoring leads may be wheeled directly into the chamber with life support functions still connected. This allows hands-on treatment at pressure in the chamber such as tracheal suctioning, starting IV's, performing serial neurologic examinations, and even defibrillation. Disadvantages in-

clude its high cost, the extra space required for compressors and volume tanks, and the fact that at least two people, the chamber operator and inside attendant, are required for its operation. Multiplace chambers become cost effective when treating 10 or more patients per day. Certain level I trauma centers and academic institutions may find the multiplace chamber advantageous, however, even if fewer patients per day are treated. This is particularly true if one anticipates treating mass casualties such as with CO poisoning and diving accidents involving several people. Critical care with its attendant multiple IV lines and monitoring is also much easier in the walk-in chamber. In 1990 the cost of a multiplace chamber with ancillary equipment ranged from about $150,000 for a relatively small, primitive chamber with a circular door to $2 million or more for a sophisticated system.

Monoplace chamber

Monoplace chambers only accommodate one individual (Fig. 10-2). The patient lies on a wheeled stretcher, which slides on rails into the chamber. Monoplace chambers typically are about 25 inches in

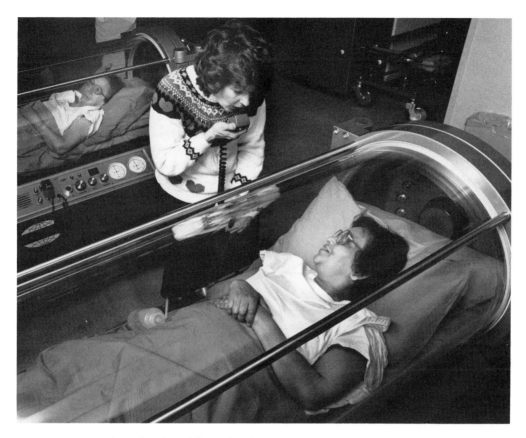

Fig. 10-2 Monoplace chambers. These chambers are pressurized with pure oxygen, and the patients do not wear masks. Patients can continue to receive IV therapy in this chamber. The apneic patient can be ventilated with a ventilator that fits inside the door. Courtesy Giovanni Orlando.

internal diameter and 7 feet long and are usually made of a clear acrylic plastic. These chambers are pressurized with pure oxygen taken directly from the hospital's standard oxygen source. It is also useful to have medical oxygen available to pressurize the chamber for training purposes. The maximum pressure attainable in most monoplace chambers is only 3 ATA, equivalent to 66 feet of seawater. For reasons of oxygen toxicity, this is the maximum pressure at which 100% oxygen can be safely breathed. Compressors, volume tanks, special fire suppression equipment, and a separate control panel are not required. Monoplace chambers can be installed in an existing patient room and operated by one attendant. Since the atmosphere in the chamber is 100% oxygen, the patient is not required to wear a mask or hood, unlike the multiplace chamber. Despite the apparent isolation of the patient in the monoplace chamber, critically ill patients requiring extensive life support equipment can be treated with this unit. Modified IV pumps deliver continuous infusions of fluids through penetrators in the chamber door. A specially designed ventilator is controlled from the outside and

can ventilate the apneic patient, although it is time and flow cycled, not volume cycled. The ECG, arterial pressure, central venous pressure, and temperature are monitored from leads and transducers within the chamber through multi-pin electrical plugs in the chamber hull. These are then displayed on standard monitors outside. Should the patient need bolus injection of a drug, it is delivered via a three-way stopcock in the IV line and pumped in using the infusion pump. In an emergency, the patient can be decompressed to the surface in less than 1 minute without any risk of decompression sickness, or the "bends," since the patient is breathing 100% oxygen. Even if cardiac arrest occurs while the patient is at pressure, there is little danger of immediate hypoxic damage, since arterial pO_2's in the patient breathing hyperbaric oxygen usually range between 1,200 and 1,800 mm Hg.

Advantages of the monoplace chamber are its relatively low cost, small space requirements, one person operation, rapid and easy installation, and no requirement for a patient mask. This is particularly useful when treating small children. The disadvantage is that multiple IV lines and life support connections must be disconnected and then reconnected through the chamber hull as the patient is placed in the chamber. Obviously, hands-on care, such as suctioning, cannot be given during treatment. An additional disadvantage is that about 10% of the patients may refuse treatment because of claustrophobia, although in some cases this can be obviated with appropriate sedation. Nearly 90% of all patients requiring HBO can be treated in monoplace chambers. The cost of installing a monoplace chamber was $115,000 in 1990, which includes the chamber cost, external monitoring gear, and the usually required ancillary equipment. Although the 100% oxygen atmosphere in the monoplace chamber presents a potential fire hazard, there has never been a fire involving a patient in the western hemisphere.

DISORDERS TREATED WITH HBO
Air embolism

When plastic surgeons operate in the neck region, air embolism is possible. Regardless of etiology, prompt recompression in the hyperbaric chamber is the only acceptable primary therapy for intra-arterial or symptomatic intravenous gas bubbles. Large amounts of gas can cause cardiac or pulmonary embarrassment, but the most common manifestations are cerebral symptoms and signs following even tiny amounts of intra-arterial air. The air can be directly or indirectly introduced into the arterial side during cardiopulmonary bypass as a result of hemodialysis or central vein catheterization and during certain neurosurgical procedures and percutaneous needle biopsy of the lung. Pulmonary overpressurization accidents (POA) occurring during scuba diving or other exposure to compressed air (e.g., escape from a submerged vehicle) can also be causal. Finally, air blown into the vagina of a pregnant woman during sex play or illegal abortion, when air is injected into the uterus, can cause fatal gas embolism. The final common pathway is intra-arterial gas, most commonly delivered to the brain. Recompression treatment is the same regardless of the cause.

Iatrogenic air embolism
Surgery

The majority of neurological deficits after open heart surgery, thoracic surgery, or other surgical procedures involving the great vessels or vessels of the neck are due to solid emboli, thrombosis, or anesthetic accidents. A small percentage of neurological problems can be attributed to the introduction of air into the vessels. If air is introduced intraarterially, the result is frequently cerebral air embolism. As little as 0.4 ml of blood-air foam delivered to the right place in the me-

dulla can be fatal. In cases where there is suspicion that air has been introduced into the circulation, an immediate trial of recompression is indicated. Therefore good clinical judgment is important, since it is not feasible to recompress every patient who exhibits neurological deficit after surgery. Stoney estimated that approximately 1 in a 1000 open heart cases produces air embolism.[82] There is a 33% fatality rate in those afflicted. Survivors usually have severe neurological deficit, if left untreated. Cerebral air embolism has also been reported after percutaneous needle biopsy of the lung. Typically in these cases, the patient suddenly loses consciousness during the procedure and may suffer seizures or a strokelike syndrome. It has also been reported in connection with hemodialysis. In these latter cases, if air is introduced intravenously, cerebral symptoms result if there is a right-to-left shunt, either though the heart or the lung. When this occurs, it is called a paradoxical embolism.

Gynecological manipulation

Occasionally, after intrauterine instrumentation, (usually an attempted self-induced abortion, especially if a catheter is used), the patient may exhibit the sudden onset of severe neurological signs and symptoms, often sudden convulsions, altered mental status, or coma. The usual working diagnosis in these patients in intracranial hemorrhage. If intravenous air reaches the cerebral circulation, it is a paradoxical air embolism, and the factor responsible is a functional intracardiac right-to-left shunt or a pulmonary shunt. Pulmonary venous air will pass into the arterial side if given in sufficient volume.

Air embolism has been reported on several occasions secondary to the insufflation of air into the vagina during sex play in pregnancy. In the pregnant patient, the vagina is quite distensible, permitting the introduction of up to 2 liters of air. The air passes through the soft, patent cervical os and dissects between the placenta and uterine wall. It is carried into the uterine veins and reaches the arterial circulation, either through intracardiac or pulmonary shunt. The history of the problem is understandably difficult to obtain, but detailed information is necessary to clarify the diagnosis.

Treatment

After ensuring an adequate airway and circulation, it is advisable to place the patient in a steep Trendelenburg's position immediately after diagnosis, for no longer than 15 minutes, regardless of the cause.[2] The hydrostatic forces generated in the exaggerated head-down position (30 to 60 degrees) tend to dilate the cerebral vasculature, both arterial and venous, and enable bubbles to pass through the capillaries more freely.

Avoid prolonging the head-down position because cerebral edema is worsened.[17] If the patient becomes asymptomatic, return to the horizontal position sooner, but the head should not be permitted to rise above the heart level. Sitting the embolism patient upright after apparent complete recovery has occasionally caused severe and sudden recurrence of signs and symptoms, which were completely resistant to subsequent recompression therapy and thus sometimes fatal. Regardless of prompt recovery, the patient should be referred for recompression therapy. Lidocaine, given in antidysrhythmic doses, has been found to ameliorate the damage caused by intravascular air.[55]

Low pressure oxygen therapy of air embolism

Recent animal studies carried out by Leitch, Greenbaum, and Hallenbeck have shown no advantage in recompressing to 165 feet of seawater (fsw) (6 ATA) breathing air, as compared with oxygen recompression to 60 (fsw) (2.8 ATA).[42] In addition, they found that once the threshold pressure of 2.8 ATA had been reached, further compression, even to depths greatly in excess of 6 ATA, did not improve cerebral blood flow as demonstrated by autoradiography. Their research also indicated that maximal bubble reduction and restoration of blood flow occurs within 8 minutes at maximum depth. Further prolongation of the time at 60 feet or greater has no effect on blood flow. Air breathing at 165 feet was found to produce a rise in intracranial pressure that remained high 90 minutes later. Oxygen-treated animals did not experience this pressure rise. Secondary embolization of the spinal cord with nitrogen emboli were also a consequence of air breathing at 165 fsw. There was no difference in the cortical evoked potentials in dogs treated at 60 fsw with oxygen compared with those treated with air at 6 ATA. Using 100% oxygen at a pressure no greater than 60 fsw (2.8 ATA) would appear to be optimal treatment, however, it must be pointed out that this work has not been substantiated in humans nor has oxygen treatment been compared with the use of 50% nitrogen/oxygen or helium/oxygen at 6 ATA.

Nevertheless, these studies have profound significance in the rationale for treating air embolism in the 3 ATA monoplace chamber, since transfer to a multiplace facility would delay treatment. Standard treatment options are explained in Table 10-1, which is now the standard multiplace treatment for air embolism and should be used for medico-legal reasons if a 6 ATA chamber is available.

Table 10-2, developed by Hart at Long Beach Memorial Hospital, may be used if a multiplace or monoplace chamber equipped with a mask for air breaks is not available. Repetitive treatment may be given if

Table 10-1

U.S. Navy Air Embolism Treatment Table[93]

Depth (ft)	Time (min)	Breathing media	Total time (min)
165	30	Air or 50% O_2-50% N_2	30
165-60	4	Air	34
60	20	Oxygen	54
60	5	Air	59
60	20	Oxygen	79
60	5	Air	84
60	20	Oxygen	104
60	5	Air	109
60-30	30	Oxygen	139
30	15	Air	154
30	60	Oxygen	214
30	15	Air	229
30	60	Oxygen	289
30-0	30	Oxygen	319

Table 10-2

Treatment Protocol Using the Monoplace Chamber[29]

Depth (ft)	Time (min)	Breathing media	Total time
66 (3 ATA)	30	Oxygen	30
50 (2.5 ATA)	60	Oxygen	90

symptoms are not completely resolved after the initial treatment. Repetitive treatment is at 2.5 ATA for 90 minutes every 8 hours for the first 24 hours, then 2.5 ATA for 90 minutes once or twice a day until symptoms are resolved or no further improvement occurs.

Burn injury

In 1988 the Committee on Hyperbaric Oxygenation of the UHMS removed *thermal burn* from a special considerations category and recommended that HBO treatment of patients with thermal burn be reimbursed by third party carriers. However, the UHMS requires that the burn patient be treated in a recognized burn-care facility according to a strict protocol.[45]

The rationale for using HBO in thermal burns is that it can maintain microvascular integrity, minimize edema, and provide the oxygen necessary to maintain tissue viability. The mechanisms include the preservation of ATP in cell membranes, as first demonstrated by Nylander and later confirmed by Yamaguchi et al,[97] who also confirmed higher levels of hydroxyproline in the healing tissues of HBO-treated animal burns.

HBO minimizes the progression of capillary occlusion, which may spread from the initial zone of coagulation by a factor of 10 during the first 2 days after injury. Edema also develops in uninjured tissue remote from the burn area; red cell aggregation and platelet thromboemboli occur. HBO decreases the inflammatory response while significantly improving blood flow in the microvasculature.[9] Controlled animal studies have shown a reduction of 30% in the extravasation of fluid in the first 24 hours with HBO treatment. HBO also reduces the generalized edema that occurs in a burn.[67] ATP levels are preserved in areas immediately below partial-thickness burn injury when HBO is used. Biopsies of burned animals have shown progression to full-thickness injury in controls while there is preservation of capillary patency and dermal elements in hyperbarically treated animals.[80,81] Although HBO does not change the bacterial flora of the burn, evidence suggests that candidal and streptococcal species are inhibited and less likely to cause infection.[30,38]

In the largest study carried out to date, Niu et al,[66] in a naval hospital in Taiwan, found that in patients with 35% to 75% total body surface (TBS) burn, 6.8% of the 117 cases in the HBO group died, compared with 14.8% of the 169 cases in the control group (p,0.028). The difference in mortality was not statistically different in less severely burned patients. They also noted that fluid resuscitation was achieved more rapidly, nasogastric feeding was initiated within the second 24 hours, and there was an acceleration of reepithelialization. The average number of hospital days was 47 in the HBO-treated group and 59 days in the control group. However, this difference was not statistically significant ($p > 0.05$). In a small control study in humans, Hart found that using a two-way (air versus oxygen, percent burn) factorial analysis of variance, the mean healing time in the control group was 43.8 days, compared with 19.7 days for the patients treated with HBO ($p < .005$).[30]

More recently, Cianci et al have reported that adjunctive HBO therapy reduced the mean length of hospitalization in patients with 18% to 39% TBS burns from 33 to 20.8 days (p, 0.012). In that study, the average cost savings per case when HBO was used was $10,850. Average HBO cost was $8,200, which was included in the total hospital charge.[13] This study was quite small, however, comprising only 16 patients.

Cianci et al also looked into the effect of HBO on the number of surgeries required in burn treatment. In patients with 40% to 80% TBS burns, matched for age, percentage, and thickness, the number of required surgeries fell from 8 to 3.7 when HBO was used (p, 0.041).[12]

In a negative clinical study by Waisbren et al, in which HBO treatment of severe burns failed to reveal either a deleterious or salutary effect on mortality, grafting was reduced by 75% in the hyperbarically treated group ($p < 0.01$).[95] They cited renal toxicity as a problem with HBO therapy, although it has not been reported by any other authors studying burn injuries, and has never been a problem with HBO treatment of any other clinical entity. Patients in the Waisbren study, however, were known to have received significant quantities of nephrotoxic antibiotics.

It is important for anyone undertaking adjunctive HBO treatment of burn patients to follow the protocols used by Hart or Cianci.[13,30]

Treatment

Treatment is usually at 2 ATA for 90 minutes twice a day, excluding the descent and ascent time.[30] This schedule was derived empirically. HBO treatment should not imediately follow burn baths, since it is extremely important to avoid chilling the patient, especially children. Be alert for oxygen toxicity if the patient receives oxygen between HBO treatments.

Crush injury and compartment syndrome

Crush injury can produce severe traumatic ischemia that compromises both limb soft tissue and circulation. The entire extremity or portions of it may undergo necrosis or require amputation. When the blood supply has been compromised, nonunions are common and are frequently associated with infection. After severe crush injury and compartment syndrome, ischemia may be due to either large vessel disruption or compromise of the microcirculation.

In case of low-tissue perfusion, hyperbaric oxygen can often maintain tissue oxygen tensions at a level that will support tissue viability. The goal is to prevent tissue oxygen tension from falling below 30 mm of mercury, at which level, effective microbial killing and fibroblast function cease.[34,59] At 2 ATA the plasma and tissue oxygen tensions are increased tenfold (i.e., 1000%). Wounds heal as a function of the oxygen tension.[23] Under hyperbaric conditions, enough oxygen is physically dissolved in the plasma to keep tissues alive despite inadequate hemoglobin borne oxygen. With increased oxygen tension, the effective diffusion distance of oxygen through tissue fluids is increased by a factor of three.[40,69] Thus compromised cells normally served by capillaries that have become blocked because of sludging or edema can be maintained by capillaries at three times the distance from the cells in question.

Edema reduction is another major effect of HBO. One of the mechanisms first described by Nylander et al[68] is the preservation by HBO of adenosine triphosphate (ATP) in the cell membrane, which allows the cell to control its osmolarity and lessens the tendency of injured tissue to shift fluid interstitially.

Strauss has shown that when a compartment syndrome is induced in the hindlimb muscles of dogs, necrosis was markedly reduced when the animals were subsequently treated with hyperbaric oxygen.[86] This was a controlled study that involved raising compartment pressure to 100 mm Hg for up to 8 hours. Technitium 99 uptake was used as an indicator of muscle necrosis. No necrosis was seen in the treated group until compartment pressure had exceeded 60 mm of mercury, but at that pressure the controls took up more than twice the technitium of normal tissue. At 100 mm Hg the necrosis in the HBO-treated group was 36% of that seen in the control animals.

The recommended treatment schedule for crush injury is three 90-minute treatments per day for the first 2 days, followed by two treatments daily for the third and fourth days, and one treatment daily for the fifth and sixth days.[83] The problem is usually resolved by the sixth day.

The concept of *warm ischemic time* is as important here as in replant surgery. If the crushed tissues are allowed to become increasingly edematous for more than 8 hours, the chances of achieving a desirable result with HBO decreases. When a patient with a severe crush injury is admitted, and the required surgery must be delayed, consideration should be given to treating the patient in the hyperbaric chamber in the interim. Treatment can then be resumed immediately after surgery. The results of HBO are often degraded by the necessarily long time (> 8 hours) that some of these patients must remain in surgery.

Increasing evidence points to reperfusion injury as a cause of tissue damage and necrosis after ischemia. Free radical formation plays a major role[22,32], triggering lipid peroxidation. Raskin et al[71] have shown that HBO can inhibit peroxidation in vitro in lung homogenate. Thom has reported that the mechanism for this effect involves the occurrence of a new termination reaction between hydroperoxyl radicals and organic radicals stabilized by π bond-charge transfer complexes with monosaturated fatty acids.[90]

Further evidence that oxygen-derived free radicals have an important effect on flaps and grafts is provided by Kaelin et al,[37] who found that treatment of free flaps with exogenous superoxide dismutase (SOD), a free-radical scavenger, increased the survival rate of normothermically stored flaps from 32% to 76%. HBO raised the survival rate of free flaps stored for 21 hours from 10% to 67%. We also have assayed SOD in split-thickness skin harvested from HBO-treated animals and have found that HBO treatment significantly increases SOD activity.

The effect of HBO on reperfusion injury has also been studied by Zamboni et al using a rat epigastric axial-pattern-flap ischemia model.[98] They found that acute HBO treatment, when administered immediately after 8 hours of global ischemia, significantly improved flap survival in animals. This effect was opposite Zamboni et al's original hypothesis that HBO therapy would exacerbate reperfusion injury by increasing oxygen-derived free radical formation. Zamboni et al also used laser Doppler flow measurement to show a significant increase in the microvascular blood flow of flaps treated both before and during reperfusion, compared with ischemic controls.[100] The mechanism for this protective effect from reperfusion injury afforded by HBO may lie in the modification of neutrophil action on the microvascular endothelium. Zamboni et al used a rat gracilus muscle intravital microscopic preparation to demonstrate that HBO treatment significantly reduced leukocyte endothelial adherence in postcapillary microvenules and inhibited the progressive microarteriolar vasoconstriction that occurs during reperfusion of ischemic skeletal muscle.[99]

Grim et al have demonstrated that HBO does not increase oxidative stress as measured by H_2O_2 determinations in the expired breath of critically ill burn patients.[26]

In a recent report, it was found that when HBO was used to arrest the progression of a skeletal muscle compartment syndrome and to obviate the need for surgical decompression, the estimated cost of management was one fourth that of patients who had their compartment syndromes surgically decompressed.[85] Although the addition of HBO to the management of a patient with crush injury may add up to $3,000 in medical expenses, this is a small fraction of the cost incurred with the potential limb-threatening complications of acute traumatic ischemia, and the overall costs are reportedly lower.

Ischemic and other problem wounds

Another area where HBO may be of value in selected patients is in the management of ischemic wounds of the lower extremity in older diabetics and the preparation of large decubiti for flap coverage. HBO enhances microbial killing by leukocytes, allowing infected and grossly purulent open wounds to be more rapidly cleaned and a good bed of granulation tissue generated in preparation for flap rotation.

Diabetic ulcers of the lower extremity pose a special problem in that a careful work-up is needed to determine whether a patient will benefit from HBO therapy. The simple appearance of the wound is *not* a useful prognostic guide. Doppler studies or angiography must first be carried out to determine if the patient has sufficient large vessel patency. A low ankle to brachial blood pressure ratio (ischemic index) signifies little chance of healing, even with HBO. If the Doppler ankle pressure is less than 75 mm Hg in a diabetic, healing is unlikely even with HBO. Before such a patient is accepted for treatment, bypass grafting or angioplasty will be required. Transcutaneous (TC) po_2 measurements are also a useful adjunct in evaluating these patients[74] (see p. 172 on TC po_2 monitoring). Those patients who did not benefit from HBO had a transcutaneous po_2 measurement of less than 30 mm of mercury when breathing air at 1 ATA.[76] Sometimes more important than the actual po_2 measurement, is a trend shown by the TC po_2. If, with HBO treatment, the TC po_2 is seen to rise consistently when measured before treatment over a 2-week period, one has presumptive documentation that microvasculature is improving. Often TC po_2 increases will be seen before clinical improvement becomes manifest. Typically, there is approximately a 2 week latency period before apparent granulation begins.[87] Infection should be controlled during this time, however. By following the TC po_2 serially during treatment, it will often be seen to rise and plateau for a week or more and then experience another rise. Periodic and intermittent increases in the TC po_2 has been documented by Sheffield et al at the School of Aerospace Medicine, USAF in San Antonio, Texas.[75]

The Committee on Hyperbaric Oxygenation of the Undersea and Hyperbaric Medical Society has adopted the Wagner classification to determine the degree of compromise in the diabetic foot.[94] Wagner Grade I lesions are superficial without penetration to deep layers. Usually, there is no indication for HBO treatment in these lesions. Grade II involves deeper ulceration that reaches tendon, bone, or joint capsule. Again, HBO may not be cost effective or necessary in this situation. However, with Grade III lesions where deeper tissues are involved and gross infection such as osteomyelitis, plantar space abscess, and/or tendonitis is present, HBO may be indicated as an adjunct. Initial and continuing debridement must not be neglected. Grade IV lesions are a near end-stage situation where there is gangrene of some portions of the toe and/or forefoot. The gangrene may be wet or dry, infected or noninfected, but in general, surgical ablation of a portion of the toe or foot is indicated. Adjunctive HBO may contribute in such cases by preserving bipedal ambulation. In Wagner Grade V, gangrene involves the whole foot or enough of the foot so that no local procedures are possible and amputation must be carried out to at least below knee level. It must be emphasized that HBO is only an adjunct and does not relieve the surgeon of aggressively managing these ulcers. One must be certain to debride all osteomyelitis, be it the os calcis or a metatarsal head. If the ulcer extends into a joint, the synovium or joint must be removed.

Baroni et al[3] reported a small series of 18 hospitalized diabetic patients with gangrene who were treated with HBO and compared them with 10, closely matched controls. In the control group, only one patient improved. Five out of 10 showed no change and 4 of 10 worsened until amputation was necessary. In the treated group, 16 out of 18 patients healed ($p,.001$). This was not a random study, however, since the controls were patients who refused HBO because of claustrophobia.

Cianci et al showed that in 39 patients with problem wounds of the lower extremity and/or limb threatening lesions, adjunctive HBO therapy combined with carefully coordinated medical and surgical care resulted in a 92% overall salvage rate.[11] The average hospital stay was 30 days and the average number of HBO treatments was 31. In this series, there was a 7-day average delay before initiation of HBO therapy. Patients averaged 25 days of HBO treatments costing $10,368 per case, with total hospital charges of $29,709 per case. These costs compare quite favorably with the cost of acute amputation, which is reported to be $26,000 to $45,000.[43,44]

Cianci points out that when additional expenditures for rehabilitation after amputation are examined, the program is extremely cost effective. Using financial data from the state of California, he showed that the total cost of rehabilitation approaches $40,000, making the total cost of amputation and rehabilitation in the range of $50,000 to $70,000.

Treatment

Treatment usually consists of exposure once a day at 2 or 2.4 ATA for 90 to 120 minutes. Initially, if the ulcers are heavily infected, treatment twice a day is sometimes given empirically.

Necrotizing fasciitis

Because of edema formation and other factors, infected tissue is usually hypoxic.[78] Sonoda et al[79] have shown that when there is extensive necrosis accompanying the infection, an occlusive endarteritis occurs. This may be the reason that necrotizing soft tissue infections are so severe.

In a hypoxic setting the polymorphonuclear leukocytes lose their ability to effectively kill bacteria, provoking a vicious cycle. Mortality averages approximately 38% in reported series and the risk is directly related to a delay in diagnosis.[89] Older patients are particularly at risk. The disease is much worse when it occurs on the trunk as opposed to the extremity. Cure of this disorder has always hinged on early diagnosis and wide surgical debridement of the infected area, along with IV antibiotic therapy.

HBO has frequently been used as an adjunct when surgery and antibiotics appear to be failing.[72,101] Use of

HBO seemed rational when an increased white cell response was required. Although most reports of HBO use have been anecdotal, Riseman et al.[73] recently described 29 patients with necrotizing fasciitis, 12 of whom received surgical debridement and antibiotics only, while the remaining 17 received adjunctive HBO in addition to debridement, surgery, and antibiotics. Both groups were similar in age, race, sex, wound bacteriology, and antibiotic regimen. The hyperbaric group was sicker, however, having more perineal involvement (53% versus 12%) and 29% of the HBO group were in shock on admission as opposed to 8% of the control group. Additionally, 47% of the HBO group were diabetic compared with only 33% of the control group. Nevertheless, mortality was 23% in the HBO group and 66% in the control group (p < 0.02). A parallel finding was that an average of only 1.2 debridements were required in the HBO group to achieve wound control versus 3.3 debridements in the control group (*p* < 0.03). Based on the results of this study, Riseman recommends the routine use of adjunctive HBO in treating necrotizing fasciitis. A serious weakness of this study, however, was that it was retrospective, not prospective. It spanned an 8-year period, and the HBO patients and controls were not randomized, since they were not treated concomitantly. Although the surgeons were varied, the infectious disease consultant was the same.

Treatment

The patients are treated at 2.5 ATA for 90 minutes at least twice a day. In Riseman's series the average number of treatments was 7.4.

Refractory osteomyelitis

The plastic surgeon is occasionally called to assist the orthopedist in eradicating chronic refractory osteomyelitis by introducing a vascularized flap into the debrided area. Experience has shown that with improved blood supply, previously refractory infections can often be halted.[54,96] In some cases, it may be worth considering adjunctive HBO in conjunction with flaps, free tissue transfer, or bone grafts.

Controlled animal studies have clearly suggested the benefit of adjunctive HBO in chronic osteomyelitis.[28,46,48,58,91] The mechanism of its action involves raising the decreased oxygen tensions found in infected bone back to normal or above normal levels presuming there is some perfusion. Infected bone may have oxygen tensions ranging from 0 to 15 mm Hg.[47,65] White blood cells require at least 30 mm Hg to be bacteriocidal,[33] while most normal tissue po_2 ranges between 30 to 40 mm of mercury. One would expect that leukocyte-killing potential would be optimal within this range. How-

ever, Mader et al[47] has shown in vitro that leukocyte-killing effectiveness can be increased by 40% when the po_2 is raised from 45 mm Hg to 150 mm Hg. Recent evidence suggests that phagocytosis is also enhanced, the effect being maximal after about 10 treatments. Tissue tensions up to 250 mm Hg or greater are possible in healthy tissue when the patient is at 2 ATA in the hyperbaric chamber. Osteoclastic activity is also enhanced, since osteoclasts are nearly 100 times more metabolically active than osteoblasts. As a result, with HBO therapy, dead bone may be more rapidly removed. Care must be taken to avoid refracture during this remodeling phase.[84] Neovascularization of the infected bone is stimulated by HBO, which is perhaps one reason long-term remissions appear to be more common, although no studies have been done in this area to confirm or refute this hypothesis.

In a long-term study, Davis et al[14] showed that 30 of 34 patients with previously refractory osteomyelitis remained disease free at a follow-up interval of 7.5 to 10.5 years. They had been treated with a vigorous combination of antibiotics, surgery, and HBO.

No single mode of therapy has been proved universally successful in the treatment of chronic refractory osteomyelitis, which makes assessing the merits of any single therapy difficult. There have been no properly controlled studies for *any* form of therapy in chronic refractory osteomyelitis in humans. It is for this reason that antibiotics are combined with surgical debridement, revascularization with flaps, and free tissue transfer with HBO.[15] The patient with chronic refractory osteomyelitis incurs an enormous cost over the course of traditional therapy. Strauss has reported on a series of his most complicated cases where before use of HBO and other aspects of the treatment program, an average of $115,000 had already been spent on each patient's care. Some of them had had osteomyelitis for as long as 50 years and had endured up to a dozen surgeries. Strauss's investment, including surgery, HBO, and hospitalization was $20,000 at the time of the study. Thus the cost generated by a management program that included HBO was approximately 20% of what had previously been spent on the patients, and their previous care had not resolved the problem. HBO treatment is expensive, ranging between $15,000 and $30,000 for a course of 60 treatments. However, when one considers the cost of failure, the added cost of HBO treatment is more acceptable.[84]

It must be pointed out, however, that despite the theoretical advantages of HBO and the encouraging clinical experience, the effects of excellent and complete debridement, intensive antibiotic coverage, and expert wound care cannot be separated from the effects of HBO. There are several reports in the literature showing remission rates of 93% or higher in previously refractory cases of osteomyelitis *without* the use of HBO.[18]

Treatment

HBO treatment typically is given twice a day while the patient remains hospitalized and then is continued once a day after the patient is discharged. This treatment schedule is empirical. Although it appears successful, more data are needed relative to dose response. Patients usually receive between 30 and 60 treatments at 2 ATA for 2 hours without an air break or at 2.4 ATA for 95 minutes, including a 5 minute air break after 45 minutes of treatment.

Radionecrosis

Although radiation oncologists have vastly improved their skills in eradicating tumors, the aftereffects of radiation in healthy tissue remain and continue to worsen during the patient's lifetime. In addition to cell death, radiation induces vascular sclerosis and hypoxia, which worsens with time.[35,41,50,52] The only previously available therapy for the breakdown of radiated tissue was excision of the necrotic area and the introduction of fresh, well-vascularized tissue in the form of flaps or free tissue transfer.

HBO, however, as a new therapy, has made possible the treatment of radiated tissue itself.[51] HBO stimulates neovascularization in the radiated area and can permanently raise tissue oxygen tensions to approximately 80% of normal before they plateau.[4,16]

Soft tissue radionecrosis

After approximately 20 to 30 HBO treatments, the previously ischemic tissue may accept grafts. For this reason the use of HBO in a sufficient number of exposures should be considered *before* elective surgery is performed. Whenever the surgeon is required to deal with significantly irradiated tissue the patient is typically treated 20 to 30 times before surgery and then given 10 or more treatments after surgery.

Treatment

Treatment typically is at 2 or 2.4 ATA for 90 to 120 minutes and is usually given once a day except when the surgeon must operate immediately in a radiated area for removal of a recurrent tumor. Although the results will not be as good as before treatment, there should be immediate HBO treatment after surgery. Treatment twice a day may be advisable under such conditions, but this recommendation is only based on empirical evidence.

Osteoradionecrosis

Tooth extraction causes 89% of all trauma-induced radionecrosis of the mandible.

In a randomized prospective study, Marx demonstrated that radionecrosis of the mandible secondary to tooth extraction in patients with an irradiated jaw could be reduced by a factor of 5, when they were pretreated with 20 HBO treatments, followed by 10 treatments after extraction.[53] By avoiding radionecrosis, savings were estimated at $40,000 per patient. Applying this method has reduced failure rates in the treatment of radionecrosis of the mandible from 92% to less than 10%.[16]

Treatment

With established mandibular radionecrosis, patients are categorized into one of the following three stages before treatment begins:

Stage 1

The patient has only 1 or 2 mm of exposed mandible intraorally, and the pannorex shows the body of the mandible to be relatively disease free.

Treatment consists of 2 or 2.4 ATA for 2 hours or 90 minutes, respectively, once a day for 30 treatments. If the wound has not closed or has not shown good signs of closing by that time, the patient is advanced to stage 2. About 15% of patients with osteoradionecrosis will respond to stage 1 treatment.

Stage 2

Failure to heal after 30 HBO treatments. In stage 2 treatment, an alveolar sequestrectomy is performed, removing all dead bone, with a good closure of the mucosa to ensure a water-tight seal. HBO treatment is continued up to 60 treatments. Again, only an additional 15% of patients will experience complete remission of stage 2 disease.

Stage 3

Dehiscence of stage 2; Orocutaneous fistula present; Pathological fracture present; Involvement of the mandible by x-ray throughout its body.

In stage 3 treatment, when there is persistent disease after 30 HBO treatments, the mandible is resected intraorally, back to bleeding bone. Soft tissue deficits are repaired at this time, with flaps or a free-tissue transfer, if necessary. Orocutaneous fistulas are closed, and the mandible is held in position with an external arch bar. HBO is continued after the procedure until all surgical wounds are healed.

Ten weeks after resection, bone grafting of the mandible is performed through a transcutaneous approach. Extreme care must be exercised to avoid even a pinhole penetration into the oral cavity, or infection will destroy the graft.

Various types of bone grafts have been used successfully, but whichever type the surgeon chooses must be in accordance with the criteria that follow:

1. The graft must be of sufficient bulk to supply

the necessary strength for successful mastication.

2. A normal contour to the jaw should be restored.

3. There must be sufficient alveolar height to support dentures.

4. There must be a documented low graft loss rate.

5. Morbidity at the donor site should be minimal.

6. The operative time required for the graft should be as short as possible for these often debilitated, elderly patients.

Vascularized rib and fibula grafts do not supply sufficient strength or bulk. Vascularized iliac bone grafts have been used successfully, but are totally dependent on their single vessel vascular supply.

Marx has achieved more than a 90% success rate using cancellous bone chips from the posterior iliac crest. Cancellous bone is packed copiously (10 ml per linear centimeter) between cribs fashioned from split allogeneic rib, wired superiorly and inferiorly across the gap to be bridged. The surgical technique must be meticulous to ensure success. It is recommended that collaboration be sought with an oral surgeon who has had specific training in this procedure.

HBO therapy is continued for at least 10 treatments to a maximum of 30 after grafting, while the external arch bar is kept in place. The bone graft should heal in about 8 weeks.

To be effective, HBO treatment must be carried out in strict accordance with published protocols, which includes the proper timing of both antibiotics and surgery.

Osteoradionecrosis and other radiation injuries can be extremely painful, disabling conditions. They are potentially fatal if major vessels are eroded. HBO, when combined with reconstructive surgery, can interrupt a long and expensive clinical course with a low incidence of serious complications.[16]

Skin flaps and grafts

The vast majority of skin flaps and grafts do not require HBO therapy. It is not recommended as an adjunct unless there is a significant element of local ischemic compromise or if the patient is a systemically compromised host. HBO can be advantageous when a skin graft is placed in an irradiated field, if there have been multiple previous skin graft failures, or if there is a known decrease in the microcirculation or systemic hypoxia. Numerous animal studies have shown the value of hyperbaric oxygen in enhancing flap and skin graft survival.* It is important that HBO be instituted as early as possible after graft placement.

Champion et al, using a rabbit model, achieved 100% survival in pedicle flaps treated with HBO, compared with areas of necrosis greater than 40% in all controls.[10] Shulman and Krohn found that full and partial thickness wounds in rats had a significantly shorter healing time when treated with HBO. Repeated skin grafting and HBO reduced the healing time of partial thickness wounds to one half that of nontreated controls. Infections were entirely absent in the groups treated with HBO despite the nonsterile conditions used while performing those surgeries.[77] Jurell and Kaijser[36] found that pedicle flaps in HBO-treated rats had significantly greater flap survival compared with controls ($p < 0.001$). The surviving area in the HBO group was approximately twice that of the control group. There was a significantly greater survival area even when HBO was delayed for 24 hours after surgery ($p < 0.01$). The sooner that HBO therapy was begun, however, the greater the increase in the surviving area.

Manson et al[49] used histochemical staining with ATP to visualize small blood vessels in the pedicle flaps of guinea pigs. They were able to demonstrate a threefold increase in the distal growth of capillaries in hyperbarically treated animals when compared with controls. These same authors have shown an increase in flap tissue glucose and a decrease in lactate in HBO-treated guinea pigs, compared with controls. Nemiroff and Lungu[61] reported that the number and size of blood vessels in the microcirculation was significantly greater in animal skin flaps treated with HBO when compared with controls ($p < 0.01$). They concluded that HBO significantly enhanced flap survival by increasing and/or maintaining the number and possibly the size of vessels within the microcirculation.

Perrins and Cantab carried out a controlled clinical study in which 48 patients were divided into either treated groups or control groups and noted complete survival of grafts in 64% of the treated group, compared with only 17% for the control group (p= 0.01).[70] The authors did not explain, however, why the overall graft survivals were so low.

Bowersox reviewed 105 patients with ischemic skin flaps or grafts where 90% of the graft patients had risk factors that were considered to be poor prognostic indicators of graft or flap survival. He found that 89% of the flaps and 91% of the threatened skin grafts were salvaged with HBO therapy. This produced an approximate 10% failure rate. Other studies have shown that failure rates can reach 67% in compromised tissue.[8] HBO should be applied as soon as one suspects that a flap is becoming ischemic. The additional HBO treatment cost of $1,500 to $5,000 is low compared with the human and financial costs of a failed flap. The Perrins study, however, shows the risks of comparing the results of different clinical series.

*References 1,25,27,56,62,64,88.

Treatment

Split thickness skin grafts are treated at 2 ATA for 120 minutes or 2.4 ATA for 90 minutes immediately after surgery and then b.i.d. for the following 3 days. Treatment is usually discontinued after the third postoperative day after a total of seven treatments. This regimen is based on experimental studies performed on animals.

Treatment of full-thickness grafts usually consists of a 2 to 2.4 ATA dive from 90 to 120 minutes twice a day. Treatment is continued for 3 to 10 days depending on the type of graft or flap and its clinical appearance.

Use of the transcutaneous po$_2$

The patient must always lie prone or supine to achieve reproducibility in the readings. They must not talk during the measurements, since it will drive up the reading. Use only a calibrated machine with a good membrane. Adequate time must be allowed for the reading to stabilize. If it fails to stabilize in about 20 minutes, suspect an error, leak, or malfunction. In diabetic patients or those with severe circulation compromise, avoid leaving the electrode in place or connected for more than 30 minutes because the heated electrode ($44°$ C) has caused skin burns in these patients. Record the TC po$_2$ and the electrical draw (heat), since it often correlates with the blood flow. Avoid placing the electrode directly over a vein or bony prominence. Unfortunately, the sole of the foot is too thick to give adequate readings. Be sure to mark the spot from which the reading is taken with indelible marker so that repeat readings can be made in exactly the same place.

The Radiometer (Model TCM3) has been approved for use in the monoplace chamber.* The electrode is plugged into a special adapter cable that can be led with an appropriate plug through the 19-pin connector passing through the door frame. The monitoring box must always be outside the chamber. Placing it inside the chamber would be an extreme fire hazard. Adapter cables may be obtained from the manufacturer. Some investigators feel that TCpO$_2$ readings made at pressure are more reliable prognostically than readings made at 1 ATA. If the reading taken at 2 ATA fails to rise over 100 mm Hg, healing will be unlikely.

---

*For anyone wishing to locate a chamber in their area, information can be obtained through the Diver's Alert Network at Duke University. If your call is not an emergency, call (919) 684-2948, an informational number available from 9:00 AM to 5:00 PM, eastern standard time, Monday through Friday. For emergencies, call (919) 684-8111, a number manned 24 hours a day, and ask for the Diver's Alert Network.

REFERENCES

1. Arturson GG and Khanna NN: The effects of hyperbaric oxygen, dimethyl sulfoxide and complamin on survival of experimental skin flaps, Scand J Plast Reconstr Surg 4:8-10, 1970.
2. Atkinson JR: Experimental air embolism, Northwest Med 62:699-703, 1963.
3. Baroni G et al: Hyperbaric oxygen in diabetic gangrene treatment, Diabetes Care 10(1):81-86, 1987.
4. Beehner MR and Marx RE: Hyperbaric oxygen induced angiogenesis and fibroplasia in human irradiated tissues. In Proceedings of the sixtyfifth meeting of the American Association of Oral and Maxillofacial Surgery, 1983.
5. Bird AD and Telfer ABM: Effect of hyperbaric oxygen on limb circulation, Lancet 1:355-56, 1965.
6. Boerema I: An operating room with high atmospheric pressure, Surgery 49:291-298, 1961.
7. Boerema I et al: Life without blood, J Cardiovas Surg 1:133-146, 1960.
8. Bowersox JC, Strauss MB, and Hart GB: Clinical experience with hyperbaric oxygen therapy in the salvage of ischemic skin flaps and grafts, J Hyperbaric Med 1:141-149, 1986.
9. Boykin JV, Eriksson E, and Pittman N: *In vivo* microcirculation of a scald burn and the progression of post-burn dermal ischemia, J Plast Reconstr Surg 66:191-198, 1980.
10. Champion WM, McSherry CK, and Goulian D: Effect of hyperbaric oxygen on survival of pedicle skin flaps, J Surg Research 7:583-586, 1967.
11. Cianci PE et al: Economic considerations on the impact of adjunctive hyperbaric oxygen in potential amputees. In Bove AA, Bachrach AJ, and Greenbaum LJ, Jr. (eds): Underwater and hyperbaric physiology IX. Proceedings of the ninth International Symposium on Underwater and Hyperbaric Physiology, Undersea, and Hyperbaric Medical Society, Bethesda, 1987.
12. Cianci PE et al: Adjunctive hyperbaric oxygen reduces the need for surgery in 40-80% burns, J Hyperbaric Med 3(2):97-101, 1988.
13. Cianci PE et al: Adjunctive hyperbaric oxygen therapy reduced length of hospitalization in thermal burns, J Burn Care Rehab 19:432-435, 1989.
14. Davis JC: [Letter] The results of refractory osteomyelitis treated with surgery, parenteral antibiotics and HBO, Clin Ortho, 205(4):310, 1986.
15. Davis JC et al: Chronic non-hematogenous osteomyelitis treated with adjuvant hyperbaric oxygen, J Bone Joint Surg. 68A:1210-1217, 1986.
16. Davis JC and Hunt TK (eds): Problem wounds: the role of oxygen, New York, 1988, Elsevier Science Publishing Co Inc.
17. Dutka AJ et al: Head-down position after air embolism impares recovery of brain function as measured by somatosensory evoked response in canines, Undersea Biomed Research, 17:64-65, 1990.
18. Esterhai JL, Jr. et al: Adjunctive hyperbaric oxygen therapy in the treatment of chronic refractory osteomyelitis, J Trauma 27(7):pp 763-768, 1987.
19. Eskew P and Myers RAM (eds): Hyperbaric chambers: a directory of hyperbaric treatment chambers in the United States and Canada, Undersea and Hyperbaric Med Soc, Bethesda, 1988.
20. Farmer JC et al: Treatment of radiation-induced tissue injury by hyperbaric oxygen, Ann Otolaryngol 87:707-715, 1978.
21. National Academy of Sciences - National Research Council: Fundamentals of hyperbaric oxygen, Washington, D.C., 1966.
22. Goddio AS: Oxygen derived free radicals in plastic surgery—theraputic interest of fighting free radicals: the superoxide dismutases, Eur J Plast Surg 12:111-116, 1989

23. Gottrup F et al: The dynamic properties of tissue oxygen in healing flaps, Surgery 95(5):527-36, 1984.

24. Gozal D et al: Necrotizing fasciitis, Arch Surg 121:233-235, 1986.

25. Greenwood TW and Gilchrist AG: The effect of HBO on wound healing following ionizing radiation. In Trapp, WC et al (eds): Proceedings of the Fifth International Congress on Hyperbaric Medicine. Volume I, Canada: Simon Frasier University, 1973.

26. Grim PS et al: Lack of measurable oxidative stress during HBO therapy in burn patients, Undersea Biomed Research vol. 17, 1989.

27. Gruber RP, Heitkamp DH, and Lawrence JB: Skin permeability to oxygen and hyperbaric oxygen, Arch Surg 101:69-70, 1970.

28. Hamblin DL: Hyperbaric oxygenation: its effect on experimental staphylococcal osteomyelitis in rats, J Bone Joint Surg 50A:1129-1141, 1968.

29. Hart GB: Treatment of decompression illness and air embolism with hyperbaric oxygen, Aerospace Med 45(10):1190-1193, 1974.

30. Hart GB et al: Treatment of burns with hyperbaric oxygen, J Surg Gynec Obstet 139(5):693-696, 1974.

31. Heikkila RE, Cabbat FS, and Cohen G: In vivo inhibition of superoxide dismutase in mice by diethyldithiocarbamate, J Biolog Chem 251:2182, 1976.

32. Hess ML and Manson NH: Molecular oxygen: friend or foe, J Mol Cell Cardiol 16:969-985, 1984

33. Hohn DC et al: The effect of oxygen tension on the microbicidal function of leukocytes in wounds and in vitro, Surg Forum 27:18-20, 1976.

34. Hutton JJ, Jr., Tappel AL, and Udenfriend S: Co-factor and substrate requirements of collagen prolene hydroxylase, Arch Biochem Biophys 118:231-240, 1967.

35. Joseph DL and Shurmrick DL: Risks of head and neck surgery in previously irradiated patients, Arch Otolaryngol 97:381-384, 1973.

36. Jurell G and Kaijser L: The influence of varying pressure and duration of treatment with hyperbaric oxygen on the survival of skin flaps: an experimental study, Scand J Plast Reconstr Surg 7:25-28, 1973.

37. Kaelin CM et al: The effects of hyperbaric oxygen on free flaps in rats, Arch Surg 125:607-609, 1990.

38. Ketchum SA III, Thomas AN, and Hall AD: The effect of hyperbaric oxygen on small first, second, and third degree burns, Surg Forum 18:65-67, 1967.

39. Kindwall EP: Hyperbaric oxygen therapy: a committee report, Bethesda, May 1977, The Undersea Medical Society.

40. Krogh A: The number and distribution of capillaries in muscle with calculations of the oxygen pressure head necessary for supplying the tissue, J Physiol 52:409-415, 1919.

41. Larson DL et al: Major complications of radiotherapy in cancer of the oral cavity and oral pharynx: a ten-year retrospective study, Am J Surg 146:531-536, 1983.

42. Leitch DR, Greenbaum LJ, and Hallenbeck JM: Cerebral air embolism I, II, III, and IV, Undersea Biomed Research 11(3):221-274, 1984.

43. Levin ME: The diabetic foot: preventing its morbidity and mortality, Medical Times 16(1):23-31, 1988.

44. Mackey WC et al: The costs of surgery for limb threatening ischemia, Surgery 99(1):26-35, 1986.

45. Mader JT: Hyperbaric oxygen therapy: a committee report, Bethesda, Md, 1989, The Undersea and Hyperbaric Medical Society, Inc.

46. Mader JT et al: Therapy with hyperbaric oxygen for experimental osteomyelitis due to Staphylococcus aureus in rabbits, J Infec Dis 138:312-318, 1978.

47. Mader JT et al: A mechanism for the amelioration by hyperbaric oxygen of experimental staphylococcal osteomyelitis in rabbits, J Infec Dis 142:915-922, 1980.

48. Mader JT et al: Potentiation of tobramycin by hyperbaric oxygen in experimental pseudomonas aeruginosa osteomyelitis. Presented at the twenty-seventh Interscience Conference on Antimicrobial Agents and Chemotherapy, 1987.

49. Manson PN et al: Improved capillaries by hyperbaric oxygen in skin flaps, Surg Forum 31:564-566, 1980.

50. Marx RE: Osteoradionecrosis part I: a new concept in its pathophysiology, J Oral Maxillofac Surg 41:283-288, 1983.

51. Marx RE: A new concept in the treatment of osteoradionecrosis part II, J Oral Maxillofac Surg 41:351-357, 1983.

52. Marx RE and Johnson RP: Studies in the radiobiology of osteoradionecrosis and their clinical significance, Oral Surg 64:379-390, 1978.

53. Marx RE, Johnson RP, and Kline SN: Prevention of osteoradionecrosis: a randomized prospective clinical trial of hyperbaric oxygen versus penicillin, JADA 111:48-54, 1985.

54. May JW, Gallico GG III, and Lukash FN: Microvascular transfer of free tissue for closure of bone wounds of the distal lower extremity, New Eng J Med 306:253-257, 1982.

55. McDermott JJ et al: Effects of treatment with lidocaine and hyperbaric oxygen in experimental cerebral ischemia induced by air embolism, Undersea Biomed Res 17 (Suppl):35-36, 1990.

56. McFarlane RM and Wermuth RE: The use of hyperbaric oxygen to prevent necrosis in experimental pedicle flaps and composite skin grafts, Plast Reconstr Surg 37:422-430, 1966.

57. Meijne NG, Schoemaker G, and Bulterijs A: The value of hyperbaric oxygen in cardiovascular surgery. In Boerema I, Brummelkamp WH, and Meijne NG (eds): First International Congress on the Clinical Applications of Hyperbaric Oxygen, Amsterdam, 1963.

58. Mendel V, Scholz H, and Nagel A: Hyperbaric oxygenation: its effect on experimental chronic osteomyelitis in rats. Presented at the Second European Conference on Hyperbaric Medicine, 1988.

59. Myllyla R, Tuderman L, and Kivirikko K: Mechanism of the prolyl hydroxylase reaction: kinetic analysis of the reaction sequence ed 2, Europ J Biochem 80:349-357, 1977.

60. Nemiroff PM: Effects of cisplatinum and hyperbaric oxygen on wound healing in mice, Undersea Biomed Research 15(suppl):40, 1988.

61. Nemiroff PM and Lungu AL: The influence of hyperbaric oxygen and irradiation on vascularity in skin flaps: a controlled study, Surg Forum 38:565-567, 1987.

62. Nemiroff PM et al: HBO and irradiation on experimental skin flaps in rats, Surg Forum 35:549-550, 1984.

63. Nemiroff PM et al: Effects of hyperbaric oxygen and irradiation on experimental flaps in rats, Otolargyngol Head Neck Surg 93:485-491, 1985.

64. Niinikoski J: Viability of ischemic skin in hyperbaric oxygen, Acta Chir Scand 136:567-568, 1970.

65. Niinikoski J and Hunt TK: Oxygen tensions in healing bone, J Surg Gynec Obstet 134:746-750, 1972.

66. Niu AKC et al: Burns treated with adjunctive hyperbaric oxygen therapy: a comparative study in humans, J Hyperbaric Med 2:75-85, 1987.

67. Nylander G, Nordstrom H, and Eriksson E: Effects of hyperbaric oxygen on oedema formation after a scald burn, Burns 10:193-196, 1984.

68. Nylander G et al: Metabolic effects of hyperbaric oxygen in post-ischemic muscle, Plast Reconstr Surg 79(1):91-96, 1987.

69. Peirce EC, II: Pathophysiology, apparatus and methods, includ-

ing the special techniques of hypothermia and hyperbaric oxygen. In Peirce EC, II (ed): Extracorporeal circulation for open heart surgery, Springfield, Ill, 1969 Charles C. Thomas Publisher.

70. Perrins DJD and Cantab MB: Influence of hyperbaric oxygen on the survival of split skin grafts, Lancet 1:868-871, 1967.

71. Raskin P, Lipman RL, and Oloff CM: Effect of hyperbaric oxygen on lipid peroxidation in the lung, Aerospace Med 42(1):28-30, 1971.

72. Riegels-Nielsen P et al: Fournier's gangrene: five patients treated with hyperbaric oxygen, J Urol 132:918-920, 1984.

73. Riseman J et al: Hyperbaric oxygen therapy for necrotizing fasciitis reduced mortality and the need for debridements, Surgery 108:847-850, 1990.

74. Sheffield PJ: Tissue oxygen measurements with respect to soft tissue wound healing with normobaric and hyperbaric oxygen, HBO Review 6:18-46, 1985.

75. Sheffield PJ: Tissue oxygen measurements in problem wounds: the role of oxygen. In Davis JC and Hunt TK (eds): Problem wounds: the role of oxygen, New York, 1988, Elsevier Science Publishing.

76. Sheffield PJ and Workman WT: Non-invasive tissue oxygen measurements in patients administered normobaric and hyperbaric oxygen by mask, HBO Review 6(1):47-62, 1985.

77. Shulman AG and Krohn HL: The influence of hyperbaric oxygen in multiple skin allografts on the healing of skin wounds, Surgery 62:1051-1058, 1967.

78. Silver IA: Tissue pO_2 changes in acute inflammation, Arch Exper Med Biol 94:769-774, 1978.

79. Sonoda A et al: Spontaneous gangrene of the scrotum and penis (Fournier's gangrene), J Dermat 7:371-375, 1980.

80. Stewart RJ et al: The effects of hyperbaric oxygen on adenosin triphosphate in thermally injured skin, Surg Forum 39:87-90, 1988.

81. Stewart RJ et al: Burn wound levels of ATP after exposure to elevated levels of oxygen. In Proceedings of the American Burn Association 21:67, 1989.

82. Stoney WS et al: Air embolism and other accidents using pump oxygenators, Ann Throac Surg 29(4):336-340, 1980.

83. Strauss MB: Role of hyperbaric oxygen therapy in acute ischemias and crush injuries - an orthopaedic prospective, The Hyperbaric Oxygen Review 2(2):87-106, 1981.

84. Strauss MB: Refractory osteomyelitis, J Hyperbaric Med 2:147-160, 1987.

85. Strauss MB: Cost-effective issues in HBO therapy: complicated fractures, J Hyperbaric Med 3(4):199-205, 1988.

86. Strauss MB et al: Reduction of skeletal muscle necrosis using intermittent hyperbaric oxygen in a model compartment syndrome, J Bone Joint Surg 65A:656-662, 1983.

87. Strauss MB et al: Salvaging the difficult wound through a combined management program. Kindwall EP (ed): In Proceedings of the Eighth International Congress on Hyperbaric Medicine, San Pedro, Calif, 1987, Best Publishing Co.

88. Tan CM et al: The effect of hyperbaric oxygen and hyperbaric air on survival of island skin flaps, Plast Reconstr Surg 73:27-30, 1974.

89. Thom SR: Hyperbaric oxyen therapy, J Intensive Care Med 4:58-74, 1989.

90. Thom SR: Molecular mechanism for the antagonism of lipid peroxidation by hyperbaric oxygen, Undersea Biomedical Research 17 (suppl) 53, 1990.

91. Triplett RG et al: Experimental mandibular osteomyelitis: therapeutic trials with hyperbaric oxygen, J Oral Maxillofac Surg 40:640-646, 1983.

92. Upton PG et al: Effects of anti-oxidants and hyperbaric oxygen in ameliorating experimental doxorubricin skin toxicity in the rat, Cancer Treatment Reports 70(4):503-507, 1986.

93. U.S. Navy Diving Manual: Navsea 00994-LP-001-9010, Washington, D.C., June 1985, Navy Deptartment.

94. Wagner FW, Jr: The dysvascular foot: a system for diagnosis and treatment, Foot Ankle 2(2):64-122, 1981.

95. Waisbren BA et al: Hyperbaric oxygen in severe burns, Burns 8:176-179, 1982.

96. Weiland AJ, Moore JR, and Daniel RK: The Efficacy of free tissue transfer in the treatment of osteomyelitis, J Bone Joint Surg 66A:181-193, 1984.

97. Yamaguchi KT et al: Effect of oxygen on burn wound tissue levels of ATP and Collagen, Undersea Biomed Research. 17 (suppl.) 65-66, 1990.

98. Zamboni WA et al: The effect of acute hyperbaric oxygen therapy on axial pattern skin flap survival when administered during and after total ischemia, J Reconstr Micro 5:343-347, 1989

99. Zamboni WA et al: The effect of hyperbaric oxygen treatment on the microcirculation of ischemic skeletal muscle, Undersea Biomed Research 17(Suppl):26, 1990

100. Zamboni WA et al: Acute effects of hyperbaric oxygen on laser doppler flow in ischemic axial skin flaps, Undersea Biomed Research 17 (Suppl):37, 1990

101. Ziser A et al: Hyperbaric oxygen therapy for Fournier's gangrene, Crit Care Med 13:773-774, 1985.

CHAPTER 11

Tendon Transfers for Reconstruction of the Hand and Wrist

Neil Ford Jones

Tendon transfer is a reconstructive technique to restore motion and/or balance to a hand with impaired function of the extrinsic or intrinsic muscle-tendon units. A functioning muscle-tendon unit is divided, mobilized, and then reinserted into another tendon or bone to substitute for the action of a nonfunctioning muscle-tendon unit. Unlike a tendon graft, the transferred donor tendon remains attached to its parent muscle. A tendon transfer also differs from a free-muscle transfer in that the neurovascular pedicle to the muscle of the transferred tendon remains intact.

There are three general indications for tendon transfers in the upper extremity. First, function may be restored to a muscle paralyzed from injuries of a peripheral nerve, the brachial plexus, or the spinal cord. Second, function may be restored after closed-tendon rupture or open injuries to tendons or muscles. Third, balance may be restored to a hand deformed by a neurological disease. Tendon transfers are performed predominantly to restore function after peripheral nerve injury. The various techniques are, therefore classified according to the specific nerve palsy that they are attempting to correct. Certain general principles apply to all transfers.[8,46,49] The relative advantages or disadvantages of nerve repair, as opposed to tendon transfer, will vary with each patient. Nerve repair or nerve grafting will usually provide return of sensibility and motor power to more proximal forearm muscles. Tendon transfers are best to restore motor function in the hand for motion controlled by more distal muscles, which are less likely to be reinnervated after proximal nerve repair. For example, after transection of the ulnar nerve at the elbow, a primary nerve repair should restore function to the flexor carpi ulnaris (FCU) and the flexor digitorum profundus (FDP) muscles of the ring

and small fingers. Some return of sensibility to the ulnar side of the hand is likely, but return of intrinsic muscle function is unlikely. Tendon transfers can be used in such cases to correct clawing of the digits and to restore power pinch. The surgeon also has to decide whether tendon transfers are more appropriate for a specific patient than other alternatives such as secondary nerve grafting, tendon grafting, tenodesis, capsulodesis, or arthrodesis.

GENERAL PRINCIPLES

Steindler first suggested that tendon transfers cannot glide through edematous or scarred soft tissues nor can they flex or extend stiff metacarpophalangeal (MCP) and proximal interphalangeal (PIP) joints. He advocated tendon transfers be delayed until "tissue equilibrium" had been restored.[49] Fractures should be healed or rigidly fixed by internal fixation. Chronic scarred skin and subcutaneous tissues or skin grafts in the projected line of pull of a tendon transfer should be resurfaced with a flap. Split thickness skin grafting to cover soft tissue defects of the hand and forearm should now be avoided if secondary tendon transfers are likely to be necessary. Delayed primary coverage is now possible using pedicled flaps like the groin flap or reverse radial forearm flap or free tissue transfers such as the lateral arm flap, radial forearm flap, and temporoparietal fascial flap. Occasionally, silicone rods can be placed either beneath or through the subcutaneous fat at the time of flap transfer to create a smooth tunnel through which a tendon transfer may be later rerouted. The span of the thumb-index finger–web space should be maintained by splinting, especially after median nerve injuries. If a secondary adduction contracture develops, this should be released by a Z-plasty, skin grafting, or transposition flap before any tendon transfer to restore opposition. A full, passive range of motion of the thumb MCP and PIP joints should be achieved by physical therapy and dynamic splinting before any tendon transfer. Preliminary capsulotomies of the MCP and PIP joints or tenolysis of adherent flexor or extensor tendons may occasionally be required.

Any muscle-tendon unit selected as a potential donor for transfer must be expendable. The sublimis tendon of the ring finger, for example, may be used to correct clawing in patients with a low ulnar nerve palsy, but it is not expendable in patients with a high ulnar nerve palsy who have no functioning profundus tendon to the ring finger. The availability of a muscle-tendon unit as a tendon transfer may also be influenced by the patient's occupation. The flexor carpi radialis (FCR), for example, may be a more appropriate transfer to provide finger extension in a blue-collar worker rather than the more conventional FCU tendon transfer. The FCU is necessary in such patients for strong flexion and ulnar deviation of the wrist, necessary in hammering. When multiple tendon transfers are required, one wrist flexor, one wrist extensor, and one extrinsic finger flexor and extensor tendon should always be retained to each digit.

The surgeon, in selecting the appropriate donor muscle-tendon, must consider not only the strength of the transferred muscle but also the strength of the paralyzed muscle, as well as the strength of the antagonist muscle. Brand has shown that the maximum potential force of a muscle is directly proportional to its physiological cross-sectional area.[7,8] It has been calculated that a muscle can produce a force of 3.65 kg per square cm of its cross-sectional area. This potential force is maximal when the muscle is at its resting length, defined as the position midway between its length when fully stretched passively and when fully contracted.

The potential amplitude or excursion of a donor muscle-tendon unit must also be sufficient to restore the specific function lost. This amplitude can be determined during surgery by applying traction to the tendon. The patient can contract the muscle voluntarily under local anesthesia, but if general anesthesia is used, the muscle must be stimulated electrically to determine its contraction. The distance from the fully stretched position to the fully contracted position is the total amplitude of the muscle-tendon unit. The finger flexors have an amplitude of 70 mm, the finger extensors, 50 mm, and the wrist flexors and extensors, 33 mm. The tenodesis effect of wrist flexion or extension may also increase the effective amplitude of a tendon transfer by as much as 25 mm. The amplitude of a do-

nor muscle can also be increased by performing an extensive release of its surrounding fascia, which is best exemplified by the brachioradialis (BR) muscle.

A tendon transfer should pass in a straight direction from the origin of the donor muscle to its new insertion. Unless tendon transfers are being performed early when there is still a chance of reinnervation after nerve repair, the recipient tendons should be divided proximal to the site of the tendon juncture to create a more direct line of pull rather than forming an angled Y-shaped juncture. Tendon transfers should only act across one joint and only perform a single function. A transfer, however, may be inserted into several recipient tendons as long as they perform the same function in adjacent digits. Finally, the donor muscle selected should preferably be synergistic with the function of the muscle to be restored or potentially retrainable by voluntary control.

Selection and timing of tendon transfers

The surgeon must determine the specific functions to be restored, select the appropriate donor muscle-tendon units, and decide on the timing of the tendon transfer. Every muscle in the forearm and hand should be tested to document whether they are functioning and have their strength graded. From this list of functioning muscles, only those that are expendable are available as donor transfers. The specific functions of the hand that need to be restored are then listed. The final step is to match the available donor muscles with the functions that need to be restored, based on the force, amplitude, and direction of the various muscles available. Arthrodesis of the wrist may even be necessary to free a wrist flexor or extensor tendon for transfer. Transfers that require postoperative immobilization with the wrist in flexion are usually performed at a first stage. Those transfers requiring postoperative immobilization with the wrist in extension are performed at a second stage.

The timing of tendon transfers may be classified as early, conventional, or late. A conventional tendon transfer is usually performed after innervation of the paralyzed muscle fails to occur by 3 months after the anticipated (or estimated) time of the reinnervation, based on a rate of nerve regeneration of 1 mm a day. Brand, Omer, and Burkhalter advocate "early" tendon transfers in certain circumstances in which a tendon transfer is performed simultaneously with the nerve repair or before the expected time of reinnervation of the muscle.[8,14,37] This "early" tendon transfer acts as a temporary substitute for the paralyzed muscle until reinnervation occurs, providing an internal splint. If reinnervation is suboptimal, the "early" tendon transfer acts as a helper to augment the power of the muscle, and if reinnervation fails to occur, it then acts as a permanent substitute.

Surgical techniques

The success of any tendon transfer depends entirely on preventing scarring or adhesions around the path of the transferred tendon. Incisions should be carefully planned before elevation of the tourniquet so that the final tendon junctures lie transversely beneath skin flaps rather than lying immediately beneath the incisions. The donor muscle should be carefully mobilized to prevent damage to its neurovascular bundle, which usually enters in the proximal third of the forearm. The transferred tendon should glide in a tunnel through the subcutaneous tissues and not cross raw bone or pass through small fascial windows. Only the distal end of the tendon should be grasped, and care should be taken to prevent dessication during surgery. Tendon junctures are performed using the Pulvertaft weave technique. The donor and recipient tendons are first sutured under normal tension with one or two nonabsorbable sutures. The tension of the transfer is then checked by observing the flexion and extension of the involved digit during flexion and extension of the wrist. The hand is immobilized after surgery in a protective position for 3 to 4 weeks, at which time gentle, active range-of-motion exercises are started, usually under the supervision of a therapist. The hand is protected for an additional 3 weeks in a lightweight protective splint.

TENDON TRANSFERS TO RESTORE EXTENSION OF THE WRIST AND DIGITS IN RADIAL NERVE PALSY

The functional deficit in radial nerve palsy is an inability to extend the wrist, to extend the fingers at the MCP joints, or to extend and radially abduct the thumb. However, the most significant disability in such patients is their inability to stabilize their wrists for grasp function. The wrist falls into flexion, which impairs the flexor power to their fingers, resulting in marked weakness of grip strength.

Tendon transfers are thus required to provide wrist extension, extension of the fingers at the MCP joints, and extension and radial abduction of the thumb (Table 11-1). Unlike the median and ulnar nerves, sensory loss after radial nerve injury is not functionally disabling unless the patient develops a painful neuroma.

The timing of tendon transfers for radial nerve palsy remains controversial. The first option is to perform an "early" tendon transfer simultaneously with repair of the radial nerve to act as a internal splint providing immediate restoration of power grip.[8,14,37] The second, more conventional option is to delay any ten-

Table 11-1

Tendon Transfers for Radial Nerve Palsy

Standard FCU transfer	FCR transfer	Boyes sublimis transfer
PT to ECRB	PT to ECRB	PT to ECRL plus ECRB
FCU to EDC	FCR to EDC	FDS long to EDC long, ring and small fingers
PL to EPL	PL to EPL	FDS ring to EIP and EPL
		FCR to APL and EPB

don transfers until reinnervation of the most proximal muscles such as the BR and extensor carpi radialis longus (ECRL) fails to occur within the calculated time limit. The chances of successful muscle reinnervation after nerve repair are much less reliable in older patients or when there are extensive nerve gaps or associated soft tissue injuries. It may be more appropriate for these patients to have all necessary tendon transfers performed early. Bevin[1] has advocated performing the three standard tendon transfers in every patient without attempting to repair the radial nerve, but this is not considered an accepted practice.

Several different tendon transfers have been reported for radial nerve palsy, but three patterns seem to have evolved.* The three patterns of tendon transfer differ only in the technique of restoring finger extension and thumb extension and abduction.† The use of pronator teres (PT) to provide wrist extension is now universally accepted. The only remaining controversy is whether to insert PT into extensor carpi radialis brevis (ECRB) alone or into both ECRL and ECRB.

Standard FCU transfer

An inverted J-shaped incision is made over the ulnar-volar aspect of the distal forearm. The FCU tendon is transected at the wrist crease and released extensively from its fascial attachments up into the proximal third of the forearm. Care is taken not to damage the neurovascular pedicle by using a second incision in the proximal forearm if necessary. The palmaris longus (PL) tendon is then transected at the wrist crease through the same distal incision and the muscle mobilized into the middle third of the forearm. An S-shaped incision is then made beginning over the volar-radial aspect of the middle third of the forearm, passing dorsally and ulnarly over the radial border of the forearm. The tendon of PT is elevated from the radius in continuity with a 2- to 3-cm strip of periosteum (Fig. 11-1). The ECRB is transected at its musculotendonous junction if there is no chance for future reinnervation of

*References 3,18,20,28,29,44,48,54.

†References 3,18,20,28,29,44,48,54.

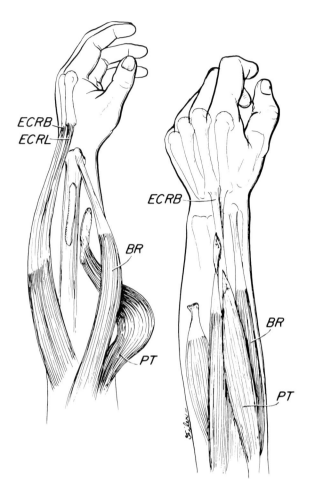

Fig. 11-1   PT to ECRB to restore wrist extension.

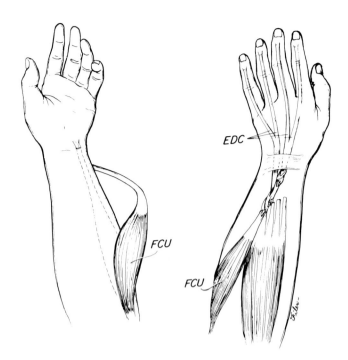

Fig. 11-2   FCU to EDC to provide finger extension.

the wrist extensors. The PT is then rerouted superficial to the BR and ECRL around the radial border of the forearm in a straight direction, ready for insertion into the ECRB. A subcutaneous tunnel is made with a Kelly clamp from the dorsal incision around the ulnar border of the forearm into the proximal incision used to mobilize FCU. The FCU tendon is passed through this subcutaneous tunnel to lie obliquely across the extensor digitorum communis (EDC) tendons proximal to the extensor retinaculum. If no return of function is to be expected in the EDC tendons, they can be transected at their musculotendonous junctions so that a more direct line of pull can be achieved.[33] Otherwise, an end-to-side juncture is performed (Fig. 11-2). The extensor pollicis longus (EPL) tendon is divided at its musculotendonous junction, removed from the third dorsal extensor tendon compartment, and passed through a subcutaneous tunnel from the base of the thumb metacarpal to the volar wrist incision (Fig. 11-3). The proper tension in radial nerve tendon transfers should be tight enough to provide full extension of the wrist and digits but without restricting full flexion of the dig-

its. The PT, under resting tension, is woven through the tendon of ECRB with the wrist in 45 degrees of extension. The distal ends of the four EDC tendons to the index, long, ring, and small fingers are then woven through the FCU tendon proximal to the extensor retinaculum. The extensor digiti minimi (EDM) is usually not included unless there is an extensor lag when proximal traction is applied to the EDC tendon to the small finger. With the wrist in neutral and the FCU under maximal tension, each individual EDC tendon is sutured to provide full extension at the MCP joint, starting with the index finger and finishing with the small finger. Tension is then evaluated by checking that all four digits extend synchronously when the wrist is palmar flexed and that all four digits can be passively flexed into a fist when the wrist is extended. Finally, the PL and extensor pollicis longus (EPL) tendons are interwoven over the radiovolar aspect of the wrist, with both tendons under resting tension with the wrist in neutral. The wrist is immobilized in 45 degrees of extension in a volar splint with the MCP joints positioned in slight flexion and the thumb in full extension and abduction.

Active flexion and extension of the fingers and thumb are started in 3½ to 4 weeks, and active exercises of the wrist begin at 5 weeks. Protective splinting is continued until 6 to 8 weeks after surgery (Fig. 11-4).

FCR transfer

Several authors have suggested that the FCU is not an expendable tendon and therefore prefer to use the FCR as the donor tendon to restore finger extension.[48,53] The advantage of using the FCR is that it preserves the important moment of flexion and ulnar deviation of the wrist, which is so important for power grip in a blue-collar worker.

The skin incision extends from the radiovolar aspect of the mid forearm coursing dorsally over the third and fourth extensor tendon compartments. The PT is transferred to the ECRB and the PL to the extensor pollicis longus (EPL) exactly as previously described in the FCU transfer. The FCR is transected at the wrist crease, mobilized approximately to the level of the mid forearm, and rerouted around the radial border of the forearm. The four EDC tendons, and if necessary, the EDQ, may be woven through the donor FCR tendon proximal to the extensor retinaculum, but frequently the extensor tendons need to be rerouted superficial to the extensor retinaculum to obtain a straighter line of pull (Fig. 11-5). To prevent a bulky tendon juncture, the small finger EDC and EDQ may be sutured side-to-side to the ring finger EDC and the index finger EDC sutured side-to-side to the long finger EDC under appropriate tension. Only the two EDC tendons to the long and ring fingers then require weaving through the FCR tendon. As with the standard FCU transfer, these tendon junctures are performed with the wrist in neutral and the MCP joints in full extension, with the FCR tendon under maximal traction. Tenodesis of the abductor pollicis longus (APL) may be necessary to prevent a collapse flexion deformity at the carpometacarpal joint of the thumb. After transection of the APL tendon in the distal forearm, it is looped around the BR, proximal to the radial styloid and sutured to itself with the thumb metacarpal held in extension with the wrist in 30 degrees of extension.

Boyes sublimis transfer

Boyes first pointed out that neither the FCU nor the FCR has sufficient amplitude (30 mm) to produce full extension of the digital extensor tendons (50 mm) without the increase in amplitude that is to the tenodesis effect of wrist flexion. Therefore Boyes advocated using the sublimis tendons to the long and ring fingers, which have an amplitude of 70 mm, to act as donor tendons to restore finger extension.[3,18] The advantages of the Boyes transfer are that it will allow simultaneous wrist and finger extension. Second, it potentially allows independent thumb and index finger extension. Finally, it does not weaken wrist flexion. However, the long and ring fingers are deprived of sublimis function, which may result in a weak grip. Harvesting the sublimis tendons may also lead to subsequent development of either a "swan neck" deformity or a flexion contracture at the PIP joint.[36]

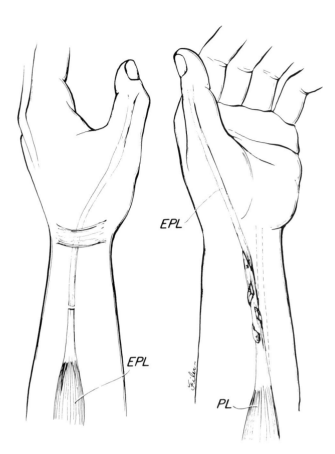

Fig. 11-3 PL to EPL to provide thumb extension.

The sublimis tendons to the long and ring fingers are exposed between the A1 and A2 pulleys, either through one transverse incision or two separate longitudinal incisions at the base of the fingers. The sublimis tendons are transected just proximal to their decussation and then withdrawn proximally through a longitudinal incision over the volar surface of the middle third of the forearm. The tendon of the PT can be transected and rerouted through this same incision as described previously. Blunt dissection on either side of the flexor profundus muscles allows a window to be excised in the interosseous membrane just proximal to the pronator quadratus (Fig. 11-6). This window should be made as large as possible, approximately 4 cm long and as wide as the interosseous space so that the muscle bellies of the two sublimis tendons can be passed through this window to minimize the development of adhesions. Thompson and Rasmussen[51] prefer to transfer the two sublimis tendons through subcutaneous tunnels around the radial and ulnar borders of the forearm (Fig. 11-7). The extensor tendons are isolated together with ECRB through a J-shaped incision passing transversely across the dorsum of the wrist and then extending proximally along the dorsum of the ulna. In

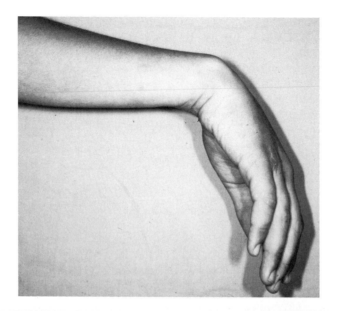

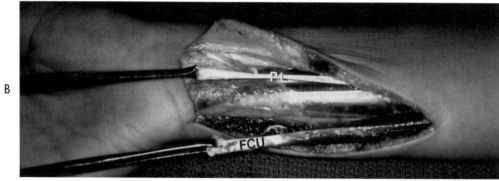

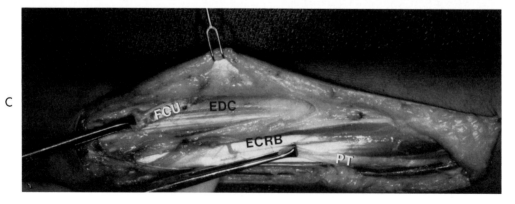

Fig. 11-4 Reconstruction of radial nerve palsy. **A,** by standard PT to ECRB. FCU to EDC and PL to longus EPL transfers (**B** and **C**) Postoperative wrist extension

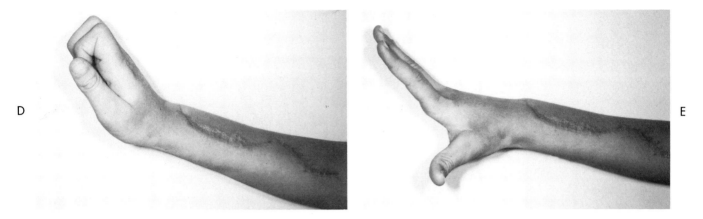

D   E

(D), and finger extension. (E).

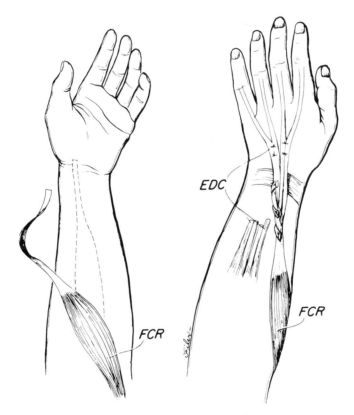

Fig. 11-5   FCR to EDC transfer.

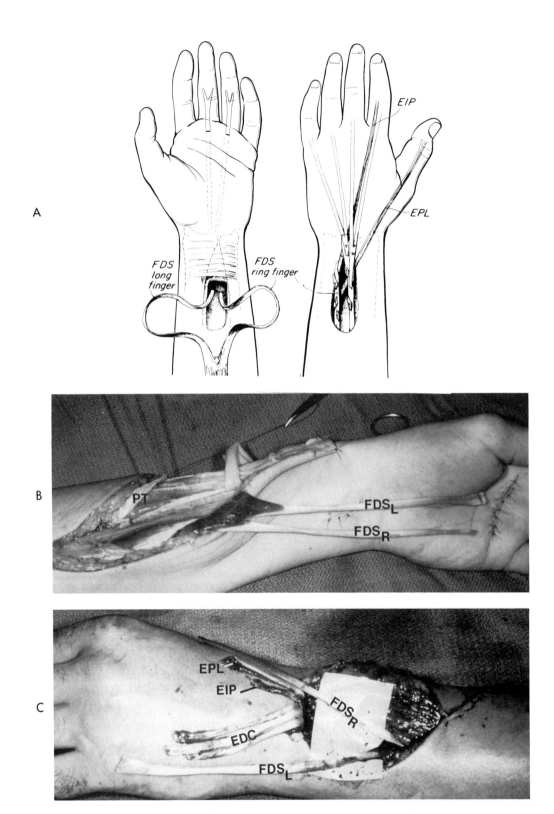

Fig. 11-6 A, B, and **C,** Transfer of the long and ring finger sublimis tendons through a window in the interosseous membrane to restore extension to EDC tendons and EIP and EPL.

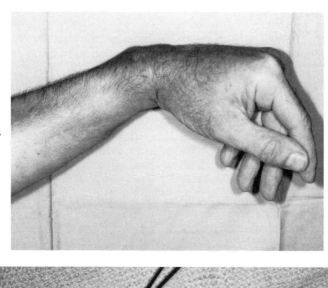

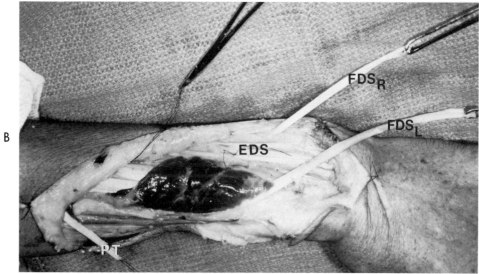

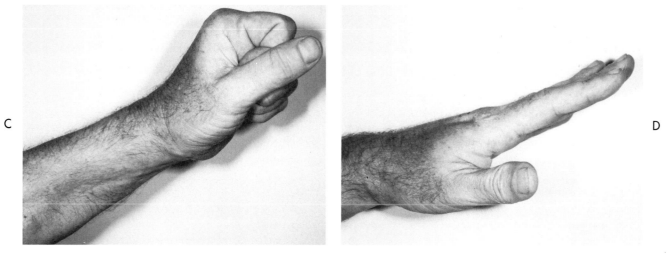

Fig. 11-7   A, In this patient with radial nerve palsy, the long and ring finger sublimis tendons were passed subcutaneously around the radial and ulnar border of the distal forearm **B,** to restore wrist extension **(C),** and finger and thumb extension. **(D).**

Boyes' original description[3] the PT was sutured to both the ECRL and the ECRB. However, to prevent excessive radial deviation after radial nerve tendon transfers, the PT should be woven end to end into the ECRB with the wrist in 30 degrees of extension. The long finger sublimis is then passed to the radial side of the profundus muscles and the ring finger sublimis to the ulnar side through the interosseous window into the dorsal incision. After transection of the EPL and EIP tendons, they are woven end to end into the ring finger sublimis tendon. Similarly, the transected EDC tendons to the index, long, ring, and small fingers are woven end to end into the long finger sublimis tendon, although this arrangement can be reversed. The tendon repairs are performed proximal to the extensor retinaculum without tension in the donor sublimis tendons but maintaining full extension at the MCP joints. The APL is transsected at its musculotendonous junction and passed through a subcutaneous tunnel from the base of the thumb into the volar forearm incision. Either the PL or the FCR are transected at the wrist crease and woven end to end into the tendon (APL) to provide thumb abduction and prevent a collapse deformity of the metcarpal. The tourniquet should be deflated before the closure of the incisions to control any bleeding from the anterior or posterior interosseous vessels.

TENDON TRANSFERS FOR MEDIAN NERVE PALSY

Median nerve injury distal to its innervation of the extrinsic flexor muscles results in loss of thumb opposition and volar sensation over the thumb, index, long, and radial half of the ring fingers.

Thumb opposition is a composite motion that occurs over three joints to position the volar pad opposite the distal phalanx of the long finger. Abduction, pronation, and flexion occur at the carpometacarpal joint, abduction and flexion at the MCP joint, and either flexion or extension at the interphalangeal (IP) joint. Approximately 40 degrees of thumb metacarpal abduction occurs at the carpometacarpal joint, and 20 degrees of the proximal phalanx abduction occurs at the MCP joint. The thumb pronates approximately 90 degrees to achieve opposition to the long finger. Extension of the IP joint is required for pulp-to-pulp pinch, whereas slight flexion of the IP joint allows tip-to-tip pinch.

Of the three intrinsic thenar muscles, the flexor pollicis brevis (FPB) muscle receives a dual innervation from both the median and ulnar nerves. The FPB muscle may remain innervated by the ulnar nerve in approximately 70% of median nerve injuries, resulting in no significant functional loss but, careful testing before surgery will reveal a decreased range of abduction and pronation.

The goal of all the various opposition tendon transfers should be to position the thumb ready for grasp rather than attempting to increase grip strength. Selection of a specific opposition transfer may, however, be influenced by the patient's requirement for either abduction or pronation.

Before any opposition transfer, patients with median nerve injuries should be instructed to prevent the development of an adduction or supination contracture of the thumb by a program of passive abduction exercises. A static splint may be used at night but usually interferes with the already compromised function of the hand if used during the day. Care should be taken to ensure that such splints abduct the thumb metacarpal rather than the proximal phalanx. Otherwise the median nerve palsy will be compounded by attenuation of the ulnar collateral ligament of the MCP joint. If the patient has an established adduction or supination contracture of the thumb, release of the thumb-index finger—web space skin, fascia over the first dorsal interosseous muscle, or even the first dorsal interosseous and adductor muscles themselves may be required before any opposition tendon transfer.

Bunnell[12] first emphasized that the pull of an opposition tendon transfer should be in an oblique direction from the MCP joint to the area of the pisiform and that second, the transfer should be inserted into the dorsoulnar base of the proximal phalanx to produce pronation. Generally, transfers that are directed along the radial aspect of the palm will produce a greater component of palmar abduction, whereas transfers that pass from the pisiform will produce both abduction and pronation. The more distal the transfer that passes across the palm, the greater the power of thumb flexion. Several methods of opposition transfer insertion have been advocated, including attachment into the dorsoulnar base of the proximal phalanx,[12,27,42,52] insertion into the abductor pollicis brevis (APB) tendon,[32] dual insertion into the APB tendon with continuation distally into the MCP joint capsule, and EPL tendon,[41] insertion into the APB, dorsal joint capsule, and adductor pollicis insertion,[21] and finally, use of a distal based EPB tendon.[40] However, a biomechanical study has shown that opposition tendon transfers inserted into the APB tendon alone will produce full abduction and pronation.[19] Therefore the more complex dual insertions should probably be restricted for combined median and ulnar nerve palsies.

The chances of reinnervation of the thenar muscles after group fascicular repair of a distal median nerve laceration should be reasonably optimistic. Therefore conventional timing of an opposition tendon transfer may only be required in those patients who fail to demonstrate signs of reinnervation within the usual calculated time interval. Timing of median nerve tendon transfers will be discussed further under high median nerve palsy.

Extensor indicis proprius (Burkhalter transfer)[15]

The extensor indicis proprius (EIP) tendon is transected through a small transverse incision just proximal to the MCP joint of the index finger. The distal stump of the EIP tendon is then repaired to the EDC tendon of the index finger to prevent extensor lag at the MCP joint. The EIP tendon is mobilized through two small transverse incisions, one proximal and one distal to the extensor retinaculum and the muscle belly mobilized through a longitudinal incision over the dorsoulnar aspect of the mid forearm. A transverse incision is made just proximal to the pisiform bone and a subcutaneous tunnel developed to connect this incision to the dorsal forearm incision. The EIP tendon is then passed subcutaneously around the ulnar border of the distal forearm superficial to the ECU tendon into the pisiform incision. The APB tendon is identified through a small flap incision over the radial aspect of the MCP joint of the thumb and a subcutaneous tunnel made connecting this incision with the pisiform incision. The tendon transfer is passed obliquely across the palm and woven into the tendon of the APB under maximum tension with the wrist in neutral and the thumb in maximal palmar abduction (Fig. 11-8). The tension of the transfer is then tested by the tenodesis effect of the wrist. Palmar flexion of the wrist should allow the thumb to be passively adducted. If dorsiflexion of the wrist produces excessive flexion or extension of the thumb at the MCP joint, this indicates that the transfer has been inserted either too far volarly or too far dorsally and should be adjusted accordingly. The thumb is immobilized in full abduction with the wrist in slight palmar flexion for 4 weeks, at which time active abduction and opposition movements are begun with protective splinting for an additional 3 to 4 weeks. The only potential disadvantage with this tendon transfer is that the EIP tendon is only just long enough to reach the APB tendon.

Ring finger flexor digitorum sublimis (Bunnell transfer)[12]

The ring finger sublimis tendon is isolated through a small transverse incision just distal to the distal palmar crease and the tendon transected between the A1 and A2 pulleys. A curved incision is made over the volar aspect of the distal forearm and the ring finger sublimis delivered into this proximal incision. The FCU tendon is split longitudinally to create a distally based strip along the radial half of the tendon. This strip is

then passed through a slit in the FCU tendon just proximal to the pisiform and sutured to itself to create a pulley (Fig. 11-9). The distal end of the ring finger sublimis tendon is passed through the pulley and an oblique subcutaneous tunnel across the palm into a flap incision over the radial aspect of the MCP joint of the thumb. All the other incisions are then closed and the tension on the tendon transfer adjusted as described previously.

Simple looping of the ring finger sublimis around the FCU tendon, rather than using a fixed pulley, rapidly becomes ineffective and the transfer becomes converted to a flexor of the MCP joint rather than a true opposition transfer. Less favored pulleys for the ring finger sublimis transfer include passing the tendon through Guyon's canal or through a window in the transverse carpal ligament.[47]

The ring finger sublimis muscle is stronger than the EIP and has greater length. However, the ring finger sublimis is not available as a donor tendon in high-median nerve injury or in low-median nerve injuries in which there have been associated injuries to the flexor tendons. The ring finger sublimis transfer should also not be selected in combined low-median and high-ulnar nerve palsies, since it is the only remaining flexor tendon in the ring finger. In low median, low ulnar nerve palsies, the ring finger sublimis may be required for correction of clawing. Finally, harvesting the sublimis tendon may result in either a flexion contracture or a "swan-neck" deformity of the donor finger PIP joint.

Palmaris Longus (Camitz transfer)[9,17,30]

This simple transfer will provide abduction of the thumb but little pronation or flexion and is particularly indicated in elderly patients with thenar atrophy attributable to carpal tunnel syndrome. A strip of palmar fascia is dissected in continuity with the distal PL tendon through a standard carpal tunnel incision in the palm, extending proximally into the distal forearm. A subcutaneous tunnel is developed from the radial aspect of the distal forearm incision along the thenar eminence into a mid-axial incision on the radial aspect of the MCP joint of the thumb. The fascial extension of the PL tendon is passed through the subcutaneous tunnel and sutured to the APB tendon under maximal tension with the wrist in neutral (Fig. 11-10).

Other opposition tendon transfers

Transfer of the abductor digiti minimi manus (ADMM)[26,31,35] may occasionally be indicated in patients with a combined median and radial nerve palsy and also in children with congenital anomalies affecting the thumb. Since the muscle originates distal to the pisi-

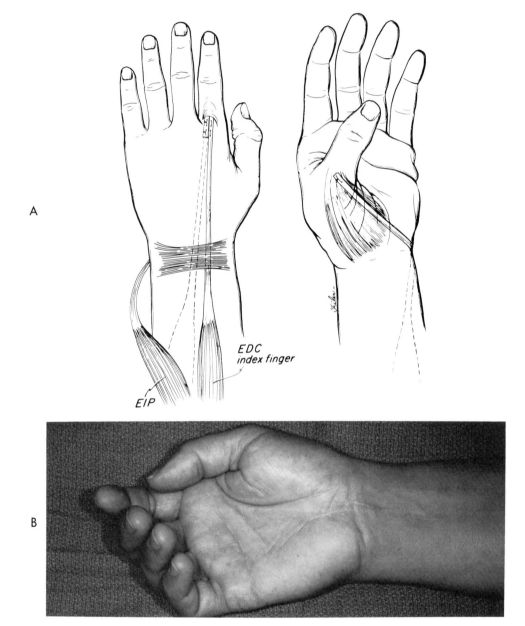

EDC
index finger

EIP

Fig. 11-8 A, Transfer of EIP subcutaneously around the
ulnar border of the distal forearm to provide thumb opposition. In this patient with thenar atrophy due to a laceration
of the motor branch of the median nerve **(B,)** EIP is mobi-

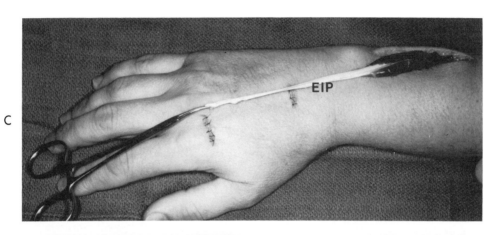

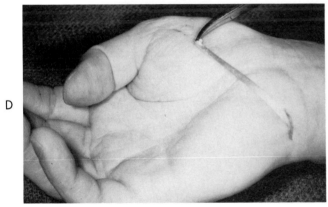

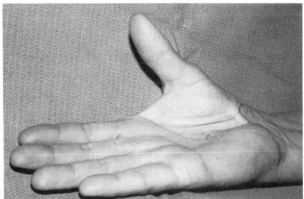

lized (**C**), and passed through a subcutaneous tunnel across the palm (**D**), to restore palmar abduction and pronation of the thumb (**E**).

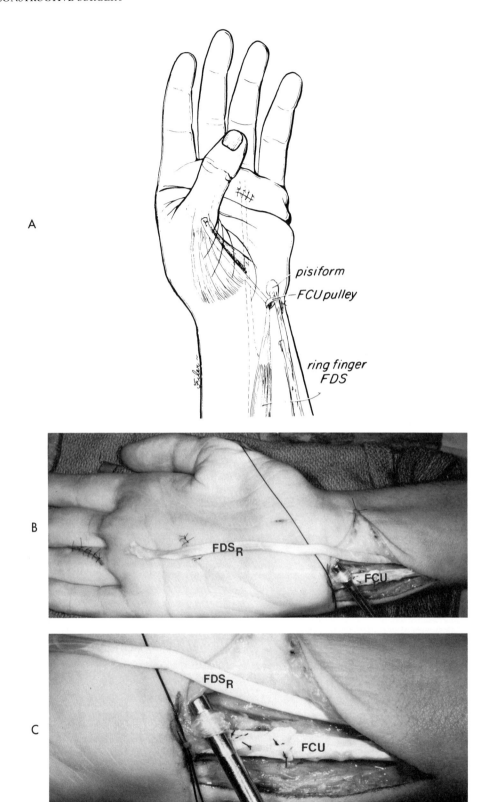

Fig. 11-9   A, Transfer of the flexor digitorum sublimis from the ring finger to restore thumb opposition. **B,** A distal-based strip of FCU provides a pulley just proximal to the pisiform and **C,** the sublimis tendon is passed obliquely through a tunnel in the palm marked by the silk suture to insert into the tendon of APB.

form, this transfer provides excellent flexion and pronation of the thumb but little palmar abduction. Through an ulnar mid-axial incision along the proximal phalanx of the small finger, the tendon insertion of ADMM is transected from the ulnar lateral band. The incision is then continued proximally along the radial aspect of the hypothenar eminence and the muscle elevated in a distal-to-proximal direction, taking care to protect the neurovascular bundle that enters the muscle just beyond the pisiform. A wide subcutaneous tunnel is dissected between the APB tendon insertion at the MCP joint of the thumb and the hypothenar incision. Hemostasis is achieved after releasing the tourniquet, and the entire ADMM muscle is rotated 180° through the subcutaneous tunnel in the palm and sutured into the APB. This transfer has been compared with turning the page of a book.[26,35]

The EPB is transected at its musculotendonous junction in the distal forearm and retrieved through an incision at the MCP joint of the thumb. This distally based tendon may then be passed through a subcutaneous tunnel obliquely across the palm to the area of the pisiform. The ECU tendon is transected at the base of the fifth metacarpal and routed subcutaneously around the ulnar border of the wrist to be interwoven with the EPB tendon.[25,40] The extensor digiti minimi (EDM) is transected over the dorsum of the MCP joint of the small finger, withdrawn into the mid forearm, and passed subcutaneously around the ulnar border of the wrist into an incision overlying the pisiform. The tendon is long enough to be passed through a subcutaneous tunnel, diagonally across the palm, to insert into the APB tendon.[43,50]

HIGH MEDIAN NERVE PALSY

The functional deficit after injury to the median nerve proximal to its innervation of the extrinsic flexor muscles consists of inability to flex the index finger at the PIP and distal interphalangeal (DIP) joints and the thumb at the IP joint in addition to loss of opposition. This is due to paralysis of all four flexor digitorum sublimis (FDS) muscles, the FDP tendons to the index and long fingers, and the Flexor pollicis longus (FPL). Patients are often still able to flex the long finger because of interconnections between the profundus tendons to the long, ring, and small fingers in the distal forearm. Therefore the two functions that need to be restored in patients with a high median nerve palsy are flexion of the IP joint of the thumb and flexion of the PIP and DIP joints of the index and long fingers, together with a conventional opposition tendon transfer.

Flexion of the IP joint of the thumb is restored by transfer of brachioradialis to the FPL (Fig. 11-11). The BR is divided at its insertion on the radial styloid and extensively mobilized from its investing fascia up into

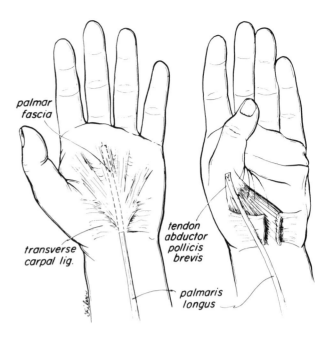

Fig. 11-10 Camitz transfer. Transfer of palmaris longus extended by a strip of palmar fascia to provide palmar abduction of the thumb.

the proximal third of the forearm so that the freed muscle can develop approximately 30 mm of excursion. If reinnervation of the FPL muscle has not occurred after repair or grafting of the median nerve, the tendon can be divided at its musculotendonous junction and woven end to end into the BR tendon. However, if there is a chance of reinnervation of the FPL, the BR tendon should be woven end to side into the FPL tendon, which remains in continuity.

Through the same volar forearm incision, the profundus tendons of the index and long fingers can be sutured side to side to the ulnar innervated profundus tendons of the ring and small fingers (Fig. 11-11). If power flexion of the index and long fingers is required, then formal transfer of the ECRL tendon to the index and long finger profundus tendons can be performed. The ECRL is transected through a small transverse incision at the base of the index finger metacarpal and passed subcutaneously around the radial border of the distal forearm into the volar incision. The profundus tendons to the index and long fingers are woven into the ECRL tendon so that with the wrist in 30° to 45° of dorsiflexion, the tips of the index and long fingers almost touch the palm. Similarly, with the wrist in full palmar flexion, the fingers will assume an almost fully extended position. Adjusting tension on this transfer using the tenodesis effect of the wrist is absolutely critical because the donor tendon ECRL has only 30 mm of amplitude, whereas the profundus tendons normally have 70 mm of excursion. If this transfer is sutured un-

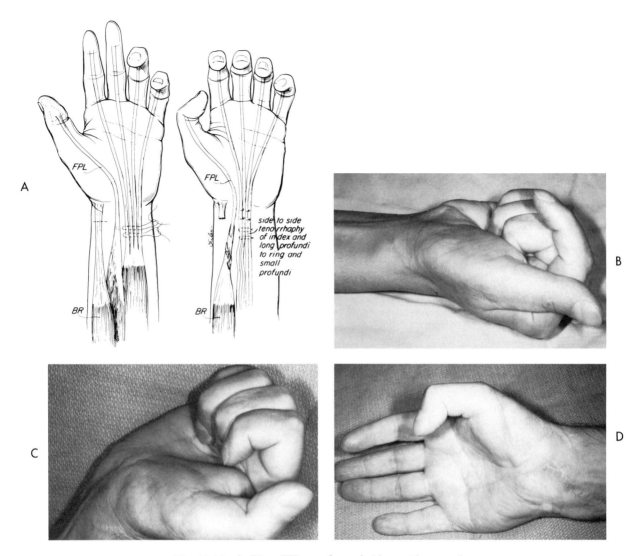

Fig. 11-11 **A,** BR to FPL transfer and side-to-side tenorrhaphy of the profundus tendons to the index and long fingers to the ulnar innervated profundus tendons to the ring and small fingers for reconstruction of a high median nerve palsy. **B,** Loss of DIP joint flexion of the index finger and IP joint flexion of the thumb in a high median nerve palsy restored by tenorrhaphy of the flexor digitorum profundus tendons in the distal forearm and BR to FPL transfer (C and D).

der too much tension, it will result in flexion contractures of these two fingers and significantly impair hand function.

The timing of tendon transfers in a high median nerve palsy remains controversial.[14] If a good primary or delayed primary nerve repair can be performed, there is a reasonable chance of reinnervation of the extrinsic flexor muscles in a young patient. Consequently, "early" BR to FPL or side-to-side repair of the index and long finger profundus tendons to the ring and small finger profundus tendons is not necessary. However, if the patient is seen late and requires secondary nerve grafting of the median nerve, then tendon transfers for restoration of thumb flexion and index and long finger flexion should be performed simultaneously with the nerve graft.

Careful observation of thumb function after either a low- or high-median nerve palsy will reveal whether an "early" tendon transfer for thumb opposition is necessary. The FPB remains innervated by the ulnar nerve in approximately 70% of median nerve injuries so that thumb function may not be significantly compromised.

crease incision and split longitudinally into two slips. The radial lateral bands of the ring and small fingers are approached through radial mid-axial incisions, and each slip of the long finger sublimis tendon is passed down the lumbrical canals of the ring and small fingers. With the wrist in neutral, each slip is sutured to the radial lateral band with the MP joints in 45° of flexion and the IP joints fully extended (Fig. 11-12). Tension is tested using the tenodesis effect of the wrist. Dorsiflexion of the wrist causes the fingers to assume the "intrinsic-plus" position. The hand is immobilized in a dorsal block splint with the wrist in slight flexion and the MP joints flexed 70 degrees for 3½ to 4 weeks. Occasionally, the long finger sublimis may be split into 3 slips should the long, ring, and small fingers need correction. With a total intrinsic palsy the sublimis tendons to the long and ring fingers are each divided into two slips and passed down the lumbrical canals to the radial lateral bands of the index long, ring, and small fingers. Brand advocates insertion of the slip to the index finger into the ulnar lateral band to provide improved three-point pinch. However, this may result in scissoring of the index and long fingers.

The disadvantages of the modified Stiles-Bunnell transfer are that the ring finger sublimis is not expendable in a high ulnar nerve palsy or a combined median-ulnar nerve palsy. Second, the transfer may result in progressive overcorrection of the claw deformity, eventually resulting in "swan-neck" hyperextension of the PIP joints. The modified Stiles-Bunnell transfer should therefore only be used in patients with mild PIP joint flexion contractures or stable fingers without passive hyperextension at the PIP joints.

Brand ECRL and ECRB transfers[5,6,8]

In an extensive series of intrinsic transfers performed in leprosy patients, Brand has convincingly documented increased grip strength. The ECRL with four plantaris tendon grafts are passed through the lumbrical canals to the radial lateral bands of the long, ring, and small fingers and to the ulnar side of the index finger into the ulnar lateral band (Fig. 11-13, A). Two short transverse incisions are made over the second dorsal extensor tendon compartment and over the radial aspect of the mid forearm to allow transection of the ECRL tendon, which is withdrawn into the mid forearm. The tendon is then rerouted around the radial border of the forearm, beneath the BR into a transverse volar forearm incision approximately 2 to 3 inches proximal to the wrist crease. Each half of a folded plantaris tendon graft is then split longitudinally to make four slips and its proximal end sutured to the ECRL tendon, projecting through the volar forearm incision. Through a 3-cm long incision just to the ulnar side of

the thenar crease, tendon-tunneling forceps are passed along the floor of the carpal tunnel to exit on the ulnar side of the volar forearm incision. The four tendon grafts are then pulled distally through the carpal tunnel into the palmar incision. The proximal tendon juncture therefore lies distal to the volar forearm incision but proximal to the transverse carpal ligament. Through radial mid-axial incisions over the proximal phalanges of the long, ring, and small fingers, the tunneling forceps are passed volar to the deep transverse intermetacarpal ligaments through the lumbrical canals into the palmar incision and the three tendon slips brought into each mid-axial incision. The tendon slip to the index finger may be tunneled through the first dorsal interosseous muscle to the radial lateral band[46] or passed through the second intermetacarpal space to the ulnar lateral band as advocated by Brand.[5,6] This will produce supination of the index finger and may provide better three-point pinch. The hand is positioned on a lead frame with the wrist extended 40 degrees, the MP joints flexed 70 degrees, and the IP joints fully extended. After taking up all the slack in the four plantaris grafts, they are sutured to the lateral bands just proximal to the PIP joints and the hand immobilized in this position for 3 weeks.

Brand originally described this intrinsic transfer as a dorsal transfer using the ECRB to activate a four-tailed plantaris graft passed from dorsal to volar through the intermetacarpal spaces (Fig. 11-13, B). The ECRB tendon is transected through a transverse incision overlying the bases of the metacarpals and withdrawn through a dorsal transverse incision at the level of the mid forearm. The four-tailed plantaris graft is sutured to the ECRB tendon and then passed distally into the wrist incision superficial to the extensor retinaculum. This places the proximal tendon juncture in unscarred tissues. The radial lateral band is identified through a mid-axial incision over the proximal phalanx of each finger and the tendon tunneler passed in a distal-to-proximal direction until it is opposite the metacarpal heads. The deep transverse intermetacarpal ligament can be felt by the nose of the tunneler, which is passed volar to the ligament. The fingers are then fully flexed and the tunneler directed dorsally through the intermetacarpal spaces into the dorsal wrist incision. Each tendon graft can be pulled distally through the intermetacarpal spaces into the mid-axial incisions. When making the tunnel to the small finger, the tunneler should be passed volar to the deep transverse intermetacarpal ligament between the ring and small finger metacarpal heads and then passed through the intermetacarpal space between the long and ring finger metacarpals. The graft to the index finger can either be tunneled through the first dorsal interosseous muscle

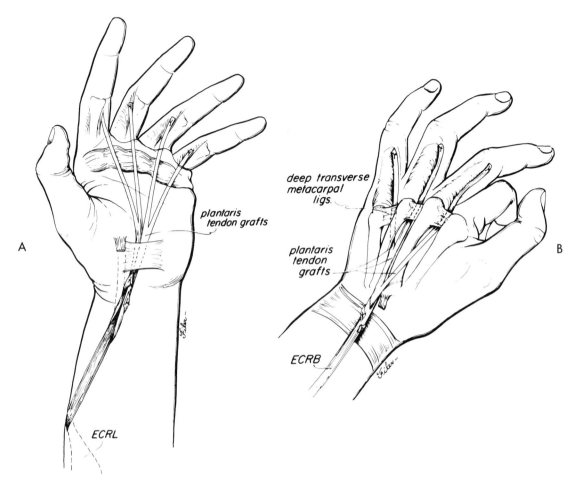

Fig. 11-13 A, Brand transfer of ECRL elongated with a 4 tailed plantaris tendon graft to restore MP joint flexion and IP joint extension. **B,** Dorsal route of the original Brand transfer using ECRB to correct clawing of the fingers.

to the radial lateral band or, as Brand suggested, through the second intermetacarpal space to the ulnar lateral band. The hand is then positioned on a lead hand with the wrist extended 45 degrees, the MCP joints flexed 90 degrees, and the IP joints extended. Slack is taken up in the four tendon grafts, and they are sutured at the resting tension of the ECRB muscle. The hand is immobilized in this same position in a volar splint for 3 weeks. Relaxation of ECRB and the tendon grafts during wrist extension is a relative disadvantage of this original dorsal routing of the Brand transfer.

Riordan[41] described a similar transfer using the FCR transferred dorsally around the radial border of the forearm and elongated with tendon grafts passed through the intermetacarpal spaces volar to the deep transverse intermetacarpal ligaments to the radial lateral bands. This transfer is mutually beneficial if there is an associated flexion contracture of the wrist. The dorsal route also forms the basis for the Fowler transfer[41] in which the EIP

and EDM tendons are each split longitudinally and passed through the intermetacarpal spaces to the radial lateral bands of the fingers. The EIP tendon controls the index and long fingers and the EDM, the ring and small fingers. Riordan,[22] in a modification of the Fowler transfer, has described splitting only the EIP tendon into two slips and passing them through the third and fourth intermetacarpal spaces to insert into the radial lateral bands to correct clawing of the ring and small fingers.

A variant of the Fowler transfer has been advocated by Blacker, Lister, and Kleinert[2] to correct the ulnar deviation of the small finger (Wartenberg's sign). The ulnar half of extensor digiti minimi (EDM) is detached, passed volar to the deep transverse intermetacarpal ligament, and sutured into the insertion of the radial collateral ligament of the MCP joint on the base of the proximal phalanx. If there is associated clawing of the small finger, it is looped under the A2 pulley and sutured back to itself (Brooks insertion).

Tendon transfers to provide adduction of the thumb

The most successful tendon transfers to restore adduction of the thumb have a transverse direction of pull across the palm, deep to the flexor tendons with insertion into the tendon of adductor pollicis (AP). Littler[24,32] has advocated transfer of the ring finger sublimis deep to the flexor tendons of the index and long fingers parallel to the transverse fibers of the AP into a drill hole just distal to the adductor insertion and has been able to document an increase in pinch strength to 71% of the opposite hand. Smith[45] used the ECRB, extended by a free tendon graft, passed through the second intermetacarpal space, and tunneled deep to the AP toward its insertion. Other tendon transfers to provide adduction of the thumb have included either the BR[38] or ECRL, elongated with a tendon graft and passed through the third intermetacarpal space to the thumb MP joint and the extensor indicis proprius, passed through the second intermetacarpal space. Combined transfers to provide both thumb adduction and index finger abduction have been recommended by splitting the EIP[38] or EDM.[57] Occasionally, arthrodesis of the IP or MCP joints of the thumb may be a simpler alternative to tendon transfers to provide strong key pinch.

Ring finger flexor digitorum sublimis[24,32]

The ring finger FDS tendon is transected between the A1 and A2 pulleys through a short oblique incision at the base of the ring finger. The sublimis tendon is then passed transversely across the palm, deep to the index and long finger flexor tendons to the ulnar aspect of the thumb MCP joint if necessary, using a short incision just to the ulnar side of the thenar crease. The transfer is either sutured to the AP tendon or passed into a drill hole through the proximal phalanx just distal to the adductor insertion and tied over a button. Tension is set with the wrist in neutral and the thumb adducted against the index finger with the sublimis tendon at its resting length. This is then tested so that with palmar flexion of the wrist, the thumb can be passively abducted. Edgerton and Brand[21] have described a variation of this transfer in which the ring finger sublimis is brought through a window in the palmar fascia and then passed subcutaneously to the adductor insertion. Obviously the ring finger cannot be used as an adductor transfer in patients with a high ulnar nerve palsy, since this would deprive the ring finger of its only remaining flexor tendon.

Extensor carpi radialis brevis[45]

The ECRB is transected through a short transverse incision over the second dorsal extensor compartment just distal to the extensor retinaculum and withdrawn through a second transverse incision just proximal to the extensor retinaculum. A small flap is then elevated over the ulnar aspect of the MCP joint of the thumb and a palmaris or plantaris tendon graft sutured to the AP tendon. Through a short transverse incision overlying the proximal third of the second intermetacarpal space, a tendon passer is used to tunnel the tendon graft deep to the AP and then dorsally through the second intermetacarpal space. After passing the tendon graft subcutaneously to the most proximal incision, it is woven into the ECRB tendon with the wrist in neutral and the thumb adducted (Fig. 11-14). Tension is then checked by tenodesis of the wrist. With palmar flexion the thumb should become strongly adducted, whereas dorsiflexion of the wrist should allow easy passive abduction of the thumb. The thumb is immobilized for 3 weeks after surgery, midway between full abduction and full adduction with the wrist in 20° to 30° of dorsiflexion.

Tendon transfers to provide index finger abduction

Restoration of strong index finger abduction is the second component required for a powerful pinch. Bunnell[13] reported transfer of the extensor indicis proprius, extended with a short tendon graft and inserted into the first dorsal interosseous tendon. Bruner[11] divided the EPB tendon over the dorsum of the thumb MCP joint and tunneled it subcutaneously beneath the EPL tendon into the first dorsal interosseous tendon.

Accessory abductor pollicis longus and free tendon graft

Neviaser, Wilson, and Gardner[34] described elongation of an accessory APL tendon with a palmaris or plantaris tendon graft transferred to the insertion of the first dorsal interosseous muscle (Fig. 11-14). A small flap is elevated over the radial aspect of the proximal phalanx of the index finger and the tendon graft sutured to the first dorsal interosseous tendon just distal to the MCP joint. The proximal end of the tendon graft is then passed subcutaneously into a transverse incision over the first dorsal extensor compartment. After opening the compartment, one of the accessory APL tendons that does not insert on the base of the thumb metacarpal is transected and interwoven into the tendon graft with the wrist in neutral and the index finger radially abducted.

HIGH ULNAR NERVE PALSY

Many surgeons fail to realize the significant functional deficit produced in patients with a high ulnar nerve palsy attributable to paralysis of the FCU and

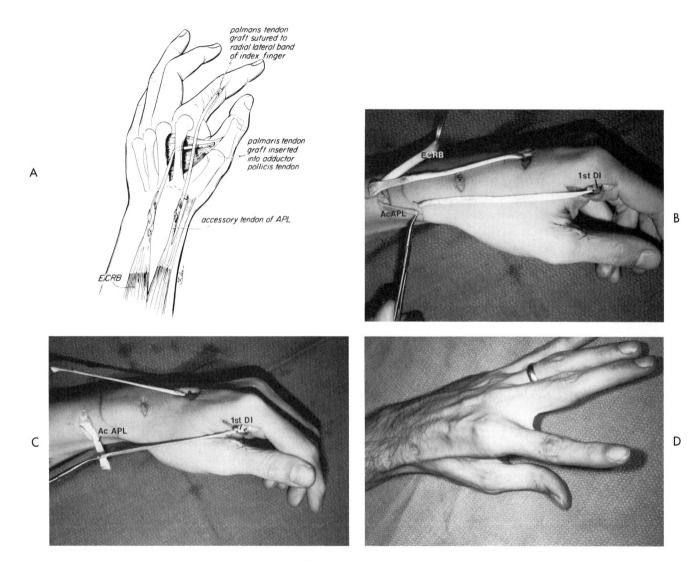

Fig. 11-14 A and **B,** Restoration of power pinch by transfer of ECRB extended by a palmaris tendon graft into the adductor pollicis insertion and transfer of an accessory tendon of APL elongated with a palmaris tendon graft into the first dorsal interosseous. Traction on the tendon grafts intraoperatively **C,** demonstrates the strong adduction of the thumb and abduction of the index finger that can be achieved after surgery **D.**

profundus tendons to the ring and small fingers. The only remaining tendons on the ulnar side of the hand are the sublimis tendon to the ring finger and the usually diminutive sublimis tendon to the small finger. Often, however, paralysis of the profundus tendons to the ring and small fingers will be masked by interconnections between these two tendons and the long finger profundus tendon in the distal forearm. If there is significant weakness of the ring and small fingers, power grip can be restored by side-to-side tenorrhaphy of the ring and small finger profundus tendons to the long finger profundus tendon. The long finger sublimis tendon can also be used as a donor tendon to restore independent profundus function to the ring and small fingers. Patients requiring strong ulnar deviation and flexion of the wrist may also require transfer of the FCR tendon to FCU.

CONCLUSION

Tendon transfers, if selected carefully and performed meticulously, can provide a gratifying improvement in function to the hand affected by radial, median, or ulnar nerve palsy.

REFERENCES

1. Bevin AG: Early tendon transfer for radial nerve transection, Hand 8:134, 1976.
2. Blacker GJ, Lister GD, and Kleinert HE: The abducted little finger in low ulnar nerve palsy, J Hand Surg 1:190, 1976.
3. Boyes JH: Tendon transfers for radial palsy, Bull Hosp Joint Dis 21:97, 1960.
4. Brand PW: Paralytic claw hand with special reference to paralysis in leprosy and treatment by the sublimis transfer of Stiles and Bunnell, J Bone Joint Surg 40B:618, 1958.
5. Brand PW: Tendon grafting illustrated by a new operation for intrinsic paralysis of the fingers, J Bone Joint Surg 43B:444, 1961.
6. Brand PW: Tendon transfers for median and ulnar nerve paralysis, Orthopedic Clin North Am 1:447, 1970.
7. Brand PW, Beach RB, and Thompson DE: Relative tension and potential excursion of muscles in the forearm and hand, J Hand Surg 6:209, 1981.
8. Brand PW: Clinical mechanics of the hand, St. Louis, 1985, The CV Mosby Co.
9. Braun RM: Palmaris longus tendon transfer for augmentation of the thenar musculature in low median nerve palsy, J Hand Surg 3:488, 1978.
10. Brooks AL and Jones DS: A new intrinsic tendon transfer for the paralytic hand, J Bone Joint Surg 57A:730, 1975.
11. Bruner JM: Tendon transfer to restore abduction of the index finger using the extensor pollicis brevis, Plast Reconstr Surg 3:197, 1948.
12. Bunnell S: Opposition of the thumb, J Bone Joint Surg 20:269, 1938.
13. Bunnell S: Surgery of the intrinsic muscles of the hand other than those producing opposition of the thumb, J Bone Joint Surg 24:1, 1942.
14. Burkhalter WE: Early tendon transfer in upper extremity peripheral nerve injury, Clin Orthop 104:68, 1974.
15. Burkhalter W, Christensen RC, and Brown P: Extensor indicis proprius opponensplasty, J Bone Joint Surg 55A:725, 1973.
16. Burkhalter WE and Strait JL: Metacarpo-phalangeal flexor replacement for intrinsic muscle paralysis, J Bone Joint Surg 55A:1667, 1973.
17. Camitz H: Ueber die Behandlung der Opposition-Slahmung, Acta Chir Scand 65:77, 1929.
18. Chuinard RG et al: Tendon transfers for radial nerve palsy: use of superficialis tendons for digital extension, J Hand Surg 3:560, 1978.
19. Cooney WP, Linscheid RL, and An KN: Opposition of the thumb: an anatomic and biomechanical study of tendon transfers, J Hand Surg 9A:777, 1984.
20. Dunn N: Treatment of lesion of the musculo-spiral nerve in military surgery, Am J Orthoped Surg 16:258, 1918.
21. Edgerton MT and Brand PW: Restoration of abduction and adduction to the unstable thumb in median and ulnar paralysis, Plast Reconstr Surg 36:150, 1965.
22. Enna CD and Riordan DC: The Fowler procedure for correction of the paralytic claw hand, Plast Reconstr Surg 52:352, 1973.
23. Fowler BS: Extensor apparatus of the digits, J Bone Joint Surg 31B:477, 1949.
24. Hamlin C and Littler JW: Restoration of power pinch, J Hand Surg 5:396, 1980.
25. Henderson ED: Transfer of wrist extensors and brachioradialis to restore opposition of the thumb, J Bone Joint Surg 44A:513, 1962.
26. Huber E: Hilfsoperation bei Medianus Slahmung, Dtsch Z Chir 126:271, 1921.
27. Jacobs B and Thompson TC: Opposition of the thumb and its restoration, J Bone Joint Surg 42A:1015, 1960.
28. Jones R: On suture of nerves and alternative methods of treatment by transplantation of tendon, Brit Med J 1:679, 1916.
29. Jones R: Tendon transplantation in cases of musculospiral injuries not amenable to suture, Am J Surg 35:333, 1921.
30. Littler JW and Li CS: Primary restoration of thumb opposition with median nerve decompression, Plast Reconstr Surg 39:74, 1967.
31. Littler JW and Cooley SGE: Opposition of the thumb and its restoration by abductor digiti quinti transfer, J Bone Joint Surg 45A:1389, 1963.
32. Littler JW: Tendon transfers and arthrodeses in combined median and ulnar nerve paralysis, J Bone Joint Surg 31A:225, 1949.
33. Moberg E and Nachemson A: Tendon transfers for defective long extensors of the wrist and fingers, Acta Chir Scand 133:31, 1967.
34. Neviaser RJ, Wilson JN, and Gardner MM: Abductor pollicis longus transfer for replacement of the first dorsal interosseous, J Hand Surg 5:53, 1980.
35. Nicolaysen J: Transplantation des M Abductor Dig V bei fehlender Oppositionsfahigkeit des Daumens. Dtsch Z Chir 168:133, 1922.
36. North ER and Littler JW: Transferring the flexor superficialis tendon: technical considerations in the prevention of proximal interphalangeal joint disability, J Hand Surg 5:498, 1980.
37. Omer GE: The technique and timing of tendon transfers, Orthoped Clin North Am 5:243, 1974.
38. Omer GE: Evaluation and reconstruction of the forearm and hand after acute traumatic peripheral nerve injuries, J Bone Joint Surg 50A:1454, 1968.
39. Parkes A: Paralytic claw fingers-a graft tenodesis operation, Hand 5:192, 1973.
40. Phalen GS and Miller RG: The transfer of wrist extensor muscles to restore or reinforce flexion power of the fingers and opposition of the thumb, J Bone Joint Surg 29:993, 1947.
41. Riordan DC: Tendon transplantations in median nerve and ulnar nerve paralysis, J Bone Joint Surg 35A:312, 1953.
42. Royle ND: An operation for paralysis of the intrinsic muscles of the thumb, JAMA 111:612, 1938.

43. Schneider LH: Opponensplasty using the extensor digiti minimi, J Bone Joint Surg 51A:1297, 1969.

44. Scuderi C: Tendon transplants for irreparable radial nerve paralysis, SGO 88:643, 1949.

45. Smith RJ: Extensor carpi radialis brevis tendon transfer for thumb adduction—a study of power pinch, J Hand Sur 8:4, 1983.

46. Smith RJ: Tendon transfers of the hand and forearm, Boston, 1987, Little, Brown & Co.

47. Snow JW and Fink GH: Use of a transverse carpal ligament window for the pulley in tendon transfers for median nerve palsy, Plast Reconstr Surg 48:238, 1971.

48. Starr CL: Army experiences with tendon transference, J Bone Joint Surg 4:3, 1922.

49. Steindler A: Tendon transplantation in the upper extremity, Am J Surg 44:260,534, 1939.

50. Taylor RT: Reconstruction of the hand: a new technique in tenoplasty, SGO 32:237, 1921.

51. Thompson M and Rasmussen KB: Tendon transfers for defective long extensors of the wrist and fingers, Scand J Plast Reconstr Surg 3:71, 1969.

52. Thompson TC: A modified operation for opponens paralysis, J Bone Joint Surg 24:632, 1942.

53. Tsuge K and Adachi N: Tendon transfer for extensor palsy of forearm, Hiroshima J Med Sci 18:219, 1969.

54. Zachary RB: Tendon transplantation for radial paralysis, Br J Surg 23:350, 1946.

55. Zancolli EA: Claw hand caused by paralysis of the intrinsic muscles: a simple surgical procedure for its correction, J Bone Joint Surg 39A:1076,1957.

56. Zancolli E: Structural and dynamic bases of hand surgery, ed 2, Philadelphia, 1979, JB Lippincott Co.

57. Zweig J, Rosenthal S, and Burns H: Transfer of the extensor digiti quinti to restore pinch in ulnar palsy of the hand, J Bone Joint Surg 54A:51, 1972.

CHAPTER 12

Soft Tissue Coverage of the Upper Extremity: Flaps and Tissue Transfer

Hani S. Matloub
N. John Yousif

Soft tissue coverage of the upper extremity is an extensively developed area of reconstructive surgery that has evolved over many years.

Soft tissue deficits usually have functional and cosmetic consequences, and proper management should affect both positively. An optimal outcome is achieved if the surgeon gives detailed attention to the problem in all of its preoperative, operative, and postoperative phases, both at the donor and recipient sites.

GENERAL CONSIDERATIONS

By definition, the various forms of soft tissue coverage exclude any deep structural bone or muscle reconstruction. Simple soft tissue coverage includes random flaps, axial flaps from the hand and forearm, and microsurgical transfers. The goals of hand coverage include appropriate matching of the lost tissue for sensory potential, skin color, functional potential such as glabrous skin, and appropriate contour in the palm and dorsum of the hand. Other considerations that influence the choice of reconstructive technique include limiting donor-site morbidity, choosing the simplest procedure with the highest success rate, and choosing procedures that facilitate postoperative therapy.

Certainly there are many options, some of which are nonsurgical. For example, a small area of tissue deficit where underlying structures are not in danger can be closed by secondary intention, usually in an area limited to 1 cm.[2]

Skin grafts, either split or full thickness, may be the appropriate choice if skin loss has occurred while preserving vascularized subcutaneous tissue. Full-thickness grafts provide better protection, better color match, less recipient site contraction, and a better potential for sensory reinnervation. Split-thickness skin grafts are useful in areas where the recipient site is not well vascularized. They may also allow for gradual diminution of the size of the defect as they contract with time, but they do not allow for sensory reinnervation as readily as full-thickness grafts, and color changes are more frequent.

SPECIFIC FLAPS AND THEIR USES

In situations where skin and subcutaneous tissue loss leave a poorly vascularized bed or where important structures are exposed, tissue transfer that imports its own blood supply is required.

Local random flaps

Local random flaps include Z-plasties, local transposition, and other types of rotation and advancement flaps from around the hand. Usually, the transposition flaps take skin from the surrounding tissue, while maintaining a wide base to perfuse the flap on the subdermal plexus. The donor site is either closed primarily or covered with skin grafts.

One of the disadvantages of this type of flap is that the surrounding tissue frequently is injured and is used for transfer. These flaps usually can cover only small defects, and the donor site must frequently be grafted.

Local advancement flaps

Several types of local advancement flaps are possible, including a volar flap and paired, or single, lateral advancement flaps. These flaps are ideal for small fingertip injuries with exposed bone. The direction of injury frequently guides the type of flap that can be used. Lateral advancement flaps are most applicable when there is residual tissue laterally. The Atasoy-Kleinert palmar advancement flap is indicated when there is residual palmar tissue. Both volar and lateral advancement flaps do not provide adequate movement to cover straight transverse amputations or fingertip injuries angled so that the volar side is shorter than the dorsal side.

Examples of Atasoy flaps are in Figs. 12-1 and 12-2.

Points to remember
1. Crossing the palmar crease is not contraindicated.
2. Tourniquet control and adequate magnification are needed while raising the flap.
3. Release of all septi and deep connections allows the greatest flap movement.

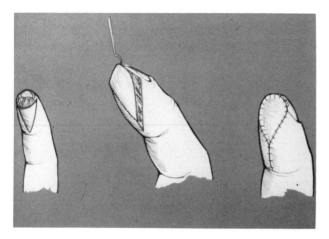

Fig. 12-1 The diagram shows advancement of a Atasoy-Kleinert palmar advancement flap. It is important to isolate and remove all the septi and deep connections to allow movement of the flap.

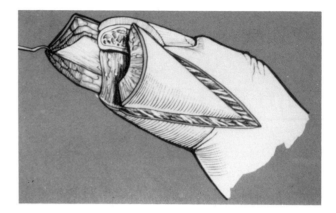

Fig. 12-2 Example of elevation of a Kutler flap. These flaps are applicable when there is excess tissue lateral to the injury.

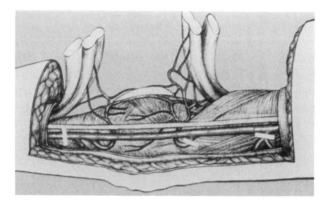

Fig. 12-3 Shows the dorsal branches to the skin of the middle phalanx. Ligatures on the dorsal branches to the proximal phalanx and PIP joint were placed and injections given through the digital artery. The dorsal branch shows its territorial perfusion.

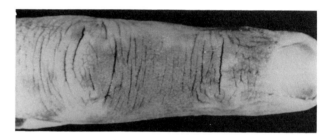

Fig. 12-4 The dark area shows the territory of the dorsal branch perfusing the cross finger flap.

4. Excessive tension must be avoided.
5. The volar V-to-Y advancement flap should have a wide body, but distally the flap should not be greater than the nail width.

Disadvantages
1. Only small areas can be covered.
2. Scar tissue may result over the palmar aspect of the fingertip.

Cross finger flap

The cross finger flap is useful when remaining palmar and lateral tissue are not available. In these cases, tissue transfer from the dorsal surface of one finger to the palmar or dorsal surface of another finger is advantageous. The blood supply to the cross finger flap, ini-

tially considered random, is in most cases provided by a branch of the palmar digital artery (Fig. 12-3). This vessel is usually located approximately 0.8 cm distal to the proximal interphalangeal (PIP) joint. The base of a cross finger flap need only include this vessel. Injections directly into this vessel showed complete coloration of the skin overlying the middle phalanx (Fig. 12-4).

The operative technique of the cross finger flap is shown in Fig. 12-5. It is important to maintain peritenon over the extensor tendon of the donor finger and to immobilize the involved digits to allow complete acceptance of a skin graft to the donor site. Limited, controlled postoperative mobilization and therapy is useful to maintain some mobility of the surrounding joints. Innervation of the flap has also been described and is possible by harvesting the contralateral dorsal branch of one digital nerve and suturing it to one of the digital nerves in the recipient finger.

Points to remember
1. Preservation of peritenon over the donor finger extensor tendon is essential.
2. A distal cutback is possible for more mobility.
3. Color match is improved by using upper extremity skin as the donor site.

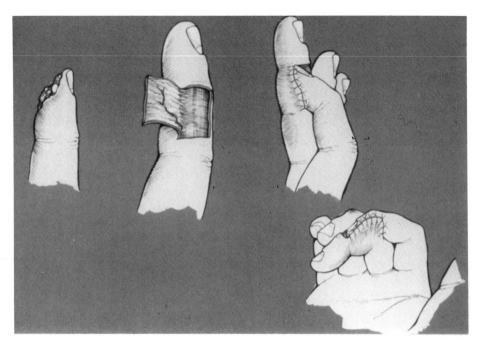

Fig. 12-5 The sequence of elevation of the cross finger flap is shown. It is important to preserve the perfusing vessels and the peritenon overlying the extensor tendon.

4. Flap innervation is possible.
5. Postoperative immobilization is important.
6. Division of the flap may be performed as early as 10 days after surgery.

Disadvantages
1. There is often inappropriate tissue match.
2. Poor color match may be more obvious in darker skinned patients.
3. A skin graft is required for the donor site, which can produce scarring, skin discoloration, and an area of depression on the dorsal surface of the digit.

Thenar flap

The thenar flap provides glabrous skin to the injured fingertip, while allowing primary closure of the donor site. The flap is usually suitable for fingertip injuries where local advancement flaps are not adequate for coverage.

Usually the flap is elevated as a radially based flap with primary closure at the base of the thumb (Figs. 12-6 and 12-7). Other designs may be used that simplify inset while still allowing primary closure.

Points to remember
1. The use of a tourniquet and magnification is advisable.
2. The digital nerves to the thumb are quite superficial and must be avoided during flap elevation.
3. The flap should be designed to avoid acute flexion of the PIP and MP joints of the finger.

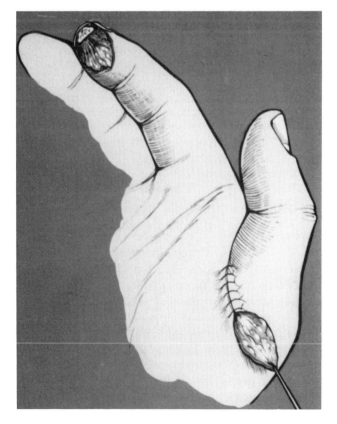

Fig. 12-6 The thenar flap is usually based radially at the base of the thumb to allow primary closure.

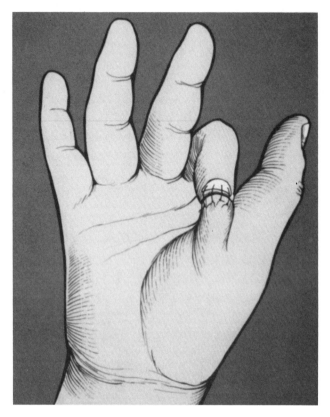

Fig. 12-7 Transposition to the injured finger should avoid excessive angulation of the metacarpal, phalangeal, and PIP joints.

4. The injured finger must be held in a flexed position with a splint.

Disadvantages
1. A stiff finger can result from prolonged immobilization in older patients.
2. Donor scar can be sensitive.
3. There can be lack of fingertip volume after surgery (Fig. 12-8).

Moberg advancement flap

This flap is used primarily to cover thumb tip amputations. The ideal patient has a soft tissue defect not exceeding 1.5 cm². Bilateral midaxial line incisions are used to elevate the volar skin, subcutaneous tissue, and both neurovascular bundles of the thumb at the level of the flexor tendon sheath. Dorsal branches of the digital arteries along the proximal phalanx should be identified and spared to prescribe blood supply to the dorsal surface of the thumb. The flap is advanced distally while flexing the thumb into the palm and resurfacing the tip defect with innervated glabrous skin (Fig. 12-9). Active extension exercises are initiated by 2 weeks.

Additional flap advancement can be obtained by in-

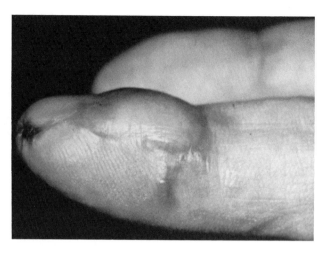

Fig. 12-8 An example of the pin-cushion effect.

cising the skin at the base of the flap, creating an island flap on both neurovascular pedicles. This can be devised as a V-Y advancement flap with primary closure of the donor site.

Points to remember
1. This flap should only be used for thumb defects.
2. Further advancement is possible as an island pedicle flap.

Disadvantages
1. There is limited advancement.
2. A flexion contracture can occur at the IP joint.
3. Dorsal thumb skin loss can occur if the dorsal vascular branches are not preserved.

Neurovascular island pedicle flap

A neurovascular island pedicle flap from the volar surface of an adjoining finger provides sensate glabrous skin closely resembling that lost on the pulp defect. This flap is transfered from one side of a finger to another digit or the thumb on one neurovascular bundle. If the recipient site is the thumb, one would usually attempt to take an area innervated by the median nerve, most likely the ulnar aspect of the middle finger. During dissection, the surgeon isolates one digital artery and nerve along with some surrounding soft tissue to provide venous drainage. The flap is then rotated in the palm and transferred to the other digit (Fig. 12-10). It is important to avoid any tension on the neurovascular bundle, which has been implicated in a slow decrease in the quality of sensibility to the flap. The common distal nerve must be dissected under magnification, proximally to avoid tension. The patency of the other distal artery in the donor and the adjacent finger must be determined with an Allen's test before flap transfer. The donor site is covered with a skin graft.

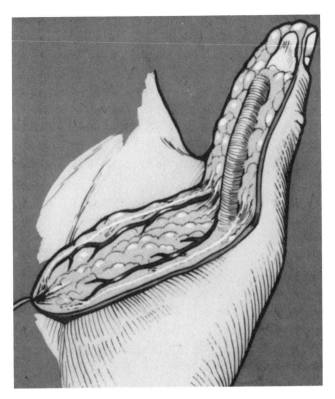

Fig. 12-9 Elevation of the Moberg flap is performed through bilateral midaxial incisions elevating both the subcutaneous tissue and the neurovascular bundles.

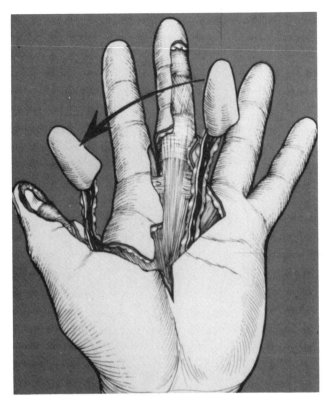

Fig. 12-10 Elevation of the neurovascular island pedicle is performed on the nonfunctional side of the digit. It is important to maintain soft tissue around the neurovascular bundle to allow venous outflow.

Points to remember

1. A digital Allen's test of the donor and adjacent finger ensures their blood flow after flap transfer.
2. The flap is usually taken from the ulnar side of the middle finger.
3. The flap must maintain soft tissue around the pedicle for venous drainage.
4. Lengthening of the nerve is important to permit flap inset without tension.

Disadvantages

1. There is often donor site depression.
2. Loss of tip sensibility on one side of the donor digit is probable.
3. Sensory reeducation is difficult in adults.
4. Venous drainage may be impaired.

Metacarpal flaps

Metacarpal flaps provide local coverage for soft tissue defects of the hand. These flaps are based on one of the dorsal metacarpal arteries, either in antegrade or retrograde fashion. The most reliable arteries dorsally are the first, second, and at times, the third dorsal metacarpal artery. The first and second metacarpal artery flaps are most frequently used. The metacarpal vessels originate from either the radial artery, the dor-

sal metacarpal arch, or at times, from the deep palmar arch. The metacarpal arteries usually course deep to the level of the extensor tendons and follow the midaxial line of the interosseous spaces toward the web space (Fig. 12-11). The vessels divide at the level of the web space into branches that run along the dorsal aspects of the two fingers adjacent to that web. Just distal to the metacarpophalangeal (MP) joint, the metacarpal arteries frequently connect to the palmar vascular system through a web space connecting vessel (Fig. 12-12).

Operative technique

The skin island is designed over the interosseous space (Fig. 12-13). The flap length may encompass the entire length of the interosseous space, while the width is usually designed to allow primary donor site closure. An incision is made along the ulnar border of the planned flap and is carried down to the fascia of the dorsal interosseous muscle. The deep fascia is included within the flap, and the metacarpal artery is identified and dissected free. The dissection then proceeds from proximal to distal or from distal to proximal, depending on the direction of elevation. The donor site can usually be closed primarily.

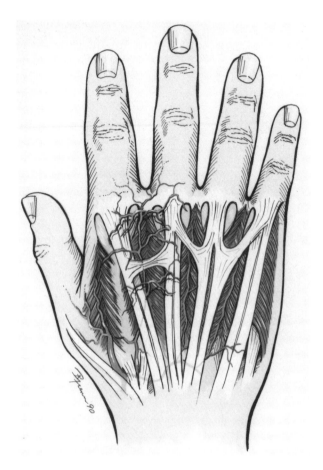

Fig. 12-11   The metacarpal arteries take a course deep to the level to the extensor tendons and follow the midaxial line of the interroseous spaces toward the web space.

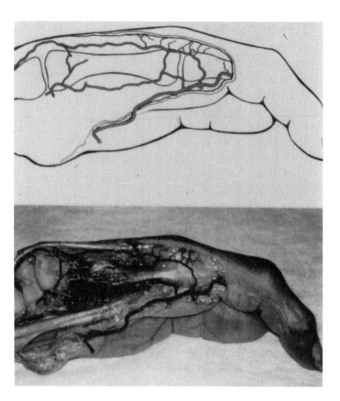

Fig. 12-12   The distal connections of the metacarpal arteries to the palmar systems allow elevation in a retrograde fashion for distal finger coverage.

The arc of rotation of the second dorsal metacarpal artery allows coverage of dorsal defects on the index or middle finger to the level of the proximal third of the middle phalanx and of the proximal phalanx on the volar surface (Fig. 12-14).

Points to remember

1. A doppler probe may not always identify the dorsal metacarpal arteries before surgery.
2. The cutaneous branches of the second dorsal metacarpal artery are found just after the artery emerges from underneath the extensor indicis tendon, an area that should be protected.
3. The connection of the second dorsal metacarpal artery, located approximately 1 cm from the web space, must be preserved when elevating a reverse flap.
4. The vessel may lie deep to the fascia and at times be surrounded by a small portion of muscle.
5. Preservation of donor-site peritenon is important for vascularization of the subsequent skin grafts.

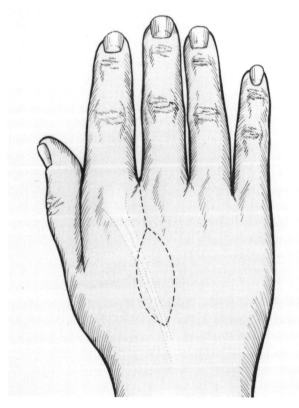

Fig. 12-13   The skin is designed over the interroseous space.

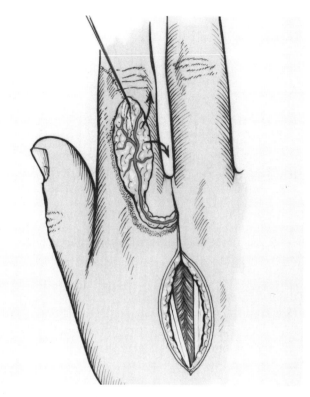

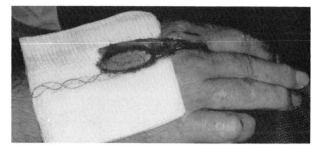

Fig. 12-15   A distally based flap on the dorsal metacarpal artery shown ready for transfer to cover a defect on the palmar side of the proximal phalanx.

Fig. 12-14   The arch of distal rotation of the second dorsal metacarpal artery allows coverage of defects of the index or middle fingers at the level of the proximal third of the middle phalanx dorsally and of the proximal phalanx palmarly.

Disadvantages

1. There may be anatomical variation in the blood supply.
2. Tissue may be hair bearing.
3. Arch of rotation may be limited.

   Examples of proximally and distally based flaps for coverage of various problems of the hand are shown in Figs. 12-15 to 12-18.

Radial forearm flap

The radial forearm flap can be used either as a reverse or axial pattern flap for coverage of soft tissue defects of the hand and forearm. This flap is based on the radial artery and its venae comitantes. An Allen's test should be performed before elevating the flap to assess the completeness of the palmar arch and the adequacy of ulnar artery blood flow to the hand. The venous outflow in a reversed flap is provided by a crossover or bridging between the two venae comitantes. For that reason, it is important to include at least one or two superficial veins.

Points to remember

1. Perform an Allen's test of both the radial and ulnar arteries.

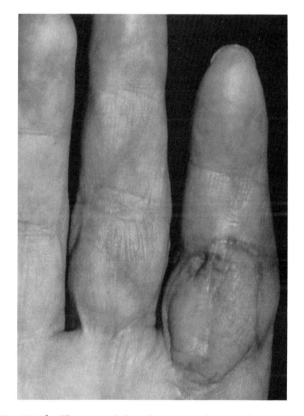

Fig. 12-16   The second dorsal metacarpal artery flap is healed approximately 4 months after surgery.

2. Peritenon over the flexor tendons must be maintained.
3. Superficial veins must be included in the reverse flap.
4. The radial forearm flap may be used as a fascial flap.

Disadvantages

1. Loss of the radial artery is probable.
2. The skin-grafted donor site is visible
3. Venous congestion is possible with the reverse flap.

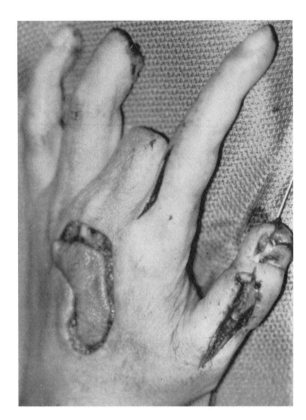

Fig. 12-17   An exposed bone graft is seen over the proximal phalanx of the left thumb and a proximally based second dorsal metacarpal artery flap is shown elevated and ready for transfer.

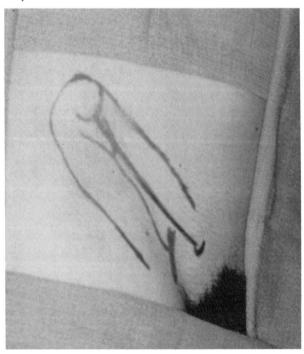

Fig. 12-19   The groin flap is based on the superficial circumflexed iliac artery, which leaves the femoral artery approximately 2.5 cm distal to the inguinal ligament.

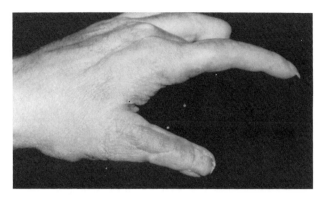

Fig. 12-18   The flap was tunneled beneath the extensor tendons of the index finger and put into place over the proximal phalanx of the thumb. The flap is healed approximately 6 months after surgery.

Distant flaps

Distant pedicle flaps, which can be used to cover hand defects, include groin flaps, cross arm flaps, chest flaps, and abdominal flaps. The groin flap is an axial pattern flap based on the superficial circumflex femoral artery and is most commonly used. This vessel leaves the femoral artery approximately 2.5 cm distal to the inguinal ligament and courses laterally over the sartorius muscle. A large amount of tissue can be elevated, lengthening the flap laterally past the anterior superior iliac spine as a nonaxial random extension. The flap can be thinned in its distal portion to improve the contour on the recipient site. Primary donor-site closure is possible, creating a well-hidden donor site scar in the groin (Figs. 12-19 to 12-23).

Advantages
1. The donor-site scar is hidden.
2. There is axial perfusion.
3. The distant pedicle flaps can cover large areas.
4. There is primary donor-site closure.

Disadvantages
1. There is excessive bulk.
2. There is often poor skin color match.
3. Dependent hand position occurs after surgery.
4. There is prolonged immobilization.

MICROVASCULAR FREE TISSUE TRANSFER

Various kinds of free tissue transfers have been described that allow the surgeon to tailor the transferred tissue to the requirements of the recipient site. Cutaneous flaps, fascial flaps, muscle flaps, and bone flaps are all available.

The cutaneous flaps most frequently used include the lateral arm, scapular, deltoid, dorsalis pedis, and sole of the foot area.

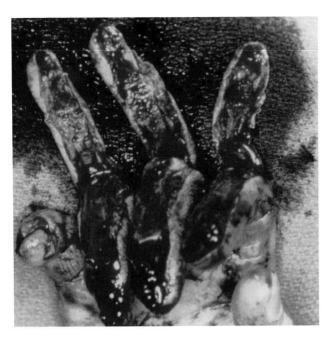

Fig. 12-20   Injury from a band saw to the dorsum of the index, middle, and ring fingers.

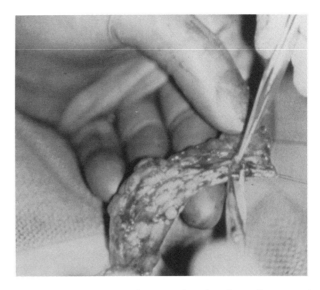

Fig. 12-21   Thinning of the groin flap distally at the time of elevation may allow better final contour while still maintaining perfusion.

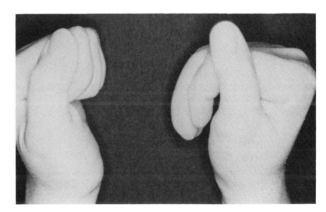

Fig. 12-23   Results of range of motion are seen 8 months after surgery and one extensor tendon release and one defatting procedure.

Lateral arm flap

The tissue overlying the lateral portion of the upper arm is supplied by the posterior radial collateral artery (Fig. 12-24). This vascular pedicle can be used to elevate a flap with a wide variety of designs, which can include skin, fascia, muscle, and bone.

The skin overlying the lateral arm varies in thickness. The distal skin overlying the lateral humeral epicondyle and the elbow in most individuals is quite thin. The skin is mobile and allows primary closure of deficits measuring up to 7 cm in width.

The flap vessels course in the lateral intermuscular septum between the triceps muscle posteriorly and the brachialis muscle anteriorly. Branches to the skin perforate the intermuscular septum and follow either a di-

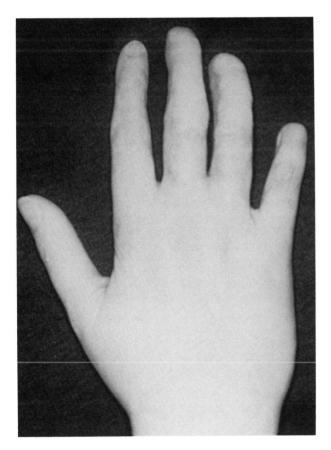

Fig. 12-22   The healed groin flap is seen over the dorsal aspect of the middle and ring fingers.

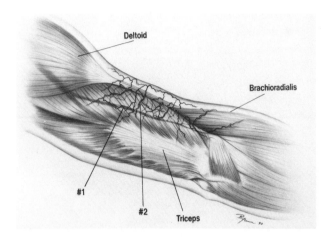

Fig. 12-24 This drawing represents a posterior view of the lateral arm. The posterior radial collateral artey (1) is shown as a shaded vessel in the lateral intermuscular septum. The main fascial cutaneous branch, (2) which exits at approximately 10 cm proximal to the lateral humeral epicondyle is also represented.

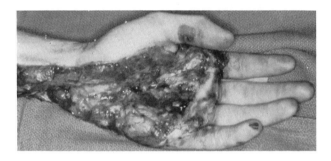

Fig. 12-26 After a grinder injury to the left palmar aspect of the hand and forearm, this patient required tendon grafts and soft tissue coverage.

rect course to the dermis or course as fascial branches, which then perfuse both the fascia and the overlying skin. The flap artery originates from the profunda brachia and has an external diameter ranging from 0.75 to 1.5 mm.

The upper portion of the flap is innervated by the antebrachial cutaneous nerve of the arm, while the antebrachial cutaneous nerve of the forearm provides innervation more distally.

Operative technique

The patient is placed in the supine position with the donor arm positioned over the chest.

The lateral intermuscular septum is identified by palpation. A point 10 cm cephalad to the lateral humeral epicondyle, over the intermuscular septum, commonly marks the location of the dominant fasciocutaneous branch in adults. The lateral intermuscular sep-

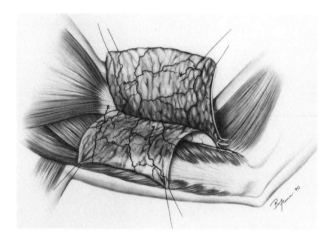

Fig. 12-25 This diagram shows the possible separation of the fascia from the subcutaneous portion of the flap.

tum represents the axis of the flap and the cutaneous paddle is centered over this area. The paddle may be moved superiorly or inferiorly along the axis depending on the amount and quality of skin desired. The use of a sterile tourniquet allows the dissection to proceed within a dry field.

The dissection is carried down to the subfascial layer over the triceps muscle and then is directed anteriorly, separating the fascia from the underlying muscle. The vessels are usually visible within the fascia at this point and can be followed behind the humerus to their origin from the profunda brachi at the base of the intermuscular septum. Care must be taken proximally to prevent injury to the radial nerve, which lies just anterior to the vascular pedicle for a short distance before entering the space between the brachialis and brachioradialis muscles.

One advantage of the lateral arm flap is that because of separate vascular leashes, its component parts can be separated and combined as necessary. Fascial flaps alone may be harvested; a sandwich flap can be made by separating fascia from skin (Fig. 12-25); anterior or posterior muscle may be included; a portion of underlying humerus may be taken; and a portion of the triceps tendon can be used. An example of a large lateral arm free flap is shown in Figures 12-26 to 12-28.

Advantages
1. The pedicle is reliable.
2. The pedicle is long.
3. There is primary donor-site closure.
4. The flap is thin.
5. Innervation is possible.
6. Composite flaps are possible.
7. Tourniquet may be used.

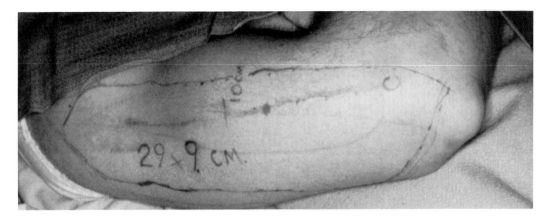

Fig. 12-27 A 29 × 9 cm lateral arm free flap was planned for the soft tissue coverage.

Disadvantages

1. Forearm nerves must be sacrificed, resulting in some loss of forearm skin sensation.
2. The lateral arm flap may be thick in some patients.
3. The diameter pedicle is small.
4. The procedure leaves an obvious scar.

Medial arm flap

A fasciocutaneous flap, which can be elevated from the medial arm, leaves a well-hidden scar. This area has been overlooked clinically because of the anatomical variations in its vascular supply. This area provides a reliable source of tissue that allows good color match for the head and neck with thin hairless skin and leaves a well-positioned donor-site scar.

Skin

The skin on the medial aspect of the upper arm in most patients is thin, quite mobile, and allows primary closure of 6 to 8 cm deficits. This area is relatively hairless in most people.

The cutaneous innervation of this flap is by the medial brachial cutaneous nerve, which runs in the subcutaneous tissue along the posterior margin of the flap.

Blood supply

The blood supply to the medial arm skin comes from a combination of vessels originating along the course of the brachial artery (Fig. 12-29). The superior ulnar collateral artery is the dominant flap vessel in 80% of patients. In the remaining 20%, either a direct cutaneous or musculocutaneous branch from the brachial artery assumes the dominant role.

When present, the superior ulnar collateral artery originates from either the profunda brachi (60%) or the brachial artery (40%). The artery accompanies the ulnar nerve along its course, giving direct cutaneous or fasciocutaneous branches to the overlying skin.

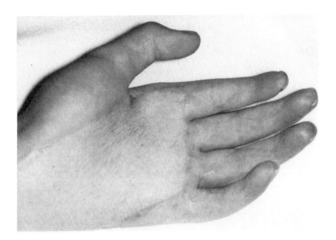

Fig. 12-28 The healed lateral arm free flap is noted, showing excellent contour at 6 months after surgery.

The primary venous drainage of this flap is through the venae comitantes, which accompany the dominant flap artery. A second drainage system does exist from the basilic vein.

Flap elevation

A line is drawn from the medial epicondyle to the posterior axial line. This forms the axis of the flap. If the upper medial arm is divided into quarters, the flap lies within the middle two quarters along this central axis.

Incisions begin at the anterior margin of the proposed skin ellipse. The dissection is carried down to the subfascial level and the flap is elevated toward the medial intermuscular septum, which separates the biceps and the medial head of the triceps muscles. Once this area is reached, the surgeon stops and takes time to determine which of the cutaneous vessels is domi-

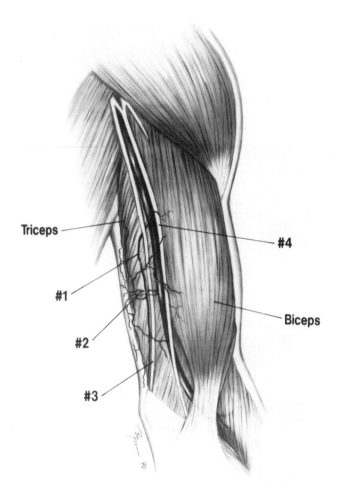

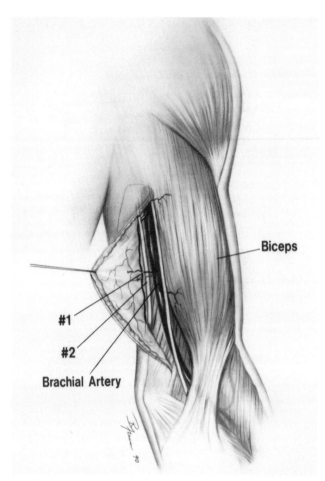

Fig. 12-29 This diagram of the medial arm area shows the superior ulnar collateral artery *(1)*, a cutaneous branch of the brachial artery *(2)*, the ulnar nerve, and *(3 and 4)*, the median nerve.

Fig. 12-30 Initial elevation of the flap is performed by an anterior incision elevated posteriorly, at which point the surgeon examines the blood supplied to the skin and determines which is the dominant vessel. The superior ulnar collateral artery is seen here *(1)* with its relationship to the ulnar nerve *(2)*.

nant and thus appropriate for use as a donor (Fig. 12-30). The artery and its accompanying venae comitantes are then carefully dissected from the brachial artery and the ulnar nerve. The lateral and posterior incisions are then completed and the flap is ready for transfer.

Advantages

1. The donor site is hidden.
2. The flap is thin.
3. There is some potential for innervation.
4. The skin is usually hairless.

Disadvantages

1. There are always anatomical variations.
2. The vessels are small.
3. The pedicle is short.

SUMMARY

The choice of reconstructive options is usually dictated by the needs of the recipient site. It is not appro-

priate to simply replace missing tissue by "filling the defect." The recipient site must be reconstructed with the simplest procedure that as closely as possible provides the structural and functional components required. It also important to remember that the hand is an aesthetic unit considered by many people to be an important part of social interaction. Therefore the final result must also be an aesthetic reconstruction.

The choice of donor sites depends on the following considerations:

1. Availability of tissue needed at the recipient site.
2. The skin quality: thin or thick, hair bearing, and color.
3. Vascular anatomy: source of perfusion, ease of dissection, pedicle length and size, and frequency of anatomical variation.
4. Tissue combinations: Can the various types of required tissue be harvested from one donor site?

5. Functional requirements at the recipient site: Is innervation needed; Is glabrous skin required; Is resistance to shearing forces necessary?

REFERENCES

1. Allen MJ: Conservative management of fingertip injuries in adults, Hand 12:257, 1980.
2. Atasoy E et al: Reconstruction of the amputated fingertip with a triangular volar flap, J Bone Joint Surg 52A:921, 1970.
3. Barton NJ: A modified thenar flap, Hand 7:150, 1975.
4. Beasley RW: Principles and techniques of resurfacing operations for hand surgery, Surg Clin North Am 47:389, 1967.
5. Berger A and Meissl G: Innervated skin grafts and flaps for restoration of sensation to anesthetic areas, Chir Plast 3:33, 1975.
6. Bossley CJ: Conservative treatment of digit amputation, NZ Med J 82:379, 1975.
7. Budo J, Finucan T, and Clarke J: The inner arm fasciocutaneous flap, Plast Reconstr Surg 73:629, 1984
8. Chang TS, Wang W, and Hsu CY: The free forearm flap—a report of 25 cases, Ann Acad Med Singapore 11:236, 1982.
9. Chase RA: Island pedicle gymnastics (discussion). In Cramer LM and Chase RA (eds): Symposium on the hand, vol 2, St. Louis, 1971, The CV Mosby Co.
10. Chase RA: Skin and soft tissue. In Atlas of hand surgery, vol 2, Philadelphia, 1984, WB Saunders Co.
11. Cohen BE and Cronin ED: An innervated cross-finger flap for fingertip reconstruction, Plast Reconstr Surg 72:688, 1983.
12. Cormacks GC and Lamberty BGH: Fasciocutaneous vessels in the upper arm: application to the design of new fasciocutaneous flaps, Plast Reconstr Surg 74:244, 1984.
13. Cronin TD: The cross finger flap: a new method of repair, Am Surg 17:419, 1951.
14. Curtis RM: Cross finger pedicle flaps in hand surgery, Ann Surg 145:650, 1957.
15. Daniel RK et al: Neurovascular free flaps: a preliminary report, Plast Reconstr Surg 56:13, 1975.
16. Daniel RK and Weiland AJ: Free tissue transfers from upper extremity reconstruction, J Hand Surg, 7:66, 1982.
17. Das SK and Brown HG: Management of lost finger tips in children, Hand 10:16, 1978.
18. Dolich BH, Olshansky KJ, and Barbar AH: Use of a cross-forearm neurocutaneous flap to provide sensation and coverage in hand reconstruction, Plast Reconstr Surg 62:550, 1978.
19. Dolmans S et al: The upper arm flap, J Microsurg 1:162, 1979.
20. Flatt AE: The thenar flap, J Bone Joint Sur 39B:80, 1957.
21. Foucher G et al: A compound radial artery forearm flap in hand surgery: an original modification of the Chinese forearm flap, Br J Plast Surg 37:139, 1984.
22. Freiberg A and Manketelow R: The Kutler repair of finger tip amputations, Plast Reconstr Surg 50:371, 1972.
23. Gilbert DA: An overview of flaps for hand and forearm reconstruction, Clin Plast Surg 8:129, 1981.
24. Godina M: Preferential use of end-to-side anastomoses in free flap transfers, Plast Reconstr Surg 64:673, 1979.
25. Grad JB and Beasley RW: Fingertip reconstruction, Hand Clin 1(4):667, 1985.
26. Haddad RJ: The Kutler repair of finger tip amputation, South Med J 61:1264, 1968.
27. Hallock GG: Refinement of the radial forearm flap donor site using skin expansion, Plast Reconstr Surg 81:21, 1988.
28. Hentz VR, Pearl RM, and Kaplan EN: Use of the medial upper arm skin as an arterialised flap, Hand 12:241, 1980.
29. Hing DN et al: Free flap coverage of the hand, Hand Clin 1(4):741, 1985.
30. Hodgkinson DJ and Shepard GH: Muscle, myocutaneous, and fasciocutaneous flaps in forearm reconstruction, Ann Plast Surg 10:400, 1983.
31. Holevich J: A new method of restoring sensibility to the thumb, J Bone Joint Surg 45:496, 1963.
32. Holm A and Zachariae L: Finger tip lesions: an evaluation of conservative treatment versus free skin grafting, Acta Orthop Scand 45:382, 1974.
33. Hoskins HD: The versatile cross-finger pedicle flap: a report of twenty-six cases, J Bone Joint Surg 42A:261, 1960.
34. House JH: Modification of volar advancement flap, ASSH Newsletter 1982:14, February, 1982.
35. Kaplan EN and Pearl RM: An arterial medial arm flap—vascular anatomy and clinical applications, Ann Plast Surg 4:205, 1980.
36. Katsaros J et al: The lateral arm flap, anatomy, and clinical applications, Ann Plast Surg 12:489, 1984.
37. Keim HA and Grantham SA: Volar flap advancement for thumb and fingertip injuries, Clin Orthop 66:109, 1969.
38. Kelsey JL et al: Upper extremity disorders: a survey of their frequency and cost in the United States, St. Louis, 1980, The CV Mosby Co.
39. Krag C and Rasmussen KB: The neurovascular island flap for defective sensibility, J Bone Joint Surg 57A:495, 1975.
40. Kutler W: A new method for fingertip amputation, JAMA 133:29, 1947.
41. Lie KK, Magargle RK, and Posch JL: Free full thickness skin grafts from the palm to cover defects of the fingers, J Bone Joint Surg 52A:559, 1970.
42. Lister GD, McGregor IA, and Jackson IT: The groin flap in hand injuries, Injury 4:229, 1973.
43. Littler JW: Neurovascular pedicle transfer of tissue in reconstruction surgery of the hand, J Bone Joint Surg 38A:917, 1956.
44. Littler JW: Neurovascular island transfer in reconstructive hand surgery. In Transactions of the International Society of Plastic Surgeons, Second Congress, London, 1960, E & S Livingstone Ltd.
45. Louis DS, Palmer AK, and Burney RE: Open treatment of digital tip injuries, JAMA 244:697, 1980.
46. McGregor IA: Less than satisfactory experiences with neurovascular island flaps, Hand 1:21, 1969.
47. McGregor IA and Jackson IT: The groin flap, Br J Plast Surg 25:3, 1972.
48. Macht SD and Watson HK: The Moberg volar advancement flap for digital reconstruction, J Hand Surg 5:372, 1980.
49. Markley JM: The preservation of close two-point discrimination in the interdigital transfer of neurovascular island flaps, Plast Reconstr Surg 59:812, 1977.
50. Matloub HS et al: The lateral arm flap in upper extremity reconstruction: an analysis of eighty cases, Plast Surg Forum 10:184, 1987.
51. May JW, Jr and Bartlett SP: Staged groin flap in reconstruction of the pediatric hand, J Hand Surg 6:163, 1981.
52. May JW, Jr and Gordon L: Palm of hand free flap for forearm length preservation in nonreplantable forearm amputation: a case report. J Hand Surg 5:377, 1980.
53. Moberg E: Discussion of the place of nerve grafting in orthopaedic surgery by Donald Brooks, J Bone Joint Surg 37A:305, 1955.
54. Morrison WA, O'Brien BM, and MacLeod A: Clinical experiences in free flap transfer, Clin Orthop, 133:139, 1978.
55. Morrison WA et al: Neurovascular free flaps from the foot for innervation of the hand, J Hand Surg 3:235, 1978.
56. Murray JF, Ord JVR, and Gavelin GE: The neurovascular island pedicle flap, J Bone Joint Surg 49A:1285, 1967.
57. O'Brien B: Neurovascular island pedicle flaps for terminal amputations and digital scars, Br J Plast Surg 21:258, 1968.

58. Posner MA and Smith RJ: The advancement pedicle for thumb injuries, J Bone Joint Surg 53A:1618, 1971.

59. Reed JV and Harcourt AK: Immediate full thickness grafts to finger tips, Surg Gynecol Obstet 68:925, 1939.

60. Reid DAC: The neurovascular island flap in thumb reconstruction, Br J Plast Surg 19:234, 1966.

61. Robbins TH: The use of de-epithelialized cross-finger flaps for dorsal finger defects, Br J Plast Surg 38:407, 1985.

62. Rose EH: Local arterialized island flap coverage of difficult hand defects preserving donor digit sensibility, Plast Reconstr Surg, 72:848, 1983.

63. Russell RC et al: Alternative hand flaps for amputations and digital defects, J Hand Surg 6:399, 1981.

64. Salaman JR: Partial thickness skin grafting of finger tip injuries, Lancet 1:705, 1967.

65. Santoni-Rugiu P: An experimental study on the reinnervation of free skin grafts and pedicle flaps, Plast Reconstr Surg 38:98, 1966.

66. Schenek RR and Cheema TA: Hypothenar skin grafts for fingertip reconstruction, J Hand Surg 9A:750, 1984.

67. Sharzer LA, Barker DT, and Adamson JE: Free composite tissue transfer in the upper extremity. In Serafin D and Buncke HJ, Jr (eds): Microsurgical composite tissue transplantation, St. Louis, 1978, The CV Mosby Co.

68. Sharzer LA et al: Clinical applications of free flap transfer in the burn patient, J Trauma 15:766, 1975.

69. Shaw DT and Payne RL: One stage tubed abdominal flaps, Surg Gynecol Obstet 83:205, 1946.

70. Shaw MH: Neurovascular island pedicled flaps for terminal digital scars—a hazard, Br J Plast Surg 24:161, 1971.

71. Shaw WW: Microvascular free flaps: the first decade, Clin Plast Surg 10:3, 1983.

72. Shepard GH: The use of lateral V-Y advancement flaps for fingertip reconstruction, J Hand Surg 8:254, 1983.

73. Smith PJ et al: The anatomical basis of the groin flap, Plast Reconstr Surg 49:41, 1972.

74. Snow JW: Use of a volar flap for repair of fingertip amputations, Plast Reconstr Surg 40:163, 1967.

75. Snow JW: Volar advancement skin flap to the fingertip, Hand Clin 1(4):685, 1985.

76. Song R et al: The forearm flap, Clin Plast Surg 9:21, 1982.

77. Song R, Song Y, and Yu Y: The upper arm free flap, Clin Plast Surg 9:27, 1982.

78. Soutar DS and Tanner NS: The radial artery forearm flap, Br J Plast Surg 37:18, 1984.

79. Stevenson TR et al: The superficial inferior epigastric artery arm flap for coverage of hand and forearm defects, Ann Plast Surg 12:333, 1984.

80. Timmons MJ et al: Complications of radial forearm flap donor sites, Br J Plast Surg 39:176, 1986.

81. Tolhurst DE, Haeseker B, and Zeeman RJ: The development of the fasciocutaneous flap and its clinical applications, Plast Reconstr Surg 71:597, 1983.

82. Upton J et al: Clinical applications of temporoparietal flaps in hand reconstruction, J Hand Surg 11A:475, 1986.

83. Wood MB, Cooney WP III, and Irons GB Jr: Upper extremity reconstruction by free tissue transfer, Minn Med 66:503, 1983.

84. Wood MB and Irons GB: Upper-extremity free skin flap transfer: results and utility as compared with distant pedicle skin flaps, Ann Plast Surg 11:523, 1983.

85. Yang G, Baoqui C, and Yuzhi G: Free forearm skin transplantation, Natl Med J China 61:139, 1981.

CHAPTER 13

The Evaluation and Management of Chronic Wrist Pain

Vernon Leroy Young
Jeffrey P. Groner
Phil E. Higgs

Almost all tasks require use of the hand. Any impairment in wrist function may have a significant impact on employment, daily living, and hobbies. Wrist problems are a major source of disability and time lost from work. However, prompt diagnosis and proper treatment can minimize cost and morbidity.

The diagnosis and management of wrist problems begin with a thorough history, physical examination, and four plain x-ray views.[161] When a definitive diagnosis is not established by this evaluation, a bone scan is obtained and the subsequent work-up is directed by its findings.

The beginning of this chapter presents a systematical approach to the diagnosis of the painful wrist following the algorithm in Fig. 13-1. Discussion of the salient features of the diagnosis and treatment of the common causes of wrist pain will follow.

HISTORY AND PHYSICAL EXAMINATION

A thorough medical history should be obtained. Pertinent information includes the patient's age, dominant hand, occupation, symptomatic hand, prior illnesses or injuries, and medications and allergies.[11,125,134,149] The onset, duration, and nature of the pain, as well as exacerbating and ameliorating factors, are noted. If the problem is the result of an injury, the time, place, and circumstances of the accident should be obtained as accurately as possible. The details of any previous treatment also should be documented.

A physical examination of the wrist begins with the patient sitting 180-degrees opposite the examining physician. An examination table is placed at a comfortable level between the patient and physician. The upper extremity is exposed from the mid-arm distally.

Examination of the wrist begins at the elbow. The medial and lateral epicondyles are palpated for tenderness. Lateral epicondylitis is often associated with wrist complaints. The elbow is put through a complete range of motion, including flexion/extension and pronation/supination of the forearm. The extremity is inspected for edema, discoloration, scars, and the amount of muscle mass is noted.

If the complaints are localized to the wrist, the hand is examined next, again inspecting for swelling, discoloration, and scars. The presence of callouses on the palmar surface of the hand should be noted and will provide information about the general level of activity performed by the hand.

Examination of the wrist is approached in a systemic fashion, beginning in an area remote from the point of maximal tenderness. The presence of abnormal motion or pain on the ulnar side of the wrist at the lunotriquetral joint is determined by the examiner. This is performed by placing the examiner's index finger on the pisiform and the thumb on the triquetrum. The examiner's opposite hand is used to stabilize the rest of the wrist. The pisiform and triquetrum are then moved back and forth in a volar/dorsal direction. Pain experienced on this test may indicate a lunotriquetral ligament injury, pisotriquetral arthritis, ulnar impaction syndrome, or a triangular fibrocartilage injury.

Testing of lunotriquetral stability is followed by palpation of the ulnar head. The distal ulna can be shifted dorsally and volarly to assess stability and the presence or absence of pain on motion. Pain with ulnar head motion can be associated with ulnar impaction syndrome, triangular fibrocartilage injuries, radioulnar joint arthritis, and subluxation or dislocation of the dis-

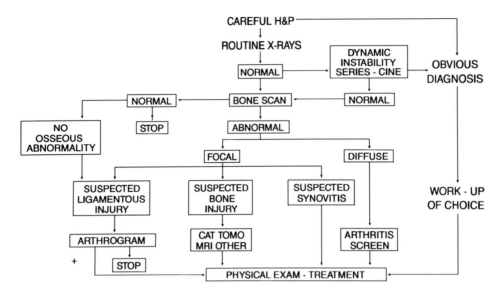

Fig. 13-1 This algorithm illustrates our approach to the evaluation of patients with wrist pain. The algorithm begins with a thorough history and physical examination followed by a four-view series of wrist x-rays. If these efforts do not establish a diagnosis, a bone scan is obtained and subsequent testing is directed by the results. This systematic approach increases the probability of establishing an accurate diagnosis.

tal ulna. The forearm is also placed through a full range of pronation and supination in an attempt to produce displacement of the ulnar head.

Examination of the ulna is followed by palpation of the lunate. The scapholunate joint lies in a line drawn almost directly distal to Lister's tubercle, and the lunate is immediately ulnar to that joint. The lunate is most easily palpated with the wrist in mid-palmar flexion. Pressure over the lunate on the dorsum of the wrist can produce pain in the presence of Kienböck disease, lunotriquetral ligament injuries, scapholunate ligament injuries, and fractures. The presence of radiocarpal arthritis involving the lunate fossa will also produce pain on palpation of the lunate.

The scaphoid is palpated dorsally next to the scapholunate joint and laterally at the anatomical snuffbox. A Watson scaphoid-shift test is helpful in diagnosing scaphoid fractures, radioscaphoid arthritis, and tears of the scapholunate ligament with scapholunate instability. The test relies on the fact that, in ulnar deviation, the scaphoid is extended more vertical relative to the carpus. The patient's elbow is supported by the examination table, and the wrist is placed in neutral flexion and ulnar deviation. The examiner's thumb stabilizes the scaphoid distal pole by placing pressure on the tubercle as the wrist is brought into radial deviation. Normally, motion of the scaphoid and lunate is linked by the scapholunate ligament, and the scaphoid rotates smoothly into a flexed position. The two bones

are no longer linked with a scapholunate ligament injury. When the examiner maintains the scaphoid in extension, the proximal pole of the scaphoid is dorsally subluxed and accompanied by a "clunk" or pain. A normal scaphoid may also produce clunking, but this is not usually accompanied by pain.

Midcarpal instability should also be evaluated by using a provocative test. Normally, movement of the triquetrum on the hamate is controlled by the volar capitotriquetral ligament. When the wrist is placed into ulnar deviation, the triquetrum is guided into the lower position on its helicoid articulation with the hamate. This forces the proximal carpal row into an attitude of slight extension. When this ligament is lax, the proximal carpal row assumes a position of flexion induced by gravity. As the wrist is axially loaded and moved into ulnar deviation, the proximal carpal row suddenly rotates dorsally, late in the ulnar deviation maneuver. This dysynchronous movement is detected by the examiner as a clunking sensation, which is painful to the patient. A similar finding may be present in the contralateral wrist but is not associated with pain.

Proceeding distally, the carpometacarpal (CMC) joint at the base of the thumb is examined. The base of the thumb metacarpal is palpated and moved passively through a full range of motion. A grind test is also performed. The thumb is grasped in one hand and the wrist stabilized with the opposite hand. The metacarpophalageal (MP) joint is slightly flexed and the phalanges used as a lever to rotate the metacarpal while pushing against the trapezium. Although pain at the metacarpal base is relatively specific for osteoarthritis at the CMC joint, pain may also be noted with de Quervain's tenosynovitis and fractures of the scaphoid, trapezium, or radial styloid.[28] Palpation of the base of the thumb metacarpal on the radiovolar aspect will often produce pain in the presence of CMC arthritis.

The grind test and examination of the CMC joint is followed by examination of the first dorsal compartment for de Quervain's stenosing tenosynovitis. The first dorsal compartment is palpated over the abductor pollicis longus (APL) and extensor pollicis brevis (EPB) tendons, and a Finkelstein's test is performed. In this test the thumb is flexed into the palm of the hand while applying an ulnar deviation force to the hand. The test is positive when the patient experiences pain in the area of the first dorsal compartment, which is usually indicative of de Quervain's tenosynovitis.

The CMC joints are examined by viewing them in a tangential manner with the wrist in slight flexion. A mass in that area is often a carpal boss, and arthritis between the bony elements of such a carpal boss can produce pain. The inflammation associated with arthritis at a carpal boss also produces tenderness on palpation.

The completion of these maneuvers will have included examination of the common points where bone and joint pathology frequently occur in the wrist. The wrist should also be placed through a full range of motion, including flexion, extension, radial and ulnar deviation, and pronation and supination. Any pain, locking, clicking, snapping, or limitation of movement should be recorded. Also, attention should be given to any mass or swelling, which may indicate a fracture, bruise, ligament injury, tenosynovitis, arthritis, infection, ganglion, or tumor.

Evaluation of the hand and wrist is completed with a neurological examination. Sensation should be documented in the median, ulnar, and radial nerve distributions.

Motor function in the intrinsic and extrinsic muscles should be evaluated by measuring two-point discrimination and Semmes-Weinstein monofilament testing.

IMAGING MODALITIES
X-ray

The history and physical examination is followed by a standard four view radiographical evaluation of the wrist. A four view wrist series includes posterior-anterior (PA), lateral, oblique, and ulnar deviation views. The x-ray tube should be placed opposite the dorsum of the hand with the palm applied to the film cassette. These routine four view x-rays can diagnose

fractures, dislocations, arthritis, Kienböck disease, static instability patterns, carpal bossing, and bone tumors. Additional diagnostic studies that may be beneficial include computerized tomography (CT), magnetic resonance imaging (MRI), arthrography, arthroscopy, blood tests, and nerve conduction studies.[93] The most efficient way to proceed is to follow the history, physical examination, and plain x-rays with a bone scan.

Scintigraphy

The scintigram (bone scan) is obtained by administering approximately 20 mCi of technetium-99 methylene diphosphonate (^{99m}TC-MDP) as a bolus by rapid intravenous injection. Images are made in three phases. The first phase is an immediate radionuclide angiogram, which is obtained in palmar or dorsal projection at 2- to 3-second intervals over approximately 30 seconds. The second phase is a blood pool image obtained immediately after the dynamic or angiogram images. The third phase of the bone scan is the delayed image, which is made 2 to 4 hours after the injection. Increased delayed phase activity is indicative of accelerated bone turnover. Magnification views and additional projections, including pinhole images, are obtained when necessary.

A bone scan will detect a fracture in nearly 100% of cases.[100] A normal scan virtually excludes the presence of a fracture. The bone scan is also approximately 95% accurate in identifying acute intrinsic ligament ruptures,[131] which are believed to be positive because of avulsion of a small bone chip at the ligament insertion. Bone scans may also be helpful in diagnosing arthritis, synovitis, epicondylitis, tenosynovitis, avascular bone necrosis, and reflex sympathetic dystrophy. Once a bone scan is obtained, the subsequent evaluation is directed by the findings of the scan and may include special views, MRI, CT, arthrography, or angiography. If the bone scan is negative and there is a low suspicion of pathology from the history and physical examination, the evaluation can be stopped and the patient followed. If a ligament injury is suspected from the history and physical examination, an arthrogram and instability series should be considered, even with a normal bone scan.

Instability series

This series of radiographs is designed to demonstrate dynamic instability patterns that only may be apparent when the wrist is placed into certain positions. The studies that may be indicated include PA, and lateral and oblique views in the neutral position, as well as in radial and ulnar deviation; lateral flexion-extension views; dorsal-volar and radial-ulnar stress views in the PA and lateral projections; and an AP closed-fist

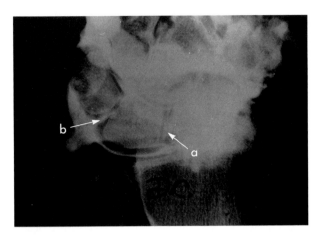

Fig. 13-2 Arthrography is useful in demonstrating the presence or absence of defects in intrinsic intercarpal ligaments, triangular fibrocartilage, and capsular structures. The arthrogram above demonstrates contrast material passing through defects in the scapholunate *(a)* and lunotriquetral *(b)* ligaments *(arrows)*. Usually there is no connection between the proximal carpal joints and the midcarpal joints. However, the frequency of defects in the intrinsic ligaments increases with age.

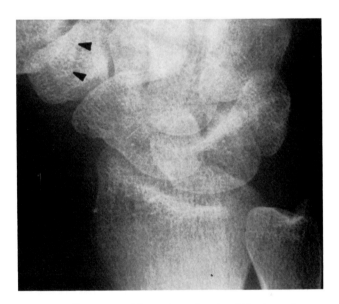

Fig. 13-3 Fractures of the volar tubercle of the trapezium *(arrows)* are frequently missed on routine wrist x-rays. The diagnosis can be established by a bone scan followed by multiple views with slightly different rotation of the wrist or a CT scan. These fractures must be ruled out in patients with unexplained pain around the base of the thumb.

view. The studies selected depend on the instability pattern suggested by the findings on history and physical examination. Cineradiographs may also be helpful in selected cases.

Arthrography

An arthrogram is the injection of contrast material into a joint space. Arthrography may use both positive radiopaque contrast material and air to produce a double contrast image. A wrist arthrogram should include injections into the radiocarpal, midcarpal, and radioulnar joints.[188] The arthrogram is helpful in demonstrating tears of the intercarpal ligaments and the triangular fibrocartilage.[57,83]

Normally there is no communication between the proximal and midcarpal joints. Positive arthrographical findings include the leakage of dye between the two carpal rows across a defect in the triangular fibrocartilage[188] (Fig. 13-2). Defects in the scapholunate and lunotriquetral ligaments and the triangular fibrocartilage may result from injury or wear. Arthrographical findings do not differentiate between degenerative and traumatic defects. Positive arthrographical findings must be correlated with the history, physical examination, bone scan, and spot films.[58,98,146]

Arthrography is often combined with an instability series that can also demonstrate dynamic instability patterns present only with certain movements.

Fluoroscopy and Special Views

If the bone scan shows an abnormality suggesting bone injury, the area of focally increased uptake can be further evaluated by a CT scan, tomography, MRI, or fluoroscopy. Fluoroscopy and special views are useful in evaluating patients who complain of popping clicking, locking, or unexplained pain. A videotape of these images provides a permanent record and allows detailed review. Spot films are beneficial in detecting subtle, minimally displaced fractures in the area of the ulnar styloid or a volar tubercle fracture of the trapezium (Fig. 13-3). Magnification views are often used in conjunction with fluoroscopy to add greater detail.

X-rays to determine ulnar variance require special positioning. The elbow is flexed 90 degrees, the shoulder is abducted 90 degrees, and the forearm is held in neutral rotation. This procedure will often require the patient to kneel with the arm on the x-ray table. The x-ray beam is centered over the distal radioulnar joint.[156] The physician may need to specially instruct the x-ray technician about the proper position to obtain this study. Failure to properly position the wrist for this x-ray can result in a 5 mm difference in the relationship between the distal radius and ulna. This view is useful in the evaluation of Kienböck disease and ulnar impingement syndromes.

Tomography

Conventional and CT are two commonly used types of tomography. Conventional tomography is used

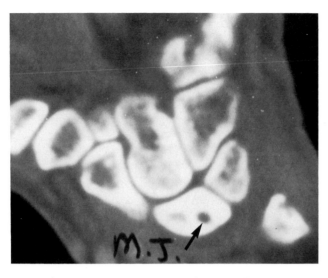

Fig. 13-4 CT scan demonstrating a lucent defect in the lunate *(arrow)*. This lucency does not communicate with a joint space, and the CT scan does not show a fracture of the "cyst" wall. The next step in evaluating this finding would be an MRI scan.

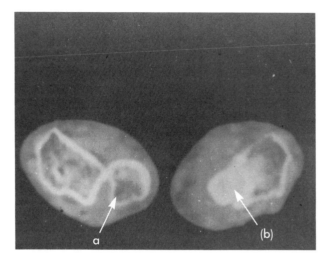

Fig. 13-5 Subluxation of the distal ulna: CT is the most accurate method of demonstrating subluxation or dislocation of the distal ulna. The CT scan above demonstrates subluxation of the left ulna *(a)* while the right ulna *(b)* maintains its normal relationship with the distal radius. Comparison of the two sides is critical because of individual variation.

less often today than CT scanning. The primary use of conventional tomography is to evaluate the healing of scaphoid fractures. It is also useful to assess the angulation of scaphoid fractures to determine if surgery is necessary and to visualize hamate hook fractures.[133] Conventional tomography may be superior to CT scanning if metallic wires or plates are present in the area being studied.

CT is good for evaluating cortical abnormalities, fracture fragments, healing of fractures, and carpal alignment.[141,170] It can be used to help localize lytic lesions associated with silicone synovitis. CT can accurately demonstrate the size and location of these lesions and is useful in determining whether a volar or dorsal approach should be used to evacuate the lytic area (Fig. 13-4).

CT is also useful to evaluate lucent defects in the carpal bones. The defects are usually detected on routine x-rays, and bone scans may demonstrate a focal area of increased activity in the region of the lesion. CT scanning can also clarify the anatomical details of lucent areas, such as bone cysts, enchondromas, and intraosseous ganglions, and their relationship to adjacent joints. CT scanning is also the diagnostic method of choice in establishing the presence of subluxation or dislocation of the distal radioulnar joint[81] (Fig. 13-5). A CT scan is better than MRI in demonstrating cortical architecture and the presence of small fractures. MRI is better in demonstrating bone marrow and soft tissue disorders.

MRI

MRI relies on radio signals emitted by hydrogen atoms of the tissues when they are excited by exposure to fluctuating magnetic fields.[144] Therefore MRI does not rely on standard radiation to generate an image. The radio signals are converted to images of the tissues by computer manipulations of the emmision data. Fat normally has a bright signal on T-1 weighted images. The T-2 images are brightest in areas that contain water. Bone and fibrous tissues such as ligaments produce a dark signal, and muscle and hyaline cartilage have an intermediate signal on both T-1 and T-2 images (Figs. 13-6, 13-7, & 13-8).

Ultrasound

Ultrasound is useful in confirming the diagnosis of an aneurysm or pseudoaneurysm of vessels supplying the wrist and hand, and it has been used to evaluate ganglion cysts. MRI is superior for both of these applications but more expensive.

Angiography

Angiography is not used to diagnose the etiology of wrist pain. However, in individuals with collagen vascular disease, angiography can be useful in defining the anatomy and directing treatment. Although it is not essential in the diagnosis of ulnar artery thrombosis, angiography can be helpful in defining the extent of occlusion and distal runoff.

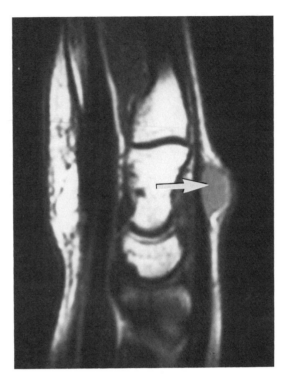

Fig. 13-6 T1-weighted MRI scan of a wrist demonstrating a dorsal wrist mass *(arrow)* with low intensity signal.

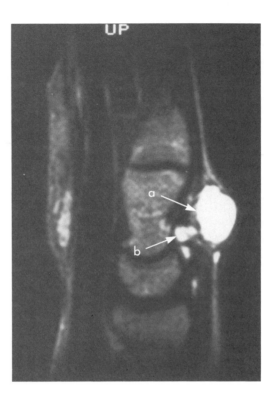

Fig. 13-7 T2-weighted MRI scan of the wrist. The mass is seen as a bright image *(a)* and a connecting stalk *(b)* connects the mass to a wrist joint. The bright image on a T2 image indicates a high water content and is consistent with a ganglion.

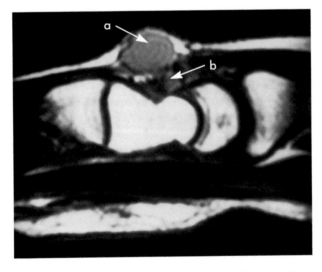

Fig. 13-8 Proton spin density MRI image of the wrist. The proton spin density has the least static and produces the sharpest MRI image. The mass *(a)* and the connecting stalk *(b)* are visible.

Electrical studies

Nerve conduction studies and electromyography are helpful in establishing and confirming the diagnosis of nerve compression, myopathies, and neuropathies. The most common compression to produce wrist or hand pain is carpal tunnel syndrome (CTS). Approximately 80% of people with CTS will have abnormal sensory nerve conduction when properly studied.[150]

Sympathetic blocks

Sympathetic blocks may be of diagnostic and/or therapeutic benefit in patients suspected of having reflex sympathetic dystrophy (RSD). This entity is characterized by constant burning pain after injury. The severity of the involvement has wide variation.

Arthroscopy

The role of arthroscopy in the management of wrist pain is evolving. Arthroscopy is performed by introducing small fiberoptic scopes and small specially designed instruments into the wrist joint through multiple stab incisions.[122] Arthroscopy has the advantage of allowing the surgeon to view wrist pathology and, in some instances, to treat the abnormality. In experienced hands it is at least as accurate as arthrography in detecting defects in the intrinsic wrist ligaments. Triangular fibrocartilage tears and areas of synovitis and chondromalacia are adequately treated with minimal morbidity through the arthroscope. The major disadvantages of arthroscopy include the expense of the equipment, the additional training and experience required to become proficient at the technique, and the need for an anesthetic.

Serology

Blood tests such as SMA-12, CBC, platelets, erythrocyte sedimentation rate, uric acid, antinuclear antibody, and rheumatoid factor are useful in diagnosing systemic problems that manifest as wrist pains.

Functional testing

Grip- and pinch-strength testing, sensory testing using monofilament fibers, and two-point discrimination are helpful in providing baseline functional data.[13,145] Selective nerve blocks and ninhydrin sweat testing are occasionally useful in diagnosing subtle neurological problems.

THE SYSTEMATICAL APPROACH

The patient with wrist or hand pain should be approached systematically. We use the algorithm outlined in Fig. 13-1. The evaluation begins with a thorough history and physical examination. If a diagnosis of glomus tumor, trigger finger, de Quervain's tenosynovitis, ganglion, or lipoma is made, treatment is initiated without further work-up. If a definitive diagnosis is not established by the history and physical examination, suspected diagnoses are noted, and the work-up proceeds with a four-view x-ray series.

Abnormal four-view series

Abnormalities detected by the four-view wrist x-ray series include static instability, fractures, arthritis, sclerotic lesions, or lucent defects in carpal bones. If a static instability pattern is demonstrated, an arthrogram is obtained to confirm the diagnosis and rule out other ligamentous defects. Definite treatment can then be undertaken. The amount of any fracture fragment displacement must be determined. Most fractures displaced 2 mm or more must be treated by open or closed reduction and internal fixation. Special x-rays such as CT, tomograms, or special views are ordered to direct treatment when displacement or reduction cannot be determined by plain films. Lucent defects and sclerotic lesions require further evaluation by bone scan, MRI, and CT, if necessary. If the results of these diagnostic studies confirm these lesions as the cause of the pain, they should be excised and the defect bone grafted. When a correlation cannot be made between the history and physical examination and the diagnostic studies, the wrist is immobilized in a long arm cast for 3 to 4 weeks and then reevaluated. Arthritic problems detected by the four-view series may be focal or diffuse. In either case the x-ray findings are correlated with the history of the immediate complaints and the physical exam, and appropriate treatment is initiated.

Normal four-view series/normal bone scan

A bone scan is obtained if the four-view series is normal, and the patient's wrist is immobilized with a long arm cast for 2 to 3 weeks if the bone scan is normal. If the patient continues to have pain while adequately immobilized, an explanation for the pain (other than pathology) in the wrist is explored. A bone, joint, or ligament injury must be ruled out by appropriate studies if the patient's symptoms improve while immobilized but recur when the cast is removed.

Normal four-view series/abnormal bone scan

A generalized synovitis, arthritis, or reflex sympathetic dystrophy is suspected when the four-view series is normal and the bone scan suggests diffuse uptake. A sympathetic block is done for diagnostic and therapeutic purposes if the history and physical examination suggests RSD. An arthritis screen is obtained and the patient referred to a rheumatologist for a suspected synovitis or arthritis.

An arthrogram and instability series are obtained if the bone scan shows a focal abnormality consistent with a ligamentous injury. The diagnosis of a ligamentous injury is confirmed and treatment proceeds accordingly when the findings of these studies correlate with the history and physical examination. If a diagnosis cannot be made from these studies, an occult fracture must be ruled out by additional studies such as spot and magnification views, CT scans, or MRI. The involved wrist is immobilized for 3 to 4 weeks if these studies fail to establish a diagnosis, and the patient is reevaluated at the end of that time.

SKIN AND SUBCUTANEOUS TISSUES

Bruises, lacerations, infections, and burns involving the subcutaneous tissues of the wrist are usually obvious. There is generally a clear history and physical examination and straightforward treatment. Painful soft tissue tumors found in the wrist include the common ganglion and less common angiomatous tumors.

Ganglions

Ganglions occasionally cause wrist pain. Pain may also be attributed to them because they are visible or palpable, while the actual source of the pain is due to some other etiology. Ganglions can occur at any age, including childhood.[97,143] They are most common in the second through the fourth decades of life and affect women almost three times more than men. Predominance in women may be due to hormonal or immuno-

Differential Diagnosis of Ganglions

WRIST GANGLIONS

NEOPLASMS/CYSTS

Xanthoma
Lipoma
Fibroma
Epidermoid inclusion cyst
Hemangioma
Lymphangioma
Osteochondroma
Synovial sarcoma
Histiocytoma
Chondrosarcoma

INFECTIONS

Tuberculosis
Fungi
Secondary syphilis

INFLAMMATION

Gout
Rheumatoid nodule
Rheumatoid extensor tenosynovitis
Bursitis

POSTTRAUMATIC

Scar
Foreign body granuloma

OTHER

Radial artery aneurysm
Anomalous muscle

logical factors affecting collagen metabolism.[10] There is no predilection to the left or right hand, racial predisposition, or association with repetitive motion or occupation.[7,187]

Although the exact origin of ganglions remains uncertain, the most popular explanation for their formation is that they are degenerative structures whose liquid contents represent the end products of myxoid change in collagen and/or connective tissue. The degeneration is believed to be a result of metaplasia or trauma. Ganglions typically originate in ligaments or tendon sheaths and subsequently communicate with the joint by rupturing into it. It is important to recognize that ganglions are not herniations from joints or tendon sheaths and that they do not contain synovium.

Dorsal wrist ganglions most often originate from the scapholunate ligament or over the trapezium and trapezoid articulations. They account for 60% to 70% of all ganglions, with the next most common site of origin (18% to 20%) being the volar surface of the wrist between the flexor carpi radialis (FCR) and brachioradialis (BR). Other sites are in the volar tendon sheath, distal interphalangeal (IP) joints and less common intertendinous, interosseous, and proximal IP joint locations. The typical ganglion is a firm, well-defined cystic tumor that is often multiloculated and filled with a viscous mucoid material. The cyst wall is smooth, white, and translucent. The lumen is connected to an underlying joint capsule or tendon sheath by a series of tortuous and intercommunicating mucin-filled ducts forming a stalk.

Ganglions, which usually appear as a knotlike mass, sometimes cause pain and weakness. Some authors have suggested that smaller ganglions may be more symptomatic than larger ones, particularly in the dorsal scapholunate complex.[6,18] Large volar wrist ganglions can produce median or ulnar nerve compression symptoms.[78,157] Ganglions can appear suddenly or over a period of several months, and spontaneous regression has been reported to occur in 40% to 60% of patients.[18,50,104] A history of antecedent trauma is common. It is important to recognize that ganglions can fluctuate significantly in size and that the efficacy of any treatment must be evaluated over several months. The diagnosis is usually straightforward and based on the presence of a firm, mobile, cystic mass in a typical anatomical location. Pain associated with ganglions is sometimes initiated by bleeding into the mass. Occult ganglions, which cannot be seen or palpated, can also be painful.[142] The diagnostic modality of choice for identifying ganglions is MRI, in which the ganglion appears as a bright shadow on the T-2 weighted images.[157] The differential diagnosis of ganglions is listed in Box 13-1. The work-up for a routine ganglion consists of a thorough history and physical examination and a four-view wrist x-ray series. Further evaluation is not necessary unless the findings are atypical.

No treatment is necessary if the ganglion is asymptomatic and the patient is not concerned about the cosmetic deformity. Nonsurgical treatments that have been recommended include bursting the ganglion with a book or digital pressure, aspiration, or aspiration plus the injection of steroids.[190] Nonoperative therapy has reportedly eliminated approximately 40% to 65% of ganglions.[120] Our results have not been this good. Aspiration with or without injection of low doses of triamcinolone are reasonable treatments as long as the patient recognizes that it is unlikely to result in permanent regression of the ganglion. Surgical excision of the ganglion with adequate anaesthesia in a bloodless field is the definitive treatment for wrist ganglions. The recurrence rate for complete cyst excision should not exceed 5% if they are excised correctly. Ganglion excision is not a small procedure. Patients should be informed of the potential risks, including prolonged pain, stiffness, and the need for postoperative immobilization for 3 to 6 weeks, as well as the attendant time missed from work.

The most common complication after excision is recurrence or development of a new ganglion. Failure to adequately debride the ligamentous origin of the cyst usually results in recurrence.

Painful soft tissue tumors of the hand and wrist

Painful tumors are less frequent and more obscure causes of wrist pain. With the exception of ganglions, soft tissue tumors in the hand and wrist are uncommon. Most of these soft tissue neoplasms do not directly cause wrist pain but may produce pain secondary to impingement on surrounding structures such as the median or ulnar nerves.

Soft tissue masses may be either benign or malignant. Malignant tumors are much rarer and are not discussed here. A number of benign and malignant tumors involving bone can also cause pain localized to the hand or wrist.

The list of soft tissue tumors found in the hand and wrist is extensive and includes ganglions, lipomas, glomus tumors, inclusion cysts, hemangiomas, leiomyomas, lymphangiomas, myxomas, giant cell tumors, fibromas, neurilemmomas, neurofibromas, aneurysms, and gouty tophi.

Glomus tumor

Glomus tumors in the wrist are uncommon. A total of four cases have been reported in the literature.[73,77] These tumors ranged in size from 2 mm to 5 cm. They were characteristically painful to palpation, and the diagnosis was usually made by finding an exceptionally painful area, localized with the point of an instrument such as a ball point pen. Tenderness is specifically localized to the tumor, while immediately adjacent areas are not tender. The tumors are often sensitive to cold, but this factor is not diagnostic. Treatment of glomus tumors, which are usually solitary, should be complete excision under tourniquet control with loupe magnification. Complete excision is curative, and malignant transformation has not been reported.

Angiolipoma

The angiolipoma is a more vascular variant of the much more common lipoma. These tumors usually present as tender, slowly growing masses, and multiple tumors are common. Two types of angiolipoma have been described. One is well encapsulated and the other infiltrating. The infiltrating variety is locally infiltrating but does not metastasize and is not considered malignant. Treatment for these tumors is surgical excision. Recurrence is rare, but formation of additional lesions is common in patients with multiple sites of involvement.

Angioleiomyoma

The angioleiomyoma is uncommon and may present as a painless mass or as a slightly tender mass that undergoes periods of paroxysmal pain believed to be associated with vascular spasm. The tumors arise from the smooth muscle of blood vessels or from piloerector smooth muscle. They are closely related to leiomyomas but are much more vascular. Treatment is excision, and recurrence is rare.

Hemangioma

Cavernous hemangiomas are rare in the hand and wrist. Superficial lesions, which are usually blue in color, are often painless and compressible. Lesions in the palm are frequently tender and, if deeply placed, may be difficult to diagnose. More superficial hemangiomas become tender if they thrombose. The preferred treatment for hemangiomas is surgical excision. Hemangiomas should not be confused with arteriovenous malformations, which are more extensive and difficult to treat.

Hemangiopericytoma

Hemangiopericytoma is a rare painful tumor derived from the same anatomical structures as the glomus tumor. Histologically the tumors demonstrate infiltration of adjacent tissues and range from clearly benign to undoubtedly malignant. The recommended treatment is a wide excision.

All of the tumors previously discussed are uncommon. However, the discovery of a slowly growing painful mass in the hand or wrist should raise the question of a vascular tumor. Although solid tumors and the less vascular variants of the aforementioned neoplasms can cause pain, they are more likely to be painless. With the exception of the glomus tumor and the hemangioma, painful masses will be difficult to diagnose accurately by a preoperative work-up. MRI and CT can be helpful in determining the extent of the tumor, but the final diagnosis is made by pathological examination.

TENDONS

Problems involving the tendons and synovium can usually be diagnosed by history and physical examination. Tenosynovitis, which is frequently the result of acute or chronic trauma,[32] is often found.

Tenosynovitis

Nonspecific tenosynovitis is a relatively common cause of wrist pain. Any of the tendons traversing the wrist may be involved. However, the first dorsal compartment tenosynovitis, de Quervain's syndrome, is the most common. de Quervain's stenosing tenosynovitis is a nonspecific, chronic inflammatory process involving the first dorsal compartment. It is often associated with overactivity or performance of repetitive tasks such as raking leaves or machine-paced manufacturing. It produces severe pain on the dorsoradial aspect of the wrist. Swelling of the first dorsal compartment, erythema, and crepitus surrounding the tendon sheath may also be present. There is tenderness of the first dorsal compartment at the level of the radial styloid and with ulnar deviation of the wrist with the thumb in flexion (Finkelstein's test). Conservative treatment consisting of immobilization or steroid injection should be attempted first. The offending activity should be avoided if possible. Immobilization with a thumb spica–polyform splint or cast for 2 to 4 weeks will usually relieve the symptoms dramatically. One or two steroid injections with a water-soluble steroid will also significantly relieve the symptoms in up to 80% of patients.[68]

Surgical treatment is reserved for failure of nonoperative methods. Release of the first dorsal compartment is performed trough a transverse or longitudinal incision overlying it. The sensory branch of the radial nerve must be identified and protected. The first dorsal compartment is often subdivided with the EPB tendon in a separate subcompartment.[91] Each tendon must be decompressed throughout the involved area. Failure to release all tendon slips can result in residual symptoms.[9]

Postoperative management consists of 3 to 4 weeks of splinting followed by restricted activities and physical therapy for 3 to 6 weeks. Tendon subluxation is an uncommon but potentially troublesome complication. A period of immobilization after release is recommended to allow some healing of the pulley and sheath.

Tenosynovitis may also involve the extensor pollicis longus (EPL), the intersection between extensor carpi radialis longus (ECRL) and extensor carpi radialis brevis (ECRB), the common extensors, and the extensor carpi ulnaris (ECU). Anatomic variations may be the cause.[31] The diagnosis can usually be established from history and physical examination. The patient is asked to forcibly contract the musculotendinous unit while the examiner provides resistance to the movement and palpates the area of the tendon. A bone scan may be obtained if the diagnosis remains unclear. A CT scan comparing the two wrists will usually be helpful if the bone scan is positive but not diagnostic. A CT will

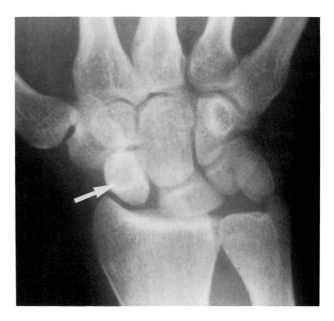

Fig. 13-9 CT of the wrist demonstrating tenosynovitis involving the right extensor carpi ulnaris tendon sheath. *(a)* The involved tendon sheath is indistinct and surrounded by soft tissue swelling. The left tendon *(b)* is sharply demarcated and no swelling is seen.

typically show edema and loss of contrast around the involved tendon, while the tendon will be sharply demarcated on the uninvolved side.

An initial trial of nonoperative treatment consisting of immobilization and steroid injections is usually attempted. Surgery is usually not necessary for nonspecific tenosynovitis involving the common digital extensors but may be necessary for treatment of ECRL, ECRB, or ECU tenosynovitis. A portion of the tunnel must be preserved to prevent subluxation of the ECU tendon after decompression of the sheath. Subluxation of this tendon is painful and difficult to correct.

LIGAMENT

Ligament injuries are a common source of wrist pain. Specific injury mechanisms, which produce ligament injuries ranging from partial tears to complete rupture, have been identified. The most common ligament injuries producing lasting wrist symptoms are those involving the scapholunate ligament, lunotriquetral ligament, and the triangular fibrocartilage. Typically the patient will relate a history of an injury that is followed by localized or diffuse pain. Patients with radial-sided ligament injuries will occasionally describe diffuse or even ulnar-sided symptoms.

An attempt should be made to accurately localize the injury to a specific anatomical structure. This is best done by a thorough and systematical physical examination of the wrist and hand.

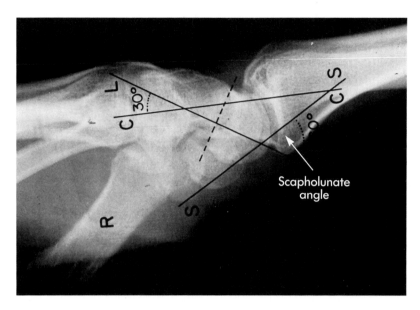

Fig. 13-10   Signet ring sign. The scaphoid assumes a more vertical position with rotary subluxation, and the scaphoid has the appearance of a signet ring *(arrow)* on the posterior-anterior x-ray.

The diagnosis of a ligament injury can usually be established by history and physical examination, while demonstrating tenderness when stressing the ligament and an arthrogram or arthroscopy. A bone scan may be helpful in ruling out coexisting pathology such as an occult fracture. Unless a static instability pattern is present, routine x-rays will be normal. Close attention should be given to the width of the scapholunate joint space. Suspicion of a scapholunate ligament injury should be raised if this interval is greater than 2 mm in width. The scaphoid should also be carefully examined in both the PA and lateral views.[115] Foreshortening of the scaphoid and a signet ring sign indicate static rotary subluxation of the scaphoid (Fig. 13-9). The scapholunate angle will be increased more than 60 degrees on the lateral view (Fig. 13-10). This angle is determined by drawing one line across the most volar aspect of the proximal and distal scaphoid and a second line through the longitudinal axis of the lunate, perpendicular to a line connecting its dorsal and volar poles. Values of 30 to 60 degrees are considered normal. A scapholunate angle of 60 to 80 degrees is suggestive of dorsal intercalated segment instability (DISI). Angles greater than 80 degrees or less than 30 degrees are indicative of carpal instability.[56]

An arthrogram is obtained by injection at three sites: the radiocarpal joint, the midcarpal joint, and the distal radioulnar joint. Normally there is no communication between these three spaces, and contrast material flowing between the radiocarpal and midcarpal joints or between the radiocarpal and distal radioulnar joints, indicates the presence of a ligamentous defect.

Arthrographical evidence of a scapholunate ligament defect associated with a history of trauma and tenderness in the scapholunate area is generally considered indicative of a ligament tear. The significance of lunotriquetral ligament and triangular fibrocartilage defects is less clear. Ulnar-sided wrist pain may be difficult to pinpoint, and leakage through either of these areas may not be related to the actual source of pain. Studies have demonstrated asymptomatic leaks across all three structures with increasing age.[105,176]

The demonstration of a lunotriquetral ligament or triangular fibrocartilage defect by arthrography should be carefully correlated with the history, physical examination, and bone scan.[56,98] Ulnar-sided arthrographical defects that are not tender on physical examination and are associated with a negative bone scan, are unlikely to be the source of the patient's symptoms. In contrast, scapholunate ligament defects may be associated with a normal bone scan but are usually tender on scapholunate ballottement and are more likely to represent an actual ligament tear.

Cast immobilization is an important diagnostic step in the management of ligament injuries and wrist pain in general. Pain attributable to a bone or joint problem is frequently substantially reduced by a period of cast immobilization. A 4- to 6-week trial of immobilization should also significantly diminish the pain of a symptomatic ligament injury. If the patient continues to have pain while immobilized, the cause of the pain is unlikely to be a fracture or ligamentous injury. Surgical intervention is unlikely to succeed in patients who continue to complain of pain while properly immobilized and should rarely be attempted. There is no reason to expect operative stabilization by arthrodesis or ligament reconstruction to be effective if cast immobilization did not eliminate or reduce the symptoms.

Carpal instability

The wrist joint comprises two rows of carpal bones stabilized by the intrinsic and extrinsic ligaments of the wrist and the geometrical shape of the individual bones.[95] The distal carpal row is tightly bound to the metacarpal bases. The proximal carpal row is primarily attached to the distal radius but is much less tightly bound. Therefore the carpus represents a linked system in which the proximal carpal row is an intercalated segment.[177] The scaphoid is a mechanical link spanning the two rows. When a mechanical system of this type is destabilized, it collapses into a zigzag configuration.[44]

The term *carpal instability* indicates a loss of the normal patterns of force transmission through the carpus, which may result from either a fracture or ligament injury. The instability may be static and identifiable on plain x-rays, or it may be dynamic and evident only with specific loading or positioning maneuvers and fluoroscopic spot studies.

Carpal instabilities may be painful and can lead to arthritis. Collapse of the carpus into a zigzag pattern may tilt the proximal intercalated segment in either a volar or dorsal direction. The dorsal pattern, DISI, is associated with a loss of radial-sided support attributable either to fracture of the scaphoid or disruption of the scapholunate interosseous ligament.[14,94,116,162,183] A volar intercalated segment instability (VISI) pattern usually results from a disruption of the lunotriquetral ligament.[67] This pattern is much rarer than DISI. Patients with instability patterns usually will relate a history of trauma with the subsequent development of wrist pain exacerbated by loading in certain positions. Physical examination often shows swelling, tenderness over the involved ligament, and detection of dysynchrous movement of the proximal carpal row.

Scapholunate dissociation is the most common cause of carpal instability. It may occur in conjunction with other carpal fractures or dislocations or may present as an isolated injury. A DISI pattern that develops from a scapholunate ligament injury may pass through a series of stages of may immediately assume one stage if the wrist sustains a sufficient degree of trauma. Most often there is a scapholunate diastasis without subluxation of the scaphoid. Gradually, with attenuation of the scaphoid's remaining ligamentous support, rotary subluxation of the scaphoid into an attitude of flexion takes place. The proximal pole of the scaphoid is no longer correctly aligned with the scaphoid fossa at the distal radius and radioscaphoid arthritis may develop.[16,27,139]

Loss of the scaphoid as the radial support for the capitate may lead to a descent of the capitate between the scaphoid and the lunate, which Watson has termed *scapholunate advance collapse,* or SLAC wrist.[79,180,181] Arthritis characteristically occurs at the scaphocapitate, capitolunate, and radioscaphoid articulations. The radiolunate joint is usually spared.

The treatment for an acute scapholunate dissociation must restore the ruptured ligaments by immobilization or open repair. The treatment of a chronic scapholunate dissociation without radioscaphoid arthritis has included ligament reconstruction, as well as intercarpal fusions and dorsal capsulodesis.[15] The best treatment for rotary subluxation of the scaphoid with radioscaphoid arthritis and for the SLAC wrist remains controversial. When the radiolunate joint has been spared in a SLAC wrist, an ulnar column fusion, resection of the proximal pole of the scaphoid, and replacement with a tendon spacer is performed.[46] A total wrist fusion is recommended if the radiolunate joint is also arthritic.

Acute ligament injuries

Carpal alignment is the most important consideration in the treatment of ligament injuries that are less than 6 weeks old. A trial of immobilization can be performed when normal alignment is present. Immobilization allows some healing at the injury site, even if the ligament injury is severe. Occasionally the carpus can be manipulated into a reduced position and stabilized by percutaneously inserted K-wires. Open reduction, direct repair of the injured ligaments, and K-wire stabilization is indicated if a closed reduction is not possible. The ruptured ligaments will heal by forming a scar if the ends can be placed closely to one another and held there for a sufficient time. The resultant scar will not have the same mechanical properties as a healthy ligament, which may lead to chronic instability and pain. An attempt at direct repair is complicated by the friability and small size of the ligamentous structures.

Chronic ligament injuries

The goal of treatment for chronic injuries is to relieve pain and prevent arthritis through the restoration of more normal carpal kinematics. Chronic injuries are unlikely to improve with immobilization alone. The presence of arthritic changes secondary to abnormal carpal mechanics is important in deciding the correct management. The destroyed articular surfaces must be removed by fusion, arthroplasty, or proximal row carpectomy. The use of silicone carpal implants to replace individual carpal bones has fallen into disfavor because of the high incidence of silicone synovitis.[27,47,159,164] The direct repair of chronic ligament ruptures is difficult. The torn ligament is usually scarred and cannot be reliably repaired. Ligament reconstruction can be attempted with a fascia lata or other tendon graft, and satisfactory short-term results have been reported in some series.

There is no consensus on the optimal treatment for chronic ruptures of the intrinsic wrist ligaments. Triscaphoid arthrodesis has been advocated by a number of authors as the treatment of choice for chronic scapholunate dissociation (Fig. 13-11). However, several recent reports have indicated a significant incidence of residual pain, decreased strength, decreased range of motion, and pseudarthrosis.[82] Lunotriquetral fusion has proved difficult and has a significant rate of nonunion as well.[132]

The treatment options for a chronic scapholunate ligament rupture should include an attempt at ligament reconstruction with a tendon graft, a dorsal capsulodesis, scaphotrapezial trapezoid arthrodesis, scapholunate arthrodesis or scaphocapitate fusion. The best treatment for chronic painful rupture of the lunotriquetral ligament appears to be a four-bone wrist fusion incorporating the common surfaces of the hamate, capitate, lunate, and triquetrum (Fig. 13-12). This procedure has a high rate of successful fusion, pain improvement, and preservation of wrist motion.

Dorsal capsulodesis has also been proposed for treatment of rotary subluxation of the scaphoid. Excellent early results have been obtained, but long-term follow-up of a large series is not yet available. Proximal row carpectomy has been used for radiocarpal arthritis and is reported to preserve movement while reducing pain. The long-term outcome of this procedure is also unknown.

The correct treatment of triangular fibrocartilage defects is controversial as well. Excision of the central portion of the TFCC with maintenance of the fibrous ring has been recommended.[127] An ulnar-shortening procedure should be performed if the defect is secondary to ulnar impingement.

The importance of the DISI and VISI classifications is to focus attention on the cause and pathomechanics of wrist instability patterns. Often these wrist instabilities are accompanied by pain from either ligamentous strain or degenerative arthritis. Occasionally an elderly patient who places low demands on the wrist will have a painless carpal collapse pattern. Under these conditions treatment is usually not indicated.

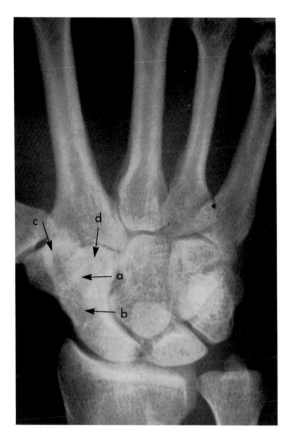

Fig. 13-11 The scapholunate angle (*arrow*) measured on the lateral wrist x-ray is increased with rotary subluxation of the scaphoid angles are considered normal, from 30 to 60 degrees; suspect, 60 to 80 degrees; and abnormal, greater than 80 or less than 30 degrees. Triscaphoid fusion. Fusion of the scaphoid, trapezium, and trapezoid (*arrow*) has been advocated for chronic scapholunate ligament injuries; however, many patients have continued wrist pain, decreased strength, and range of motion after successful arthrodesis. This has resulted in trials of several new procedures whose outcome is unclear at this time.

Ulnar impingement syndrome

Chronic ulnar pain in a patient with positive or neutral ulnar variance may represent ulnar impingement syndrome. An ulna, which is long in comparison with the radius, places pressure against the triangular fibrocartilage and lunate, causing pain at these sites.[128] Chondromalacia of the lunate and the articular surface of the ulna may develop. Lunate cysts are often present on plain radiographs. These patients may have symptoms of a torn lunotriquetral ligament or triangular fibrocartilage.[132] An assessment of ulnar variance should be obtained on a PA view with the shoulder abducted 90 degrees, the elbow flexed 90 degrees, the forearm fully pronated, and the hand on the x-ray cassette. A bone scan will often demonstrate increased lunate and distal ulnar uptake. Arthrograms may show leakage of

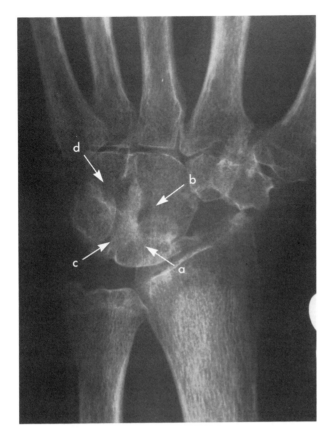

Fig. 13-12   In a four-bone wrist fusion the lunate *(a)*, capitate *(b)*, triquetrum *(c)*, and hamate *(d)* are fused together. This procedure has a high fusion rate; however, patients often have residual pain and decreased range of motion and strength.

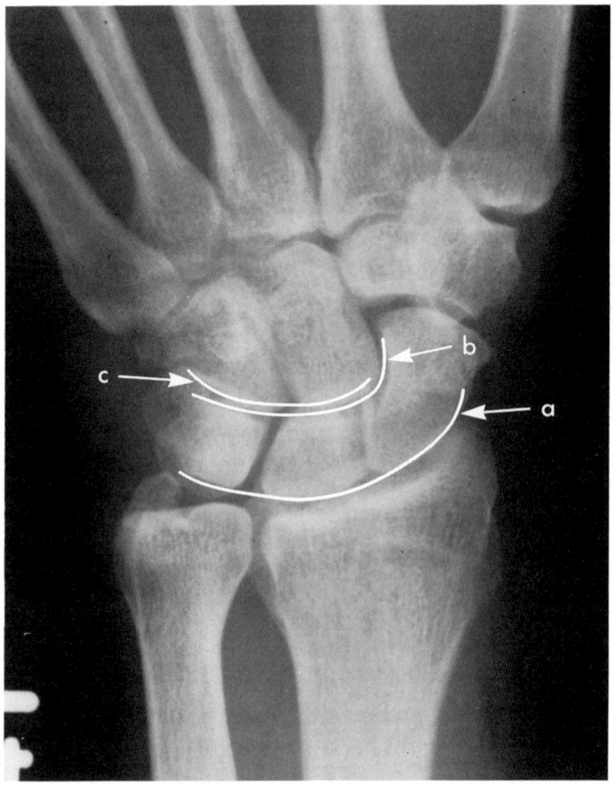

Fig. 13-13   Three congruent arcs are visible on the posterior-anterior x-ray of the wrist. The first arc *(a)* is formed by a line linking the proximal articular surfaces of the scaphoid, lunate, and triquetrum. The second arc *(b)* is formed by the distal articular surfaces of these bones. The third arc *(c)* is formed by the proximal articular surfaces of the capitate and hamate.

contrast at either the lunotriquetral or triangular fibrocartilage complex (TFCC). When there is positive ulnar variance, the most effective treatment is ulnar shortening, possibly combined with triangular fibrocartilage debridement.[17,127] Asymptomatic defects in the TFCC are common, and a careful physical examination is essential in the diagnosis of ulnar impingement/TFCC tear syndromes.[161]

Dislocations

Dislocations of individual carpal bones, carpal rows or units, or the entire carpus can occur after significant trauma.* The position of loading is usually with the wrist in the dorsiflexed position. The history is often striking and involves the application of a significant force. Dislocation of the entire carpus may also occur secondary to a systemic synovial disease such as rheumatoid arthritis, in which there is a marked laxity of ligamentous structures.[112,121,136,167] Dislocation of the carpus in relation to the lunate is called a perilunate

*References 1, 33, 60, 72, 76, 89.

dislocation. The pattern of force transmission across the carpus involves stages of progressive perilunate instability.[75,101,102,103] In the first stage, scapholunate dissociation results from disruption of the scapholunate and radioscapholunate ligaments. In the second stage, dislocation of the midcarpal joint occurs at the capitolunate articulation through the poorly reinforced space of Poirier, the weakest area of the volar wrist capsule. In the third stage, lunotriquetral dissociation occurs with disruption of the intrinsic lunotriquetral and extrinsic radiolunotriquetral ligaments. In the fourth stage, there is a complete dislocation of the lunate into the carpal canal. Force transmission proceeds from the radial to the ulnar aspect of the wrist. Variations in outcome may occur if the force is transmitted across the waist of the scaphoid rather than through the scapholunate articulation. Under these circumstances, a transscaphoid fracture with a perilunate dislocation results.[175] A fracture across the neck of the capitate may accompany the scaphoid waist fracture. Rotation of the proximal capitate fragment with the scaphoid fracture is

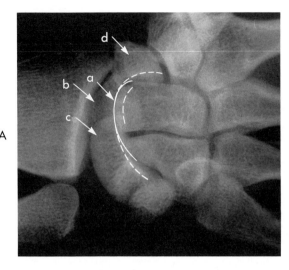 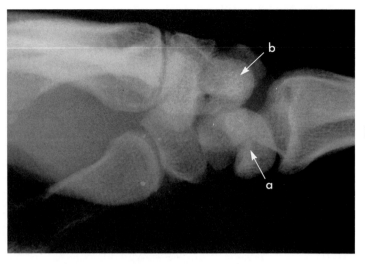

Fig. 13-14 **A,** Posterior-anterior view of the wrist with trans-scaphoid perilunate dorsal dislocation. The capitate *(a)* overlaps the proximal pole of the scaphoid *(b)* and the lunate *(c)*. The proximal fragment of the scaphoid has remained in the radial fossa with the lunate. The distal fragment has moved dorsally with the rest of the carpus. The midcarpal arc *(broken line)* is no longer congruous, and the distal carpal arc *(solid line)* overlies the midcarpal arc. **B,** Lateral view of the wrist with a dorsal perilunate dislocation. The lunate *(a)* has remained in the lunate fossa of the radius, and the remainder of the carpus *(b)* has dislocated dorsally.

called the *scaphocapitate syndrome*. Similarly, the lunotriquetral ligament may be spared and the triquetrum can be fractured.

A spectrum of dislocations involving fractures of various carpal bones, displacement of the lunate volarly or dorsally, or dislocation of the lunate in combination with displacement of the carpus may be seen.* The most important element in treating these injuries is recognition of the fractures. Radiographic confirmation of an uninjured capitate must be obtained in all scaphoid fractures. Gilula et al note that radiographically, the carpus represents three discrete congruent arcs. The first arc is formed by a line linking the proximal articular surfaces of the scaphoid, lunate, and triquetrum. The second arc is the distal articular surfaces of these bones. The third arc is at the proximal articular surfaces of the capitate and hamate (Fig. 13-13). If these arcs are incongruent, or if there is any variation in the intercarpal joint spaces, further evaluation is necessary.[57,59]

The treatment of carpal dislocations requires reduction and immobilization sufficient to allow healing to occur. Often these goals require open reduction and internal fixation with a K-wire.[61] Percutaneous K-wire or internal fracture fixation techniques must also be used if closed reduction of the dislocated carpal bones or fracture fragments can be obtained but is not stable[50,75,89,107,148] (Fig. 13-14 and 13-15).

Pain at the distal wrist level may be due to CMC dislocations (Fig. 13-16). These injuries are accompa-nied by pain and swelling that may initially be diffuse but gradually localize to the specific area of injury. Clinical suspicion is usually necessary to make the diagnosis, since the injury may not be apparent on routine x-rays. Oblique views are often helpful, and the bone scan will be positive. Fracture dislocations require a CT scan to fully assess the involvement of the articular surface. The treatment should consist of reduction and immobilization for 4 to 5 weeks. K-wire fixation and open reduction are also occasionally necessary* (Fig. 13-17).

BONE

Bone lesions, which include fractures, tumors,[51,96] cysts, and sclerotic, avascular areas, cause wrist pain.

Osteoid osteoma

Osteoid osteoma is a common benign bone tumor that rarely occurs in the carpus.[45,55] The scaphoid is most frequently involved, however, osteoid osteomas have been reported in all carpal bones. The primary complaint is pain localized to the affected bone and/or adjacent joint. The pain is frequently worse at night and is typically relieved by aspirin. Swelling overlying the affected bone is also common. The radiographic appearance is typical. Four-view wrist x-rays reveal a lucent defect with a central granular opacity and a peripheral sclerotic margin (Fig. 13-18). The diagnosis

*References 23, 24, 29, 30, 41, 71, 113, 156, 182.

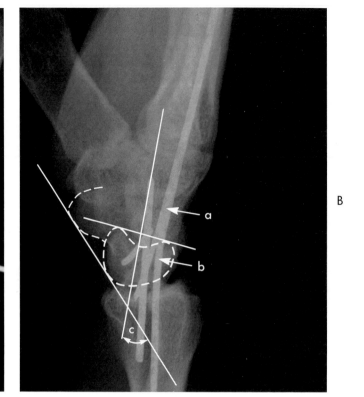

Fig. 13-15 **A,** Posterior-anterior view of the wrist with perilunate dislocation **B,** Lateral view of the wrist after reduction and internal fixation of a perilunate dislocation. The capitate *(a)* sits in normal relationship to the lunate *(b)*. The lunate is in neutral relationship *(tilt)* to the capitate and radius. The scapholunate angle *(c)* is normal.

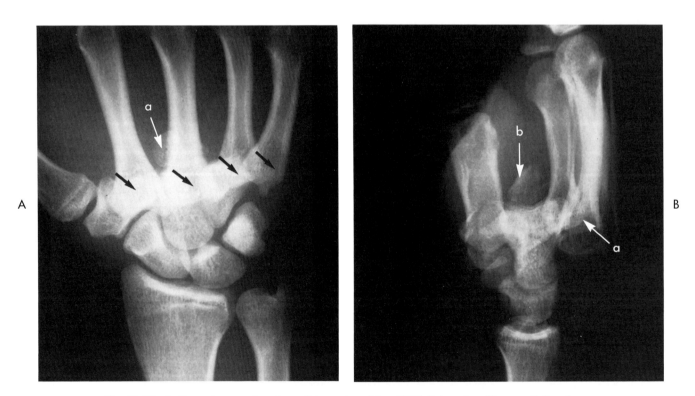

Fig. 13-16 **A,** Posterior-anterior view of the wrist with a CMC dislocation. The parallelism between the articulation of the metacarpals to the fingers and the carpal bones is lost. The metacarpal bases *(arrows)* overlay the carpal bones. There is an associated fracture of the base of the long finger metacarpal *(a).* **B,** Lateral view of the wrist with a CMC dislocation. The metacarpals *(a)* are dorsal to and proximal to their articulation with the distal carpal row. There is an associated fracture of the base of the long finger metacarpal with a large fragment *(b)* articularly with the capitate.

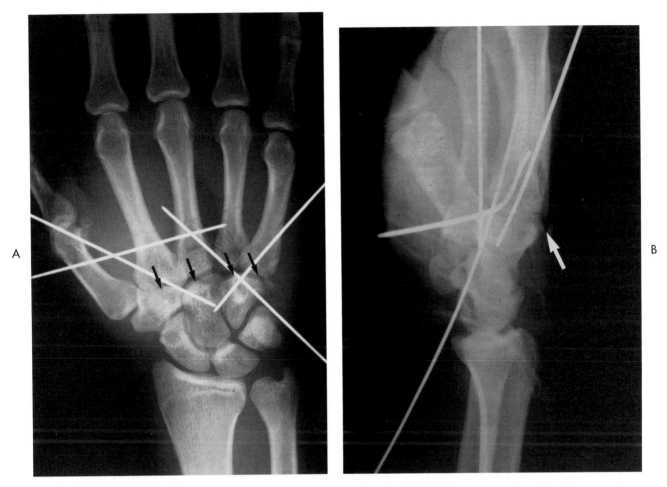

Fig. 13-17 **A,** Posterior-anterior view of the wrist after reduction and internal fixation of CMC dislocation. The parallelism between the metacarpals and their corresponding carpal articulations has been restored *(arrows).* The joints have a normal width, and the articular surfaces are parallel. **B,** Lateral view of the wrist after reduction and internal fixation of a CMC dislocation. The metacarpals have a normal relationship with the corresponding carpal bones. A small fracture fragment *(arrow)* overlays the distal capitate.

can usually be established by a typical history and the radiographic appearance. In the rare instance that pain is absent or atypical or the radiographic features are not diagnostic, CT, MRI, and bone scan should be obtained to confirm the diagnosis. Treatment consists of complete excision of the nidus and bone grafting of the resultant defect. Pain relief is usually obtained and recurrence is rare.

Bone cysts

Radiolucencies within bones are not true cysts but usually areas of fibrosis or intraosseous ganglions. Patients with these problems sometimes have a history of wrist pain or tenderness over the involved bone. Although plain radiographs can demonstrate the lesion, a full evaluation of the defect may require a bone scan, CT, and MRI (Figs. 13-19, 13-20, and 13-21).

The patient will often benefit from curettage and bone grafting of the defect if a CT scan shows communication with the outer surface of the bone (Fig. 13-22). The defect is usually best left untreated and followed by routine radiographs if a communication is not demonstrated between the lucent area and the joint space and the T2-weighted MRI image does not demonstrate a high water content. The lesion is probably a ganglion if the lucent area has a high water content on the T2-weighted MRI image (Fig. 13-21).). Removal and bone grafting frequently result in relief of pain. If the area appears to be solid on both the CT scan and MRI, with a corresponding focal area of increased uptake on bone scan, the lesion is usually fibrotic bone. Excision and bone grafting will usually relieve the pain. Fractures through the wall of bone cysts can also produce pain and can usually be demonstrated

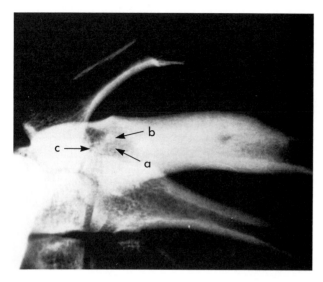

Fig. 13-18 Radiographically, osteoid osteomas are characterized by a lucent defect *(a)*, a central granular opacity *(b)*, and a peripheral sclerotic margin *(c)*.

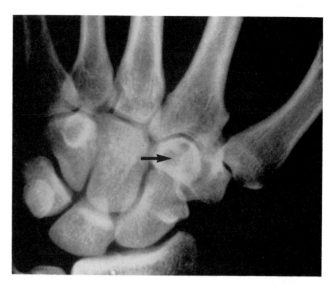

Fig. 13-19 Posterior-anterior x-ray of a lucent defect in the trapezoid. The plain x-ray demonstrates a lucency *(arrow)* but is otherwise nondiagnostic.

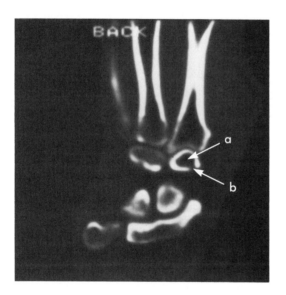

Fig. 13-20 CT scan of lucent defect in the trapezoid. This CT scan shows the location of the lucent area *(a)* and a communication within the joint *(b)*.

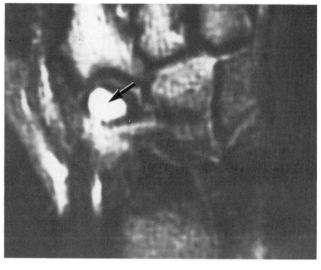

Fig. 13-21 MRI of lucent defect in the trapezoid. The T2-weighted image shows the lucent area filled with water-density material consistent with an interosseous ganglion.

by CT. An arthrogram is also usually obtained to exclude ligament injury as an alternate cause of pain.

Carpal boss

A carpal boss is a bony overgrowth located at the base of the index or long finger metacarpal and their respective carpal articulations. Most carpal bosses are congenital and asymptomatic. They occur approximately twice as frequently in women and become symptomatic after the third or forth decade. Carpal

bosses present clinically as either a painless mass on the dorsum of the hand or as wrist pain. Patients who have a painless mass on the dorsum of the hand are concerned about the nature and significance of the mass, which is usually firm and immobile. Those with pain are usually older and will often notice the pain as the result of injury or employment involving repetitive motion. The asymptomatic carpal boss does not require treatment. Those that are painful usually have developed degenerative arthritis between the opposing

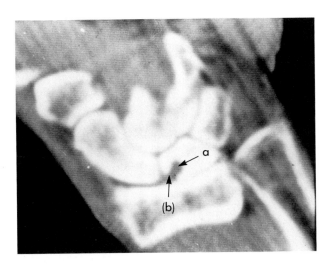

Fig. 13-22 CT scan of the lunate. This CT scan shows a lucent area in the lunate *(a)* and demonstrates that it communicates with the scapholunate joint *(b)*.

bony spurs. The diagnosis can be established by a history of pain localized to the area of the boss and a positive bone scan (Fig. 13-23). Routine x-rays usually demonstrate the bony overgrowth but may fail to indicate whether the boss is responsible for the wrist pain (Fig. 13-24). Treatment consists of removing the bony overgrowth, down to normal articular cartilage. Osteophytes at the articulating carpal bone may also be present and should be removed. A ganglion is present in about 30% of carpal bosses. It is important to establish both the diagnosis of a ganglion and a carpal boss before treatment, since removal of the ganglion without treatment of the carpal boss is unlikely to completely resolve the patient's symptoms.

Fractures

Occult fractures of the carpal bones are a relatively common cause of wrist pain.[20] Stresses to the hand are transmitted through the wrist and, to some extent, the linked array of the carpus predisposes it to certain types of injury with extreme loading in various positions. The carpal blood supply is delicate and enters a given bone at specific sites that may be disrupted during injury, resulting in avascular necrosis. Bony injuries heal by the relatively slow process of medullary callus formation.

The scaphoid is the most commonly injured carpal bone, accounting for approximately 50% of carpal bone fractures.[92] Anatomically, the scaphoid represents a link, bridging the proximal and distal rows, and it is frequently subjected to significant stresses in this location.

The circulation of the scaphoid is derived from three groups of blood vessels originating at different

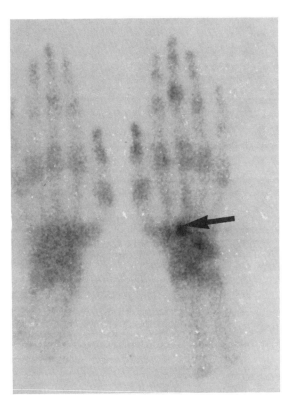

Fig. 13-23 Bone scan of a symptomatic carpal boss. The bone scan shows increased uptake in the area of the carpal boss *(arrow)*. This is consistent with degenerative arthritis between the opposing bone spurs. The bone scan also excludes other sources of pain such as CMC arthritis, occult fracture, and ligament injuries.

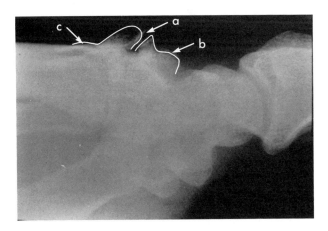

Fig. 13-24 Lateral wrist x-ray. Demonstrating a carpal boss *(a)*, originating from the capitate *(b)*, and long finger metacarpal *(c)*.

levels of the radial artery or its superficial palmar branch and converging toward the scaphoid. The vascular systems have been designated as the volar lateral, the distal, and the dorsal components. Taleisnik and Kelly demonstrated that the lateral-volar–scaphoid

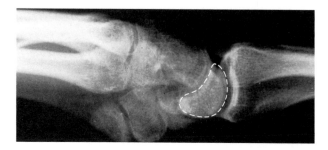

Fig. 13-25 Lateral wrist x-ray shows a DISI deformity. The key to this diagnosis is dorsal tilting of the concave surface of the lunate. The wrist must be in neutral position with the forearm to properly evaluate lunate angulation.

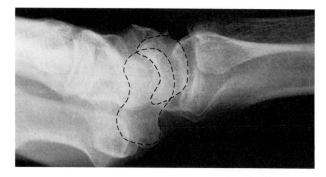

Fig. 13-26 Lateral wrist x-ray shows a VISI deformity. The concave surface of the lunate points (tilts) volarly and the scaphoid has rotated with the lunate to assume an abnormally vertical orientation. The wrist must be in neutral alignment with the forearm to properly assess lunate angulation.

group of vessels originating from the radial artery appears to be the most important source of intraosseous circulation and is the primary blood supply to the proximal two thirds of the scaphoid.[160] Vessels also enter the bone from the dorsal ridge at the waist of the distal tuberosity as branches from the dorsal scaphoid vessel. The distal arterial group is the smallest of the three and provides circulation to the tuberosity of the scaphoid. Oblitz and Hobbelstein found that 13% of cadaver specimens had no vascular perforations proximal to the waist, and 20% had only a single foramen,[65] which indicates that the majority of the nutrient vessels enter the scaphoid at or distal to the waist. Therefore any fracture proximal to the waist of the scaphoid could leave the proximal fragment without circulation, increasing the potential for avascular necrosis.

The most common mechanism of injury in scaphoid fractures is extreme dorsiflexion of the wrist in either radial or ulnar deviation.[43] Fractures result from a compressive blow or from direct impingement of the scaphoid against the dorsal lip of the radius. Most often the tensile forces are concentrated along the ulnar concave surface of the scaphoid waist. A variety of other carpal injuries can occur with increasing dorsiflexion, including fracture of the capitate, scapholunate dissociation, perilunate dislocation, and fracture of the radial side of the triquetrum.[172,173]

A scaphoid fracture is suspected when the patient gives a history of having fallen against a dorsiflexed hand. The most consistent finding on physical examination is tenderness in the anatomical snuff-box. This pain is accentuated by supination and pronation against resistance. Confirmation of the diagnosis is dependent on radiographic demonstration of a scaphoid fracture. Tomograms may be necessary. The radiographic evaluation for a scaphoid fracture begins with a four-view wrist series.[39,66] A thumb spica cast may be applied and the scaphoid x-rayed again in 2 weeks if routine x-rays are negative and the injury is less than 2 weeks old. At the end of 2 weeks, a bone scan should be obtained if the fracture is still not apparent on routine x-rays and the physical examination is still suggestive of a fractured scaphoid.[54] A CT scan is obtained if the bone scan is positive and plain films are normal. Ultrasound has been used to diagnose scaphoid fractures as well but is less reliable than radiographic diagnosis.

The presence of associated DISI (Fig. 13-25) or VISI (Fig. 13-26) may rarely be associated with a scaphoid fracture and signifies a significant ligamentous injury.[111,116] These injuries should be further evaluated because early treatment of the instability by internal fixation of the carpal bones in proper alignment can minimize the long-term disability. Failure to do this may result in chronic ligamentous instability, which may require intercarpal fusions or total wrist fusion with substantial disability. Similarly, nonunion of the scaphoid is more likely to occur under these circumstances.

Nondisplaced fractures typically can be treated with cast immobilization. If there is displacement of more than 1 mm at the fracture site, internal fixation is recommended. Angulation at the fracture site must also be corrected. The patient may develop a DISI collapse pattern if the scaphoid is allowed to heal with volar angulation. Plain tomograms or a CT scan should be obtained if any question exists as to whether angulation or displacement is present (Fig. 13-27).

The radiographic appearance of proximal pole avascular necrosis is controversial. A standard radiograph of the proximal pole cannot establish the presence or absence of vascularity. MRI studies are the best noninvasive means of determining bone vascularity (Fig. 13-28). Currently, the best method of assessing the vascularity of the proximal pole of the scaphoid has been punctate bleeding from the bone at the time of surgery.[63]

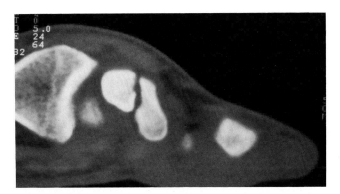

Fig. 13-27   CT scan of scaphoid fracture with displacement of fragments and volar rotation of the distal fragment. Failure to recognize this can result in malunion with a humpback deformity with chronic pain and decreased motion.

Russe categorized scaphoid fractures into three groups and evaluated their frequency, demonstrating that 20% occur in the proximal one third, 70% in the middle one third, and 10% in the distal one third.[65] Baumann and Campbell classified fractures into five types and found that 11% involved tuberosity; 9.7% were in the proximal one third; 40.3% were transverse; 36% were horizontal oblique; and 2% were vertical oblique fractures[12] (Fig. 13-29).

The treatment of scaphoid fractures is based on the location of the fracture fragments and their stability.[36] Unstable scaphoid fractures typically require surgical intervention. Displacement of the fracture fragments also indicates the degree of carpal instability. Cooney stated that fractures with greater than 1 mm displacement, a lunocapitate angle greater than 15 degrees, or a scapholunate angle greater than 45 degrees are unstable and should be treated surgically.[4]

Fractures in the middle one third are the most common type of scaphoid fracture, constituting 60% to 80% of all scaphoid fractures (Fig. 13-30). Delayed union or nonunion may occur, although most large series indicate that union occurs in 85% of all fresh middle third fractures if these are treated properly. Transverse fracture lines are subjected to greater stress from tight joint capsules and ligaments. Such injuries necessitate complete immobilization to achieve healing. One cause of delayed union or nonunion with middle third fractures is a lack of recognition of associated carpal instability manifest by DISI or, less commonly, a VISI pattern. These instability patterns may represent a partially reduced transscaphoid perilunate dislocation and require close evaluation.

Horizontal oblique fractures of the scaphoid are oblique to the long axis of the bone. These are typically stable and heal with 8 weeks of immobilization.

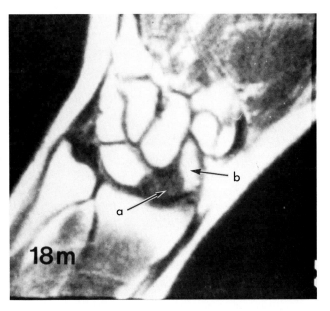

Fig. 13-28   This MRI scan of a scaphoid fracture shows decreased signal in the proximal pole of the scaphoid (a) on a T1-weighted image consistent with avascularity of this fragment. The distal pole of the scaphoid (b) and other carpal bones are bright on this image, which is consistent with normal vascularity.

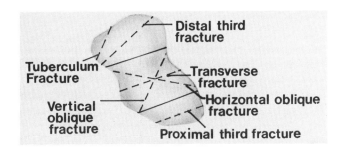

Fig. 13-29   Classification of scaphoid fractures. Scaphoid fractures have been classified according to anatomical location and orientation to the horizontal and longitudinal axes of the bone.

Transverse fractures are perpendicular to the long axis of the scaphoid and are subjected to greater shear forces because of their oblique relationship to the line of load transmission across the carpus. These require immobilization for 12 weeks.

Vertical oblique fractures of the scaphoid are parallel to the long axis of the forearm and are the most susceptible to shear forces. These fractures are unstable and commonly require internal fixation.

Fractures of the proximal third show a high incidence of nonunion and avascular necrosis of the proximal fragment related to the retrograde vascularity of this segment (Fig. 13-31). The incidence of avascular

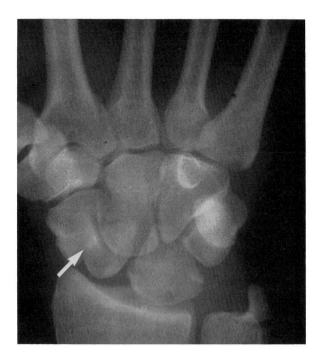

Fig. 13-30 Fracture of middle one third of the scaphoid *(arrow)* with significant displacement of fragments on posterior-anterior view.

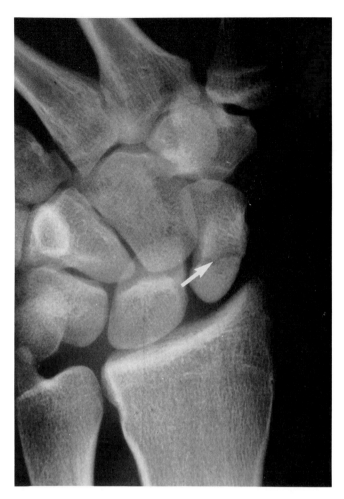

Fig. 13-31 Fracture of the proximal one third of the scaphoid in near anatomical alignment on the posterior-anterior view.

necrosis in proximal pole fractures has ranged from 14% to 39% in different series.[65] Determination of the vascularity by standard radiographic techniques or biopsy is unreliable. Green has demonstrated that direct observation of punctate bleeding at the time of surgery is the best predictor of vascularity.[63] MRI can also demonstrate vascularity and its role in predicting healing is currently being evaluated in longitudinal studies. These fractures require 12 weeks or longer to heal.

Fractures of the distal third are usually extraarticular and stable (Fig. 13-32). They generally heal promptly and are best treated by plaster immobilization in a short arm–thumb spica cast. Others believe that all scaphoid fractures, except for minor tuberosity fractures, should be treated initially with a long arm cast.

Controversies in the management of scaphoid fractures persist regarding the indications for surgery, the type of operation, and the management of nonunion or malunion. There are varied opinions in the literature regarding the position and length of immobilization for treatment of scaphoid fractures. Stable acute scaphoid fractures will heal if immobilized in a thumb spica cast for a sufficient time. Stewart reported a union rate of 95% in 436 scaphoid fractures treated with a short arm–thumb spica cast.[154] Anatomical studies have shown scaphoid motion with pronation and supination in a short arm cast. This motion is apparently transmit-

ted through the attachments of the volar radiocarpal ligaments to the scaphoid. In addition, there is a potentially disruptive action from the APL and the EPB if the thumb is not properly immobilized. A Swedish study demonstrated a statistically significant reduction in the healing time for patients immobilized in a long arm cast compared with those treated with a short arm cast.[19] The recommendation for the duration of immobilization has also varied depending on the type of fracture and its location and degree of stability. Displaced fractures are more likely to be associated with nonunion and require long periods of immobilization.

The most significant factor contributing to nonunion is an inadequate period of immobilization (Fig. 13-33). Accurate radiographic demonstration of bridging trabeculae across the fracture is essential to determine union. This is not always easy to demonstrate, and if a question exists after routine x-rays, fluoroscopically directed spot films, tomograms, or CT scans can

The Evaluation and Management of Chronic Wrist Pain **235**

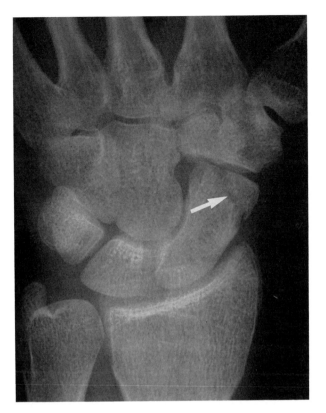

Fig. 13-32 Fracture of the distal one third (tubercle) of the scaphoid with minimal displacement on the posterior-anterior view.

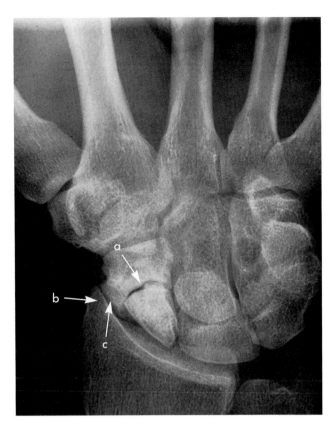

Fig. 13-33 Posterior-anterior view shows nonunion of a fracture of the middle one third of the scaphoid. Features consistent with a nonunion include sclerosis of the fracture margins *(a)*, spurring of the radial styloid *(b)*, and joint narrowing (degenerative arthritis) *(c)*.

resolve the dilemma. Displacement can recur during the first 6 to 8 weeks of treatment, and radiographic evaluation should be frequent during this time.

Scaphoid fracture healing is considered delayed if it has not ocurred after 4 months of adequate immobilization. Some factors predisposing to delayed union include late diagnosis, inadequate immobilization, and inadequate reduction.[90] Treatment of delayed unions is divided between bone grafting and internal fixation versus prolonged immobilization and electrical stimulation. A delayed union with sclerosis on both sides of the fracture site or cavitation of the fragments along the fracture line requires a more aggresive surgical approach. Most patients with delayed unions that have not healed within 6 months of nonsurgical treatment require surgical intervention.

The use of electrical stimulation for delayed union has been reported to result in union in 80% to 85% of cases. Frykman reported healing in 35 of 44 ununited scaphoid fractures at least 6 months old, with long arm-cast immobilization and pulsed electromagnetical field stimulation. The mean interval to healing was 4.3 months.[54]

Union of the scaphoid is dependent on many prerequisites, including early diagnosis, accurate fracture

reduction, adequate immobilization of any fragments, and an intact blood supply.[111,185] The location of the fracture and the stability of the fragments are contributing factors. Bone grafting and internal fixation is necessary to achieve union in these cases. The natural history of an untreated scaphoid nonunion is generally the development of severe degenerative arthritis.[174] In studies of patients with untreated scaphoid nonunions, eventual arthritic involvement occurs in almost all cases.[140] Bone grafting in these patients will not improve the arthritic changes and is contraindicated.

Numerous techniques have been advocated for the treatment of a nonunion, including a volar onlay bone graft, dorsal onlay bone graft, dorsal peg grafting, and compression with various types of screws.[38,40,178] Union rates after surgical treatment of distal and middle third nonunions is about 64%, using a variety of techniques. Displaced nonunions have a postoperative-union rate of 65% in comparison with the union rate for nondisplaced fracture nonunions.

Our current method of managing nonunions consists of obtaining an MRI study to preoperatively assess

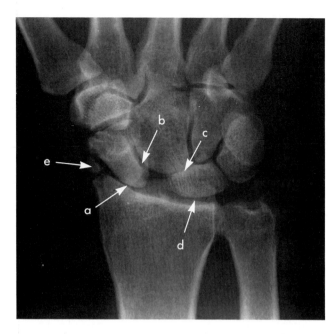

Fig. 13-34 Posterior-anterior view of SLAC wrist deformity. There has been loss of the radial support of the capitate, which has resulted in proximal migration of the capitate between the scaphoid and lunate. This ultimately leads to degenerative arthritis between the radius and scaphoid *(a)*, the capitate and scaphoid *(b)*, and the capitate and lunate *(c)*. The radio-lunate joint *(d)* is usually spared. There is an associated radial styloid fracture *(e)*.

the vascularity of the proximal pole. The proximal pole is also observed for punctate bleeding at the time of surgery. Volar or dorsal bone grafting is used in conjunction with internal fixation, which is followed in the immediate postoperative period with electrical stimulation and long arm-cast immobilization. In selected cases, vascularized bone grafts are being used, but at the present time, our series is too small to advocate the generalized use of this technique.[64,87]

The Herbert screw has been advocated since its introduction in 1984 in the operative management of scaphoid fractures and for bone grafting of malunions and nonunions.[70,178] This method uses a screw with threads of different pitch and size at each end. The technique requires a special jig, which is designed to assist in fragment stabilization, alignment, and screw insertion. Early reports indicated the Herbert screw provided rigid fixation of scaphoid fractures and, because of the associated compression, resulted in earlier and more frequent unions. Several studies reported union rates of approximately 80%. In recent years, the initial enthusiasm for this technique has decreased, since its use has become more widespread. Use of the device requires experience to achieve the 80% success rate. Mechanical studies have also shown that the actual compression generated by the Herbert screw is less

than first believed. Fracture site compression, however, should be achieved with the jig before placement of the screw, rather than relying on the compressive force generated by the screw. Other types of compression screws that may generate higher compression forces than the Herbert screw are also available. There is no conclusive data indicating any superiority of the Herbert screw over other means of internal fixation, but when used properly in experienced hands, all of these devices have been successful.

The vast majority of scaphoid fractures can be managed nonsurgically.[36] Stable fractures can be adequately treated with a long or short arm–thumb spica cast. Long arm casts are reserved by some for patients with potentially unstable fractures. The key to success lies in immobilization of the wrist until fracture union has been demonstrated radiographically. Unstable fractures should be stabilized by percutaneous pinning combined with closed or open reduction. The Herbert screw is one means of obtaining rigid internal fixation, however, we believe this device should be reserved for cases of unstable scaphoid fractures and nonunion of the scaphoid. The most common causes of treatment failure are the inability to diagnose a fracture, displaced or angulated fracture fragments, associated ligamentous instability, and inadequate immobilization. The outcome of improper treatment is often the development of radiocarpal arthritis resulting in SLAC wrist deformity (Fig. 13-34).[91]

Triqetral fractures constitute approximately 20% of carpal fractures and are usually associated with other carpal injuries. An avulsion fracture of the dorsal surface is the most common triquetral fracture (Fig. 13-35). These fractures are caused by traction, and the resulting bony fragment is usually small. This diagnosis should be suspected in a patient with a history of wrist trauma who has tenderness over the dorsum of the triquetrum. A bone scan should be obtained if routine x-rays fail to demonstrate the fracture. If there is a focal area of increased uptake in the region of the triquetrum, further evaluation should include multiple oblique views, spot films, or CT scanning. Treatment comprises short arm-cast immobilization for 4 to 6 weeks. Nonunions are rare.[42]

Fractures of the main body of the triquetrum are less common (Fig. 13-36). These are usually nondisplaced or minimally displaced and are also treated successfully with 4 to 6 weeks of cast immobilization. It is important to remember that triquetral fractures are often associated with other carpal injuries, and careful attention should be given to the rest of the carpus to exclude coexisting pathology.

Hamate fractures constitute approximately one fifth to one third of all carpal bone fractures. The hamate hook or body may be injured. Fractures of the hamate hook are among the most difficult to diagnose and they are frequently overlooked because they are not readily visible on routine wrist x-rays. These fractures usually result from sports injuries involving tennis, baseball, golf, and squash in which the patient may sustain a direct blow to the hypothenar eminence, transmitted through a raquet or club handle and resulting in the fracture. This fracture can also result from falls on the ulnar aspect of the wrist and hand.

The onset of pain or an ill-defined tenderness begins while playing the sport or right after a fall. There is usually vague tenderness to palpation over the hook of the hamate. Painful resisted abduction of the small finger may be present. Ulnar nerve symptoms consisting of either altered sensation or weakness in the interosseous muscle can also result from these fractures because of direct injury to the nerve or bleeding into Guyon's canal. Routine wrist x-rays are usually negative. Although some of these fractures can be demonstrated on a carpal-tunnel view of the wrist, the surest way to make the diagnosis is to obtain a bone scan, which will have increased uptake in the area of the hamate when a fracture is present. The anatomical details of the fracture are defined by CT. The standard treatment for hook fractures is excision of the bony fragment.[110]

Fractures of the body of the hamate also are present with ulnar-sided wrist pain (Fig. 13-37). These fractures are usually oblique and stable and heal within 4 to 6 weeks of adequate immobilization. Percutaneous or open fixation techniques are indicated for displaced fractures and symptomatic nonunions.[80,165] They may not be visible on routine x-rays, but their diagnosis can be confirmed or ruled out by a bone scan. If the bone scan is positive, the anatomical details of the fracture can be clarified with either detailed spot films or CT scanning.

Fractures of the capitate are rare and can exist as either isolated fractures of the body or neck of the capitate or in combination with fractures of other carpal bones, especially the scaphoid. The mechanism of injury is usually either a direct blow to the dorsum of the wrist or a hyperextension injury to the wrist joint. Isolated fractures can involve either the body or neck of the capitate. These fractures are managed by cast immobilization if they are not displaced. Reduction and internal fixation should be performed if the fracture is displaced. Undisplaced nonunions without arthritis should be treated with a trial of long arm-cast immobilization and electrical stimulation. Open reduction, bone grafting, and internal fixation may become necessary.[108]

The scaphocapitate syndrome consists of fractures of the neck of the capitate and waist of the scaphoid, with rotation of the proximal capitate fragment (Fig.

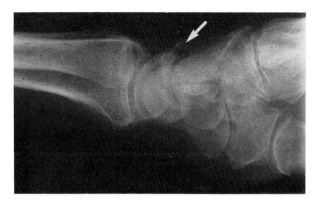

Fig. 13-35 Dorsal chip fractures of the triquetrum are best visualized on the lateral of the four-view series. The avulsed fragment is seen as a small chip overlying the dorsal aspect of the triquetrum *(arrow)*.

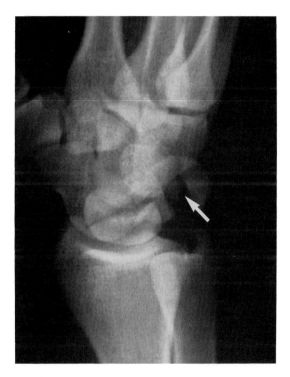

Fig. 13-36 Fractures of the body of the triquetrum are often minimally displaced and difficult to visualize, requiring multiple views, bone and CT scans.

13-38). This is a variant of the transscaphoid perilunate dislocation. These injuries are often missed because the capitate fracture is not appreciated. The capitate must be carefully evaluated with all scaphoid waist fractures. Closed or open reduction and internal fixation is required for all fractures displaced by 2 mm or more.

Fractures of the lunate are among the rarest of all carpal bone fractures, constituting 0.5% to 6.5% of all fractures affecting the wrist[18,27,163] (Fig. 13-39). Frac-

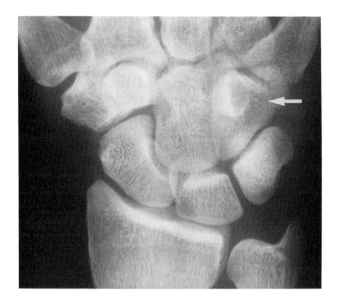

Fig. 13-37 Fractures of the body of the hamate are often minimally displaced and hard to visualize *(arrow).* Multiple views and bone scans may be required to identify and characterize these fractures.

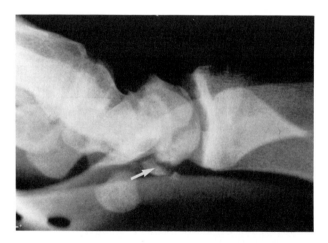

Fig. 13-39 Fractures of the lunate are usually best visualized on the lateral of four-view wrist series. They often involve the dorsal or volar pole of the lunate as seen above.

tures of the body, as well as the volar and dorsal lips of the bone, have been reported.

It is theorized that multiple subclinical compression fractures of the lunate are the cause of Kienböck disease. Multiple fractures are seen in Kienböck disease, and these progress in severity as the lunate collapses and fragments.

The treatment of large fragments should ensure an accurate reduction, which may necessitate open reduction and internal fixation. Small fragments should be treated by closed reduction and cast immobilization.

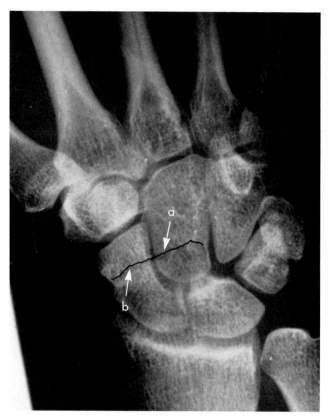

Fig. 13-38 Fractures of the capitate *(a)* are often associated with fractures of the scaphoid *(b).* This combination is called the Scaphocapitate Syndrome, and it is imperative that scaphoid fractures be ruled out in every case of capitate fracture.

Late excision of the fragments is necessary if the symptoms persist.

Fractures of the trapezium are rare.[53] We have treated four fractures of the tubercle of the trapezium. The mechanism of the injury is usually a combination of hyperextension and axial compression, which may represent a variant of the Bennett's fracture. There is generally a history of trauma followed by pain at the base of the thumb. Routine radiographs often do not demonstrate the fracture (Fig. 13-40). Bone scans show increased uptake in the area of the fracture and CT will outline its anatomy.

Fractures of the trapezoid are extremely rare. Their diagnosis can occasionally be established with routine x-rays but may require a bone and CT scan. These fractures can be treated with a short arm cast if they are only minimally displaced. They are frequently associated with fractures to the base of the metacarpals when displaced and then require open reduction and internal fixation or arthrodesis of the CMC joint.

Fractures of the pisiform result from a direct blow (Fig. 13-41). The diagnosis usually can be established

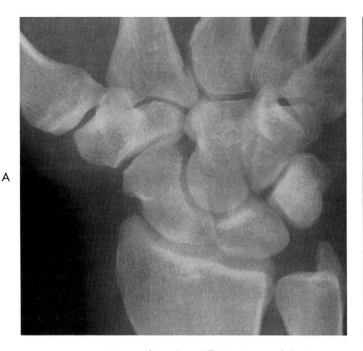
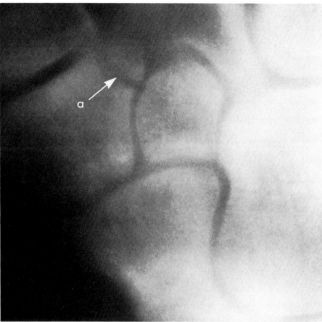

Fig. 13-40   **A** and **B,** Fractures of the trapezium may not be visualized on the four-view wrist series because the fracture line is not profiled *(a)*. CT will demonstrate these fractures *(b),* but a high degree of suspicion is needed to pursue the diagnosis.

by the presence of localized pain over the pisiform, with the fracture confirmed by x-ray.

Avascular necrosis of the pisiform has been reported.[99] Pisotriquetral instability and arthritis may result from a variety of causes.[126] The patient's hypothenar pain is exacerbated by all of these entities and by direct pressure over the pisiform, and treatment consists of pisiform excision.

Occult fractures are not normally visible on routine wrist x-rays. Fractures that are particularly likely to be overlooked include those in the tubercle of the trapezium, scaphoid, hook of the hamate, and ulnar styloid. The diagnosis of an occult fracture requires a high index of suspicion. A bone scan should be obtained if the history includes an injury mechanism compatible with a fracture; the physical examination reveals unexplained tenderness; and the routine x-rays do not demonstrate a fracture or dislocation. The bone scan will be positive in almost all fractures. This should be followed by special x-ray views, CT scans, or fluoroscopy to outline the fracture.

SCLEROTIC LESIONS

Kienböck disease, or avascular necrosis of the lunate, is a relatively common cause of wrist pain. Various etiologies have been proposed, but no definite cause has been established. Currently the most widely accepted hypothesis is that repetitive compressive forces alter the internal bony architecture, resulting in

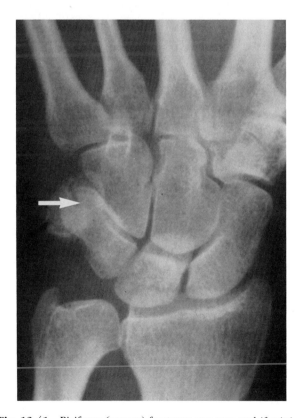

Fig. 13-41   Pisiform *(arrow)* fractures are rare and if minimally displaced, difficult to visualize on the four-view series.

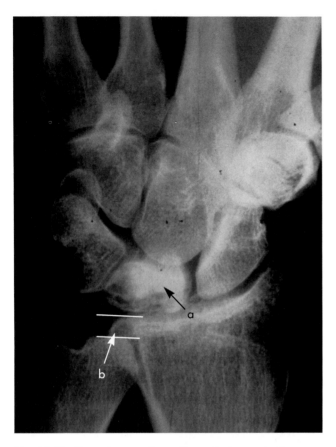

Fig. 13-42   Posterior-anterior radiograph demonstrating stage 3 Kienböck disease *(a)* and an ulnar minus ulnar variant *(b)*.

avascularity of the lunate and subsequent necrosis. The shape of the lunate may predispose the bone to the development of this condition.[138] The presence of an ulnar negative variant, an ulna that is short with respect to the distal radial articular surface, may also be important in the etiology of Kienböck disease (Fig. 13-42). The shortened ulna results in an increase in the compressive forces applied to the lunate by the radius. Nonetheless, Kienböck disease may also occur in wrists with neutral or positive ulnar variance.[119] Approximately 50% of the normal population has neutral ulnar variance and about 20% has negative ulnar variance. Approximately 80% of patients with Kienböck disease have negative ulnar variance.

The symptoms of Kienböck disease typically consist of vague wrist pain exacerbated by activity. There is often a history of trauma or work requiring repetitive wrist motion. There is tenderness over the lunate on physical examination. Confirmation of the diagnosis is made by imaging techniques. Kienböck disease has been classified in five stages. Stage 0: the patient has wrist pain with tenderness over the lunate, a normal x-ray, and a positive bone scan and MRI[5]; stage 1: the lu-

nate may appear normal on a plain x-ray or contain a coronal fracture, which is best seen on the lateral view; stage 2: the lunate is sclerotic but retains its general shape; stage 3: plain x-rays show lunate collapse or fragmentation without radiocarpal arthritis. Stage 3 includes 3A, in which the scaphoid position is normal and 3B, in which there is fixed rotary subluxation of the scaphoid; stage 4: there is collapse and fragmentation of the lunate with perilunate arthritis.

The treatment of Kienböck disease is controversial and evolving. In early Kienböck disease, immobilization of the wrist in a short arm cast may resolve the symptoms. Some authors have suggested the addition of electrical stimulation.[85] In stages 2 and 3, joint leveling maneuvers, such as ulnar lengthening of radial shortening, is indicated. These procedures are relatively straightforward. However, ulnar lengthening does require a bone graft and may also need a prolonged period of immobilization for healing.[3,117,158,169] A variety of procedures for treating patients with neutral or positive ulnar variance and stages 1, 2, or 3 of Kienböck disease have been suggested. All seek to diminish the stress loads placed on the lunate. Triscaphe arthrodesis, scaphocapitate fusion, ulnar shortening, and other procedures have been proposed.

The treatment options for stage 4 disease are limited. A proximal row carpectomy may be performed if the articular surfaces of the lunate fossa and proximal capitate are normal. Scaphocapitate fusion with lunate excision and total wrist fusion have all been recommended. We do not advise the use of a silicone lunate prosthesis for Kienböck disease, since there is a 50% incidence of silicone synovitis.[2,25] The role of vascularized bone grafts is currently being investigated. However, at this time there is not enough information available to recommend their use.

Avascular necrosis may also occur in carpal bones other than the lunate and may be idiopathic, posttraumatic, secondary to systemic disease, or related to steroid administration.[48,99,171,186]

Infections

Chronic osteomyelitis and septic arthritis are rare causes of undiagnosed wrist pain. The diagnosis of chronic osteomyelitis can usually be established by radiographic findings of bony erosions, which can be confirmed by appropriate cultures. Cultures of biopsied tissue, such as synovium or bone, is most likely to be positive. Treatment consists of debridement of all sequestrae, combined with appropriate antibiotic therapy. Bone grafting or intercarpal fusion may become necessary if bone destruction has been extensive.[109,152]

Septic arthritis represents a surgical emergency and is rarely the cause of obscure wrist pain. The diagnosis should be suspected if there is a history of acute wrist pain, swelling, and tenderness. There may be a history of penetrating trauma. Radiographs will usually show joint effusions and may also indicate joint space narrowing if a loss of articular cartilage has already taken place. Treatment consists of exposure and irrigation of the joints, proper cultures, antibiotics, and immobilization. Even with early, aggressive treatment, cartilage loss and subsequent arthritis are common.

ARTHRITIS

Osteoarthritis and rheumatoid arthritis are the two most common forms of arthritis involving the hand and wrist. Osteoarthritis most commonly affects the IP joints of the fingers and the CMC joint of the thumb. CMC joint arthritis is typically a disease of middle-aged women; the etiology of which is unknown. Patients have progressively increasing pain in the base of the thumb, which is tender to palpation and a positive grind test. There is subluxation and dislocation of the joint as the disease progresses. X-rays usually demonstrate narrowing of the joint between the trapezium and the first metacarpal and may also show spur formation on the trapezium between the first and second metacarpal (Fig. 13-43). Arthritis may also involve the scaphotrapezial and trapeziotrapezoid joints. Radiographic findings do not correlate well with the symptomatology. Further testing is unnecessary if the history, physical examination, and radiographic findings are consistent with CMC arthritis. A bone scan will demonstrate increased uptake in the area of the CMC joint to rule out other pathology or if there is a question about the diagnosis.

Treatment of osteoarthritis of the first CMC joint should begin with nonsurgical measures, including thumb spica splinting and nonsteroidal, antiinflammatory drugs. This regimen may provide sufficient relief for many patients to continue their normal activities and employment. An intraarticular steroid injection, which usually provides temporary relief of the symptoms, can also be given.

Surgical intervention is recommended if nonoperative treatment is unsuccessful. Partial or complete excision of the trapezium and replacement with either an autogenous tissue spacer or a silicone implant is one option. Fusion is usually reserved for complex cases in which there is paralysis, disease in additional joints of the thumb, or for those patients in need of a strong stable metacarpal.[26] Treatment of patients with multiple joint involvement must be individualized, usually fusing two joints and replacing one with a prosthesis to retain some movement. Isolated trapeziometacarpal disease can be treated with a distal trapezial hemiresection and placement of a tendon or fascial spacer.[69]

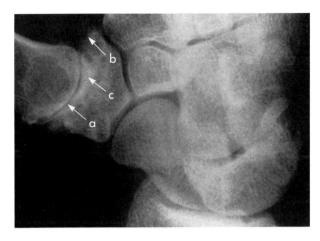

Fig. 13-43 Radiograph of the carpometacarpal joint of the thumb involved with osteoarthritis. There is joint narrowing *(a)*, spur formation *(b)*, and sclerosis *(c)*.

Complete excision of the trapezium is necessary when the scaphotrapezial articulation is involved.

Currently, silicone joint spacers are only recommended for older, less active individuals. Silicone synovitis has been reported with implant wear and breakage.[54,130,148] If a silicone spacer is used, patients should be informed of this risk and followed at yearly intervals with an examination and x-rays. Other complications of silicone joint arthroplasty at the CMC joint include dislocation, fracture of the implant, and erosion. Pain relief and mobility are usually acceptable with this arthroplasty.

Resection of the trapezium and replacement with either a tendon or fascial, autogenous-tissue spacer result in movement, pain relief, and strength comparable with that obtained after silicone joint spacer placement.[22] The tendons of palmaris longus (PL) and plantaris, the tensor fascia lata or temporalis fascia are all potential autogenous tissue spacers. Some authors advocate reconstruction of the first intermetacarpal ligament with a slip of the APL or FCR or a free tendon graft[22,184] to prevent dislocation of the implant. The cosmetic result of both of these procedures is usually excellent. The main long-term complaint of patients after either procedure is decreased strength and residual pain. Specific complaints may include difficulty in opening jars, pushing buttons, or opening car doors that have button release locks, which require pushing with the thumb.

Rheumatoid arthritis is a destructive process that usually involves the MP joints and radiocarpal joints more often than the IP joints. The patient typically has a history of swelling and tenderness in the involved joints. Radiographic characteristics may include ulnar head and styloid erosion, scaphoid and trapezial erosions with joint narrowing, zigzag deformity with radial deviation of the metacarpals and ulnar deviation of the fingers, ulnar translocation of the carpus, scapholunate dissociation, VISI deformity, and eventual palmar subluxation or dislocation of the carpus. The diagnosis can be confirmed by a positive latex fixation test. The initial treatment of rheumatoid arthritis is usually managed by a rheumatologist. Surgical intervention can involve multiple arthroplasties and fusions at various joints.[118]

CUMULATIVE TRAUMA DISORDERS

Upper extremity complaints associated with jobs requiring repetitive motion have become epidemic in American industry. Historically, these problems are post-World War II phenomena and seem most closely related to the speed of production and constant performance of repetitive tasks over long periods.[79]

This problem has been viewed and treated in the past as a group of distinct entities, including CTS, tennis elbow, and de Quervain's stenosing tenosynovitis and synovitis. Recent studies suggest that these are only manifestations of a larger, less specific problem directly related to the repetitive nature of the tasks being performed. Research in poultry workers performing low-load, high-repetition jobs demonstrated that almost two thirds of the workers had upper extremity symptoms. Questioning and examination of these individuals revealed a spectrum of findings ranging from mild aching, nocturnal swelling, and numbness to well-defined entities, including CTS and tennis elbow. The most striking finding was the large number of symptomatic individuals with some positive physical findings, who could not be labeled with a clear-cut diagnosis. This may indicate that exposure to repetitive tasks over time produces a generalized injury to muscle, tendon, ligaments, synovium, cartilage, and nerves manifest by pain, swelling, and neurological symptoms.[129] One or more tissue types or anatomical areas may be susceptible in a given individual, and, in this instance, a clear diagnosis of CTS or tennis elbow may develop. A larger group remains symptomatic but has normal x-rays, nerve conduction studies, blood tests, and physical examinations. The one common factor in almost all of these employees is exposure to repetitive motion. This problem has been documented in almost every industrial setting ranging from computer terminal operators to meat cutters and aircraft or automobile assembly-line workers. Currently there is no clear solution to the problem. Suggested solutions have included job rotation, ergonomic modification of work stations, pre-work exercise, and limited repetition.[8,114,135] All of these interventions have been beneficial in selected situations, but only automation has eliminated the problem. The work-up of these patients should include a thorough history and physical examination, routine x-rays, nerve conduction studies, and blood tests to exclude arthritis. Clear-cut syndromes should be treated. Although symptomatic individuals without a definite diagnosis will benefit from prolonged periods of rest from 2 to 6 months, some are never able to return to a repetitive-motion job.

REFERENCES

1. Aitken AP and Nalebuff EA: Volar transnavicular perilunar dislocation of the carpus, J Bone Joint Surg 42A(6):1051, 1960.
2. Alexander AH, et al: Lunate silicone replacement arthroplasty in Kienbock's disease: a long-term follow-up, J Hand Surg 15A:401, 1990.
3. Almquist EE: Kienbock's disease, Clin Orthop Rel Res 202:68, 1986.
4. Amadio PC et al: Scaphoid malunion, J Hand Surg 14A(4):679, 1989.
5. Amadio PC, Hanssen AD, and Berquist TH: The genesis of Kienbock's disease: evaluation of a case by magnetic resonance imaging, J Hand Surg 12A(6):1044, 1987.
6. Angelides AC and Wallace PF: The dorsal ganglion of the wrist: its pathogenesis, gross and microscopic anatomy, and surgical treatment, J Hand Surg 1:228, 1976.
7. Angelides AC: Ganglions of the hands and wrists. In Green DP (ed): Operative hand surgery, ed 2, New York, 1988, Churchill-Livingstone.
8. Armstrong TJ et al: Ergonomics considerations in hand and wrist tendinitis, J Hand Surg 12A(5):830, 1987.
9. Arons MS: DeQuervain's release in working women: a report of failures, complications, and associated diagnoses, J Hand Surg 12A(4):540, 1987.
10. Barnes WE, Larson RD, and Posch JL: Review of ganglia of the hand and wrist with analysis of surgical treatment, Plast Reconstr Surg 34:570, 1964.
11. Barr WG and Blair SJ: Carpal tunnel syndrome as the initial manifestation of scleroderma, J Hand Surg 13A(3):366, 1988.
12. Baumann JU and Campbell RD, Jr: Significance of architectural types of fractures of the carpal scaphoid and relation to timing of treatment, J Trauma 2:431, 1962.
13. Bell-Krotoski J and Tomancik E: The repeatability of testing with Semmes-Weinstein monofilaments, J Hand Surg 12A(1):155, 1987.
14. Berger RA et al: The scapholunate ligament, J Hand Surg 7(1):87, 1982.
15. Blatt G: Capsulodesis in reconstructive hand surgery: dorsal capsulodesis for the unstable scaphoid and volar capsulodesis following excision of the distal ulna, Hand Clin 3(1):81, 1987.
16. Blevens AD et al: Radiocarpal articular contact characteristics with scaphoid instability, J Hand Surg 14A(5):781, 1989.
17. Boulas HJ and Milek MA: Ulnar shortening for tears of the triangular fibrocartilaginous complex, J Hand Surg 15A:415, 1990.
18. Boyes JH: Bunnell's surgery of the hand, ed 5, Philadelphia, 1970, JB Lippincott Co.
19. Broome A, Cedell CA, and Colleen S: High plaster immobilization for fracture of the carpal scaphoid bone, Acta Chir Scand 128:42, 1964.
20. Bryan RS and Dobyns JH: Fractures of the carpal bones other than lunate and navicular, Clin Orthop Rel Res 149:107, 1980.
21. Burgess RC: The effect of rotatory subluxation of the scaphoid on radio-scaphoid contact, J Hand Surg 12A(5):771, 1987.
22. Burton RI and Pellegrini VD, Jr: Surgical management of basal joint arthritis of the thumb, Part II: ligament reconstruction with tendon interposition arthroplasty, J Hand Surg 11A(3):324, 1986.

23. Cain JE, Jr, Shepler TR, and Wilson MR: Hamatometacarpal fracture-dislocation: classification and treatment, J Hand Surg 12A(5):762, 1987.

24. Carroll RE and Carlson E: Diagnosis and treatment of injury to the second and third carpometacarpal joints, J Hand Surg 14A(1):102, 1989.

25. Carter PR, Benton LJ, and Dysert PA: Silicone rubber carpal implants: a study of the incidence of late osseous complications, J Hand Surg 11A(5):639, 1986.

26. Cavallazzi RM and Spreafico G: Trapezio-metacarpal arthrodesis today why? J Hand Surg 11B(2):250, 1986.

27. Cetti R, Christensen SE, and Reuther K: Fracture of the lunate bone, Hand 14(1):80, 1982.

28. Chen SC: Scaphoid compression test, J Hand Surg 14B(3):323, 1989.

29. Chen VT: Dislocation of carpometacarpal joint of the little finger, J Hand Surg 12B(2):260, 1987.

30. Chen VT: Dislocation of the carpometacarpal joint of the thumb, J Hand Surg 12B(2):246, 1987.

31. Cheng JCY and Hung LK: An unusual cause of wrist pain, J Hand Surg 7B(2):221, 1986.

32. Chun S and Palmer AK: Chronic ulnar wrist pain secondary to partial rupture of the extensor carpi ulnaris tendon, J Hand Surg 12A(6):1032, 1987.

33. Coll GA: Palmar dislocation of the scaphoid and lunate, J Hand Surg 12A(3):476, 1987.

34. Conway WF et al: Translunate, palmar perilunate fracture-subluxation of the wrist, J Hand Surg 14A(4):635, 1989.

35. Cooney WP et al: Difficult wrist fractures, Clin Orthop Rel Res 214:136, 1987.

36. Cooney WP, Dobyns JH, and Linscheid RL: Fractures of the scaphoid: a rational approach to management, Clin Orthop Rel Res 149:90, 1980.

37. Cooney WP, Dobyns JH, and Linscheid RL: Nonunion of the scaphoid: analysis of the results from bone grafting, J Hand Surg 5(4):343, 1980.

38. Cooney WP et al: Scaphoid nonunion: role of anterior interpositional bone grafts, J Hand Surg 13A(5):635, 1988.

39. Corfitsen M, Christensen SE, and Cetti R: The anatomical fat pad and the radiological "scaphoid fat stripe," J Hand Surg 14B(3):326, 1989.

40. Cosio MQ and Camp RA: Percutaneous pinning of symptomatic scaphodi nonunions, J Hand Surg 11A(3):350, 1986.

41. De Beer J de V et al: Multiple carpo-metacarpal dislocations, J Hand Surg 12(B)(1):105, 1989.

42. De Beer J de V and Hudson DA: Fractures of the triquetrum, J Hand Surg 12B(1):52, 1987.

43. Delime E, Detter PA, and Ferghney RE: Pathomechanics of the fracture of the carpal navicular, J Trauma 4:96, 1964.

44. Dobyns JH, Linscheid RL, and Cooney WP III: Injuries to the wrist. In Lamb DW, Hooper G, and Kuczynski K: Practice of hand surgery, Boston, 1990, Blackwell Scientific Publications.

45. Doyle LK et al: Osteoid osteoma of the hand, J Hand Surg 10A(3):408, 1985.

46. Eaton RG, Akelman E, and Eaton BH: Fascial implant arthroplasty for treatment of radioscaphoid degenerative disease, J Hand Surg 14A(5):766, 1989.

47. Ekfors TO et al: Cycstic osteolysis induced by silicone rubber prosthesis, Arch Pathol Lab Med 108:225, 1984.

48. Ferlic DC and Morin P: Idiopathic avascular necrosis of the scaphoid: Preiser's disease? J Hand Surg 14A(1):13, 1989.

49. Fernandez DL and Ghillani R: External fixation of complex carpal dislocations: a preliminary report, J Hand Surg 12A(3):335, 1987.

50. Flynn JE: Hand Surgery, Baltimore, 1982, Williams & Wilkins.

51. Frassica FJ et al: Aneurysmal bone cyst: clinicopathologic features and treatment of ten cases involving the hand, J Hand Surg 13A(5):676, 1988.

52. Freeland AE and Finley JS: Displaced vertical fracture of the trapezium treated with a small cancellous lag screw, J Hand Surg 9A(6):843, 1984.

53. Frykman GK et al: Treatment of nonunited scaphoid fractures by pulsed electromagnetic field and cast, J Hand Surg 11A(3):344, 1986.

54. Ganel A et al: Bone scanning in the assessment of fractures of the scaphoid, J Hand Surg 4:540, 1979.

55. Ghiam GG and Bora FW: Osteoid osteoma of the carpal bones, J Hand Surg 3A(3):280, 1978.

56. Gilula LA and Weeks PM: Post-traumatic ligamentous instabilities of the wrist, Radiology 129:641, 1978.

57. Gilula LA et al: Roentgenographic diagnosis of the painful wrist, Clin Orthop Rel Res 187:52, 1984.

58. Gilula LA et al: Wrist arthrography: the value of fluoroscopic spot viewing, Radiology 146:555, 1983.

59. Gilula LA: Carpal Injuries: analytic approach and case exercises, AJR 133:503, 1979.

60. Goldberg B and Heller AP: Dorsal dislocation of the triquetrum with rotary subluxation of the scaphoid, J Hand Surg 12A(1):119, 1987.

61. Green DP and O'Brien ET: Open reduction of carpal dislocations: indications and operative techniques, J Hand Surg 3(3):250, 1978.

62. Green DP and O'Brien ET: Classification and management of carpal dislocations, Clin Orthop Rel Res 149:55, 1980.

63. Green DP: The effect of avascular necrosis on Russe bone grafting for scaphoid nonunion, J Hand Surg 10A(5):597, 1985.

64. Guimberteau JC and Panconi B: Recalcitrant non-union of the scaphoid treated with a vascularized bone graft based on the ulnar artery, J Bone Joint Surg 72A(1):88, 1990.

65. Gumucio CA et al: Management of scaphoid fractures: a review and update, South Med 82(11):1377, 1989.

66. Gunther SF: Dorsal wrist pain and the occult scapholunate ganglia, J Hand Surg 10A:697, 1985.

67. Hankin FM et al: Carpal instability with volar flexion of the proximal row associated with injury to the scaphotrapezial ligament: report of two cases, J Hand Surg 13B(3):298, 1988.

68. Harvey FJ, Harvey PM, and Horsley MW: DeQuervain's disease: surgical or nonsurgical treatment, J Hand Surg 15A(1):83, 1990.

69. Helal B and McPherson I: Replacement of the trapezium with a silicone elastomer universal small joint spacer, J Hand Surg 14B:456, 1989.

70. Herbert TJ and Fisher WE: Management of the fractured scaphoid using a new bone screw, J Bone Joint Surg 66:114, 1984.

71. Ho PK et al: Complex dorsal dislocation of the second carpometacarpal joint, J Hand Surg 12A(6):1074, 1987.

72. Holdsworth BJ and Shackleford I: Fracture dislocation of the trapezio-scaphoid joint-the missing link, J Hand Surg 12B(1):40, 1987.

73. Jablon M, Horowitz A, and Bernstein DA: Magnetic resonance imaging of a glomus tumor of the fingertip, J Hand Surg 15A(3):507, 1990.

74. Jasmine MS, Packer JW, and Edwards GS Jr: Irreducible trans-scaphoid perilunate dislocation, J Hand Surg 13A(2):212, 1988.

75. Johnson RP: The acutely injured wrist and its residuals, Clin Orthop Rel Res 149:33, 1980.

76. Jones JA and Pellegrini VD Jr: Transverse fracture-dislocation of the trapezium, J Hand Surg 14A(3):481, 1989.

77. Joseph FR and Posner MA: Glomus tumors of the wrist, J Hand Surg 8A(6):918, 1983.

78. Kerrigan JJ, Bertoni JM, and Jaeger SH: Ganglion cysts and car-

pal tunnel syndrome, J Hand Surg 13A(5):763, 1988.

79. Kiesler S and Finholt T: The mystery of RSI, American Psychologist 43(12):1988.

80. Kimura H et al: An unusual coronal fracture of the body of the hamate bone, J Hand Surg 13A(5):743, 1988.

81. King GJ et al: Computerized tomography of the distal radioulnar joint: correlation with ligamentous pathology in a cadaveric model, J Hand Surg 11A(5):711, 1986.

82. Kleinman WB and Carroll C: Scapho-trapezio-trapezoid arthrodesis for treatment of chronic statis and dynamic scapho-lunate instability: a 10-year perspective on pitfalls and complications, J Hand Surg 15A:408, 1990.

83. Kricun ME: Wrist arthrography, Clin Orthop Rel Res 187:65, 1984.

84. Kristensen SS and Soballe K: Kienbock's disease—the influence of arthrosis on ulnar variance measurements, J Hand Surg 12B(3):301, 1987.

85. Kristensen SS, Thomassen E, and Christensen F: Kienbock's disease—late results by non-surgical treatment, J Hand Surg 11B(3):422, 1986.

86. Kristensen SS, Thomassen E, and Christensen F: Ulnar variance determination, J Hand Surg 11B(2):255, 1986.

87. Kuhlmann JN et al: Vascularized bone graft pedicled on the volar carpal artery for non-union of the scaphoid, J Hand Surg 12(B):2:203, 1987.

88. Kupfer K: Palmar dislocation of scaphoid and lunate as a unit: case report with special reference to carpal instability and treatment, J Hand Surg 11A(1):130, 1986.

89. Kuur E and Boe AM: Scaphoid-trapezium-trapezoid subluxation, J Hand Surg 11B(3):434, 1986.

90. Langhoff O and Andersen JL: Consequences of late immobilization of scaphoid fractures, J Hand Surg 13B(1):77, 1988.

91. Leslie BM, Ericson WB, and Morehead JR: Incidence of a septum within the first dorsal compartment of the wrist, J Hand Surg 15A(1):88, 1990.

92. Leslie IJ and Dickson RA: The fractured carpal scaphoid, J Bone Joint Surg 63B(2):225, 1981.

93. Linn MR, Mann FA, and Gilula LA: Imaging the symptomatic wrist, Clin Orthop Rel Res 21(3):515, 1990.

94. Linscheid RL et al: Traumatic instability of the wrist, J Bone Joint Surg. 54A(8):1612, 1972.

95. Linscheid RL: Kinematic considerations of the wrist, Clin Orthop Rel Res 202:27, 1986.

96. Louis DS, Hankin FM, and Braunstein EM: Giant cell tumour of the triquetrum, J Hand Surg 11B(2):279, 1986.

97. MacCollum MS: Dorsal wrist ganglions in children, J Hand Surg 2:325, 1977.

98. Manaster BJ, Mann RJ, and Rubenstein S: Wrist pain: correlation of clinical and plain film findings with arthrographic results, J Hand Surg 14A(3):466, 1989.

99. Match RM: Nonspecific avascular necrosis of the pisiform bone: a case report, J Hand Surg 5(4):341, 1980.

100. Matin P: Bone scintography in the diagnosis and management of traumatic injury, Semin Nucl Med 13(2):104, 1983.

101. Mayfield JK, Johnson RP, and Kilcoyne RK: Carpal dislocations: pathomechanics and progressive perilunar instability, J Hand Surg 5(3):226, 1980.

102. Mayfield JK: Mechanism of carpal injuries, Clin Orthop Rel Res 149:45, 1980.

103. Mayfield JK: Patterns of injury to carpal ligaments—a spectrum, Clin Orthop Rel Res 187:36, 1984.

104. McEvedy BV: The simple ganglion: a review of modes of treatment and an explanation of the frequent failures of surgery, Lancet 1:135, 1956.

105. Mikic SD: Age changes in the triangular fibrocartilage of the wrist joint, J Anat 126:367, 1978.

106. Minami A et al: Correlation between clinical results and carpal instabilities in patients after reduction of lunate and perilunar dislocations, J Hand Surg 11B(2):213, 1986.

107. Minami A, Ogino T, and Minami M: Limited wrist fusions, J Hand Surg 13A(5):660, 1988.

108. Minami M et al: Nonunion of the capitate, J Hand Surg 12A(6):1089, 1987.

109. Minkin BI et al: Mycobacterium kansasii osteomyelitis of the scaphoid, J Hand Surg 12A(6):1092, 1987.

110. Mizuseki T et al: Lateral approach to the hook of hamate for its fracture, J Hand Surg 11B(1):109, 1986.

111. Monsivais JJ, Nitz PA, and Scully TJ: The role of carpal instability in scaphoid nonunion: casual or causal? J Hand Surg 12B(2):201, 1986.

112. Moore DP and McMahon BA: Anterior radio-carpal dislocation: an isolated injury, J Hand Surg 13B(2):215, 1988.

113. Mueller JJ: Carpometacarpal dislocations: report of five cases and review of the literature, J Hand Surg 11A(2):184, 1986.

114. Muffly-Elsey D and Flinn-Wagner S: Proposed screening tool for the detection of cumulative trauma disorders of the upper extremity, J Hand Surg 12A(2):931, 1987.

115. Nakamura R et al: Method for measurement and evaluation of carpal bone angles, J Hand Surg 14A(2):412, 1989.

116. Nakamura R: Reduction of the scaphoid fracture with DISI alignment, J Hand Surg 12A(6):1000, 1987.

117. Nakamura R, Imaeda T, and Miura T: Radial shortening for Kienbock's disease: factors affecting the operative result, J Hand Surg 15B(1):40, 1990.

118. Nalebuff EA, Feldon PG, and Millender LH: Rheumatoid arthritis in the hand. In Green DP (ed): Operative hand surgery, ed 2, 1988, Churchill Livingstone.

119. Nathan PA and Meadows KD: Ulna-minus variance and Kienbock's disease, J Hand Surg 12A(2):777, 1987.

120. Nield DV and Evans DM: Aspiration of Ganglia, J Hand Surg 11B(2):264, 1986.

121. Norbeck DE Jr et al: Traumatic longitudinal disruption of the carpus, J Hand Surg 12A(4):509, 1987.

122. North ER and Thomas S: An anatomic guide for arthroscopic visualization of the wrist capsular ligaments, J Hand Surg 13A(6):815, 1988.

123. Nunn D: Trans-triquetral mid-carpal dislocation, J Hand Surg 11B(3):432, 1986.

124. O'Hara JJ and Stone JH: Ulnar neuropathy at the wrist associated with aberrant flexor carpi ulnaris insertion, J Hand Surg 13A(3):370, 1988.

125. Ogilvie C and Kay NRM: Fulminating carpal tunnel syndrome due to gout, J Hand Surg 13B(1):42, 1988.

126. Paley D, McMurtry RY, and Cruickshank B: Pathologic conditions of the pisiform and pisotriquetral joint, J Hand Surg 12A(1):110, 1987.

127. Palmer AK et al: Partial excision of the triangular fibrocartilage complex, J Hand Surg 13A(3):391, 1988.

128. Palmer AK: Triangular fibrocartilage complex lesions: a classification, J Hand Surg 14A(4):594, 1989.

129. Pedowitz RA and Toutounghi FM: Chronic exertional compartment syndrome of the forearm flexor muscles, J Hand Surg 13A(5):694, 1988.

130. Pellegrini VD Jr and Burton RI: Surgical management of basal joint arthritis of the thumb, Part I: long-term results of silicone implant arthroplasty, J Hand Surg 11A(3):309, 1986.

131. Pin PG et al: Role of radionuclide imaging in the evaluation of wrist pain, J Hand Surg 13A(6):810, 1988.

132. Pin PG et al: Management of chronic lunotriquetral ligament tears, J Hand Surg 14A(1):77, 1989.

133. Posner MA and Greenspan A: Trispiral tomography for the evaluation of wrist problems, J Hand Surg 13A(2):175, 1988.

134. Prince H, Ispahani P, and Baker M: A Mycobacterium malmoense infection of the hand presenting as carpal tunnel syndrome, J Hand Surg 13B(3):328, 1988.

135. Punnett L: Upper extremity musculoskeletal disorders in hospital workers, J Hand Surg 12A(5):858, 1987.

136. Rayhack JM et al: Posttraumatic ulnar translation of the carpus, J Hand Surg 12A(2):180, 1987.

137. Reinus WR et al: Arthrographic evaluation of the carpal triangular fibrocartilage complex, J Hand Surg 12A(4):495, 1987.

138. Ribbans WJ: Kienbock's disease: two unusual cases, J Hand Surg 13B(4):463, 1988.

139. Ruby LK et al: The effect of scapholunate ligament section on scapholunate motion, J Hand Surg 12A(5):767, 1987.

140. Ruby LK, Stinson J, and Belsky MR: The natural history of scaphoid non-union, J Bone Joint Surg 67A(3):428, 1985.

141. Sanders WE: Evaluation of the humpback scaphoid by computed tomography in the longitudinal axial plane of the scaphoid, J Hand Surg 13A(2):182, 1988.

142. Sanders WE: The occult dorsal carpal ganglion, J Hand Surg 10B:257, 1985.

143. Satku K and Ganesh B: Ganglia in children, J Pediatr Orthop 5:13, 1985.

144. Seeger LL: Physical principles of magnetic resonance imaging, Clin Orthop Rel Res 244:7, 1989.

145. Seror P: Phalen's test in the diagnosis of carpal tunnel syndrome, J Hand Surg 13B(4):383, 1988.

146. Shigematsu S et al: Arthrography of the normal and posttraumatic wrist, J Hand Surg 14A(2):410, 1989.

147. Siegert JJ, Frassica FJ, and Amadio PC: Treatment of chronic perilunate dislocations, J Hand Surg 13A(2):206, 1988.

148. Sollerman C et al: Silastic replacement of the trapezium for arthrosis—a twelve year follow-up study, J Hand Surg 13B(4):426, 1988.

149. Spencer JD: Amyloidosis as a cause of carpal tunnel syndrome in haemodialysis patients, J Hand Surg 13B(4):402, 1988.

150. Spindler HA and Dellon AL: Nerve conduction studies and sensibility testing in carpal tunnel syndrome, J Hand Surg 7(2):260, 1982.

151. Stahl S and Reis ND: Traumatic ulnar variance in Kienbock's disease, J Hand Surg 11A(1):95, 1986.

152. Stark RH: Group B B-hemolytic streptococcal arthritis and osteomyelitis of the wrist, J Hand Surg 12A(2):296, 1987.

153. Stern PJ: Transscaphoid-lunate dislocation: a report of two cases, J Hand Surg 9A(3):370, 1984.

154. Stewart MJ: Fractures of the carpal navicular: a report of 436 cases, J Bone Joint Surg 36A(6):998, 1954.

155. Steyer CM and Blair WF: Measuring ulnar variance: a comparison of techniques, J Hand Surg 14A(4):607, 1989.

156. Storm JO: Traumatic dislocation of the fourth and fifth carpometacarpal joints: a case report, J Hand Surg 13B(2):210, 1988.

157. Subin GD, Mallon WJ, and Urbaniak JR: Diagnosis of ganglion in Guyon's canal by magnetic resonance imaging, J Hand Surg 14A(4):640, 1989.

158. Sundberg SB and Linscheid RL: Kienbock's disease—results of treatment with ulnar lengthening, Clin Orthop Rel Res 187:43, 1984.

159. Swanson AB et al: Failed carpal bone arthroplasty: causes and treatment, J Hand Surg 14A(2):417, 1989.

160. Taleisnik J and Kelly P: The extraosseous and intraosseous blood supply to the scaphoid bone, J Bone Joint Surg 48A:1125, 1966.

161. Taleisnik J: Clinical and technologic evaluation of ulnar wrist pain, J Hand Surg 13A(6):801, 1988.

162. Taleisnik J: Scapholunate ligament excision (letter to editor), J Hand Surg 13A(5):790, 1988.

163. Teisen H and Hjarbaek J: Classification of fresh fractures of the lunate, J Hand Surg 13B(4):458, 1988.

164. Telaranta T et al: Bone cysts containing silicone particles in bones adjacent to a carpal silastic implant, Skeletal Radiol 10:247, 1983.

165. Terrono A, Ferenz CC, and Nalebuff EA: Delayed diagnosis in non-union of the body of the hamate: a case report, J Hand Surg 14B(3):329, 1989.

166. Terry DW and Ramin JE: The navicular fat stripe: a useful roentgen feature for evaluating wrist trauma, AJR 124:25, 1975.

167. Thomsen S and Falstie-Jensen S: Palmar dislocation of the radiocarpal joint, J Hand Surg 14A(4):627, 1989.

168. Trumble T et al: Intercarpal arthrodesis for static and dynamic volar intercalated segment instability, J Hand Surg 13A(3):384, 1988.

169. Trumble T et al: A biomechanical comparison of the methods for treating Kienbock's disease, J Hand Surg 11A(1):88, 1986.

170. Ueba Y et al: Computed radiography (Fuji) as a diagnostic tool for carpal disease, J Hand Surg 14A(2):408, 1989.

171. Urman JD et al: Aseptic necrosis presenting as wrist pain in SLE, Arthritis Rheum 20(3):825, 1977.

172. Van Schil P and De Smet C: Simultaneous fracture of carpal scaphoid and trapezium, J Hand Surg 11B(1):112, 1986.

173. Vender MI et al: Acute scaphoid fracture with scapholunate gap, J Hand Surg 14A(6):1004, 1989.

174. Vender MI et al: Degenerative change in symptomatic scaphoid nonunion, J Hand Surg 14A(4):514, 1987.

175. Viegas SF and Hoffmann FJ: Palmar lunate dislocation with a dorsal scaphoid fracture variant, J Hand Surg 13A(3):440, 1988.

176. Viegas SF and Ballantyne G: Attritional lesions of the wrist joint, J Hand Surg 12A(6):1025, 1987.

177. Volz RG, Lieb M, and Benjamin J: Biomechanics of the wrist, Clin Orthop Rel Res 149:112, 1980.

178. Warren-Smith CD and Barton NJ: Non-union of the scaphoid: Russe graft vs. Herbert screw, J Hand Surg 13B(1):83, 1988.

179. Watson HK and Brenner LH: Degenerative disorders of the wrist, J Hand Surg 10A(6):1002, 1985.

180. Watson HK and Ballet FL: The SLAC wrist: scapholunate advances collapse pattern of degenerative arthritis, J Hand Surg 9A(3):358, 1984.

181. Watson HK and Ryu J: Evolution of arthritis of the wrist, Clin Orthop Rel Res 202:57, 1986.

182. Watt N and Hooper G: Dislocation of the trapezio-metacarpal joint, J Hand Surg 12B(2):242, 1987.

183. Weber ER: Biomechanical implications of scaphoid waist fractures, Clin Orthop Rel Res 149:83, 1980.

184. Weilby A: Tendon interposition arthroplasty of the first carpo-metacarpal joint, J Hand Surg 13B(4):421, 1988.

185. Wilton TJ: Soft-tissue interposition as a possible cause of scaphoid non-union, J Hand Surg 12B(1):50, 1987.

186. Wounlund J and Lohmann M: Aseptic necrosis of the capitate secondary to Gaucher's disease: a case report, J Hand Surg 14B(3):336, 1989.

187. Young L, Bartell T, and Logan SE: Ganglions of the hand and wrist, South Med J 81(6):751, 1988.

188. Zinberg EM et al: The triple-injection wrist arthrogram, J Hand Surg 13A(6):803, 1988.

189. Zook EG, Kucan JO, and Guy RJ: Palmar wrist pain caused by ulnar nerve entrapment in the flexor carpi ulnaris tendon, J Hand Surg 13A(5):732, 1988.

190. Zubowicz VN and Ishii CH: Management of ganglion cysts of the hand by simple aspiration, J Hand Surg 12A(4):618, 1987.

CHAPTER 14

Wound Healing: Practical Aspects

Paul Y. Liu
Elof Eriksson
Thomas A. Mustoe

The recent formation of an international society dedicated to the study of wound healing is a reflection of increased interest and accelerated research in this field in recent years. Although the basic cellular events have been dogmatically set down in many textbooks, the practicing surgeon is often faced with many seemingly unrelated scientific facts that may or may not have anything to do with how wounds are actually treated.

This chapter takes a more "how to" approach in regard to the problematic wound, including an algorithm for diagnosis and treatment. The discussion of the healing phase alludes to recent, basic scientific discoveries and their potential clinical application. The chapter references are meant to serve as a compendium for readers who seek more detailed explanations.

DIAGNOSIS

Wounds may arise from systemic, regional, or local conditions, and although all of these wounds share certain characteristics, there is a need to be specific in identifying the particular aspect of problematic wound healing. For example, radiation wounds do not reepithelialize well, while keloids are characterized by an overabundance of collagen. Thus differences in wound etiology are useful not only for classification schemes but also to suggest different approaches in the care of these problems. Addressing the underlying conditions that predisposed the patient to problem wound healing is a necessary adjunct to the treatment of the wound itself.

Systemic etiologies

Conditions that predispose a patient to problematic wound healing include age; malnutrition; diabetes mellitus; metabolic derangements, such as hypoxia, iron deficiency, scurvy, lathyrism, lysyl oxidase/hydroxylase, or procollagen protease deficiency; cancer, including chemotherapy and radiation; rheumatoid arthritis; anemia; steroid therapy; acquired immunodeficiency syndrome (AIDS); sepsis; and neurological impairment. An indepth discussion of each is beyond the scope of this chapter, but certain diagnoses require greater discussion, since they shed light on the basic cellular and biochemical events that occur during the wound-healing process.

Aging

Aging skin is thinner, less elastic, and has less collagen in the dermis. It is associated with longer healing times and decreased tensile strength.[40] However, as a result, older people usually heal with little scarring, perhaps secondary to the decreased inflammatory response and decreased collagen production. For example, keloids are virtually nonexistent in the elderly. The rate at which aged skin reepithelializes is diminished by a factor of 2.[29] Nutrient blood flow is diminished by regression and disorganization of the dermal capillary network. A recent study demonstrated that in aging mice, infusions of macrophages from young animals restored wound-healing potential to normal.[57]

Infants and children usually heal very well, but recent work suggests that fetuses heal best of all.[1] It has been suggested that this is due to more plasticity and less committed differentiation by the cells involved in the healing process versus other factors such as better nutrition or more avid cellular proliferation.

Diabetes

Diabetes is a multifactorial problem with both mechanical and metabolic derangements. In the United States, diabetics constitute between 5% to 20% of all hospitalized patients at any time, [39]with type II, or adult-onset diabetes, being more common. The pathophysiological mechanism behind problematic wound healing seen in diabetics may be the result of decreased tissue oxygenation secondary to both microangiopathy and peripheral vascular disease.[16] Other investigators have failed to demonstrate an appreciable difference in the po_2 gradient between arterial blood and skin in diabetic and nondiabetic patients. Another mechanism contributing to tissue ischemia may be the shift in the o_2-dissociation curve brought on by a higher percentage of glycosylated hemoglobin, which holds on to oxygen more avidly than normal hemoglobin. Capillary basement-membrane thickening and increased permeability may also contribute to the pathophysiology, although as Hunt pointed out, this is seen in "normal" wound healing as well.[31] Mechanical effects include neuropathy leading to repetitive trauma and subsequent inability to heal. Goodson and Hunt showed that decreased collagen synthesis correlated with insulin deficiency and also that insulin is important in the early, inflammatory phase of wound healing.[26,27]

There are also specific defects in leukocyte function leading to an increased susceptibility to wound infections. It has been postulated that elevated serum glucose levels hamper not only polymorphonuclear neutrophil leukocyte adherence and chemotaxis[3,4] but also phagocytosis and intracellular killing.[17] One of the largest studies, involving the prospective study of 23,649 postoperative patients found that the infection rate in diabetics was 10.7%, compared with the overall infection rate of 1.8% in all patients.[11] Most evidence points to optimal management of serum glucose levels.[43]

It is also important to remember the estimate that as much as 5% of the population of the United States may have undiagnosed diabetes.[14] Thus when dealing with a problematic wound, the diagnosis of diabetesshould be considered even when not previously suspected.

Metabolic diseases

Rather than detailing the ribosomal hydroxylation of proline and lysine residues and subsequent collagen crosslinking, there is a need to recognize or rule out the diseases and conditions that fall under the heading of metabolic diseases when dealing with wound-healing problems. Much work has been done to delineate the role and importance of various cofactors and enzymes in the wound-healing process, including ascorbate, iron, oxygen, α-ketoglutarate, and hyaluronate.[38,64,65] In addition, maximizing the patient's nutritional status, with special attention given to protein (D,L-methionine), vitamins A and C, zinc, iron, phosphorous, thiamine, and ri-

boflavin, has been shown to facilitate the healing process.[50]

Wound healing is an anabolic process involving new protein synthesis. Any condition that places the patient in a catabolic state, such as major surgery, has the potential to impair healing. Good, healthy nutrition is therefore important during this time and also is frequently overlooked.

Steroid therapy

Steroid therapy includes both local and systemic therapy. Steroids reduce the inflammatory response to wounding as well as fibroplasia. The resulting deficiencies in epithelialization and contraction are reversed by vitamin A in animals.[5] Also, systemic immunocompromise occurs via dampened inflammation and fibroblast migration.[18]

Immunocompromised illness

The category of immunocompromised illness is quite broad, including not only patients with immune-specific deficiencies like AIDS but also seriously ill patients with depressed immune function, such as multisystem organ failure.

The human immuno-deficiency virus (HIV) targets T lymphocytes, rendering some types of cell-mediated immunity virtually useless and making the host vulnerable to a myriad of pathogens. Patients with AIDS come to surgery for a variety of reasons, usually for venous access procedures or for biopsies of organs involved in opportunistic infections. Yet the real impact of this disease on wound healing can be seen in its spread to all segments of society. Specific defects in T-cell immunity have been shown to have significant effects on wound strength and collagen deposition.[48] In addition, T-cells elaborate many cytokines and other factors critical to wound healing. Currently, this is an area of active research.

Regional etiologies

Regional etiologies affect the local environment of the wound by impacting on the availability of the substrates needed to affect wound healing. They also affect build-up of toxic metabolites like free-oxygen radicals and include diminished arterial inflow (peripheral vascular disease [PVD]) and venous hypertension.

Trophic ulcers and arterial insufficiency

Ischemic ulcers are a regional manifestation of systemic disease. Part of the work-up for a patient with this kind of wound involves a thorough investigation into the status of the coronary and cerebral blood flow and adequate treatment of the underlying systemic disease. In addition, we discuss a variety of conditions under this heading, since they all share common pathophysiology, and treatment is mainly concerned with maximizing marginal arterial inflow. It is our opinion that diagnosing these problematic wounds are unnecessarily complicated by arbitrary classification schemes.

Ischemic ulcers can be diagnosed by their appearance and by understanding the pathophysiology behind their creation. The typical "punched out" ulcer craters are quite deep, with prominent heaped-up edges that usually do not appear to be inflamed. They occur most frequently over bony prominences and in the feet, which have the most diminished blood flow. They occur when repetitive skin traumas do not receive enough trophic factors and oxygen to effect repair. The skin is cool and mottled and may exhibit other areas of impending or actual ulceration. Granulation tissue is sparse or absent. Doppler flow studies of the affected limb may demonstrate markedly reduced flow states, with ankle:brachial indices in the range of 0.1 to 0.3.[51] In patients with severe atherosclerosis and noncompliant vessels, particularly diabetics, the Doppler indices may be misleading, with values approaching 1.0 despite obvious local tissue hypoxia and nonhealing ulcers. In some cases, angiography may be necessary to confirm the diagnosis. The patient may complain of claudication symptoms even at rest and may have a variety of other systemic diseases, such as hypertension, diabetes, or congestive failure, which exacerbate the nonhealing state.

In addition, other ischemic states may be induced pharmacologically with drugs like ergotamine or epinephrine, causing vasospasm similar to Reynaud's phenomenon or chemical vasculitis. The underlying systemic condition in these patients must be determined and offending agents, such as pharmacopeia and smoking, eliminated.

Venous hypertension

Most clinicians can recall their first exposure to a nonhealing venous stasis ulcer. The size, amount of associated exudation, and condition of the surrounding skin, with edema, scaling, and varicosities make venous ulcers memorable. Affected limbs may show brawny induration with hyperpigmentation and swelling, termed *lipodermatosclerosis.* This is secondary to chronic fibrosis or hemosiderin deposition in the dermis. Venous ulcers, which tend to occur on the medial aspect of the lower leg, are more shallow and lack the regular outlines seen in arterial insufficiency ulcers. They are frequently present in patients with a history of prior deep venous thrombophlebitis as part of a postphlebitic syndrome. Patients often have a history of leg trauma and postinjury swelling without having a definite diagnosis of thrombophlebitis. However, diagnosing venous ul-

cers should not depend on the appearance or history alone. Systemic problems should be considered, including connective tissue diseases like rheumatoid arthritis or inflammatory bowel syndrome. These two conditions are associated with pyoderma gangrenosum, which may be confused with venous stasis ulcerations. They are distinguished by undermined purplish edges and characteristic skin "bridging" in the wound itself. Arterial insufficiency should also be ruled out in these patients, using Doppler ultrasonography. Palpating pedal pulses as an indicator of blood flow is often inaccurate. The presence or absence of diabetes should be determined. The diagnosis can usually be made with considerable confidence on clinical grounds by a history of leg swelling associated with lipodermatosclerosis and adequate arterial inflow.

Distinct from arterial insufficiency ulcers, venous ulcers are frequently heavily contaminated with both aerobic and anaerobic bacteria, which occasionally can give rise to cellulitis, osteomyelitis, or even sepis requiring hospitalization and intravenous antibiotic therapy.[24]

We agree with Falanga and Eaglestein that the term *venous stasis ulcer* should be abandoned.[20] It has been shown that venous hypertension, not the mere enlargement of dermal venous capillaries with subsequent venous pooling, is responsible for the skin alterations leading to ulceration.[8] Local tissue ischemia may again play a role, as in arterial ulcerations, but the pathophysiology is different. Transcutaneous oxygen tensions in affected limbs do confirm a hypoxic environment,[45] but this may be secondary to the accumulation of a pericapillary fibrin layer formed when unmitigated venous pressure allows fibrinogen to ooze from distended venules into the surrounding dermis.[8] This fibrin layer then prevents the free transfer of oxygen and other trophic factors into the wound.

Local injury

Local injury may be the result of trauma with skin and/or soft tissue loss or a sequelae of localized therapy.

Burns

It is important to assess the total surface area of burn involvement using the rule of nines and also the depth of the burn wound. It is helpful to know the mechanism of injury for diagnosis and treatment planning. High-voltage electrical, flame, or prolonged scald burns and chemical burns not immediately treated with copious saline irrigation tend to be more serious and may have full-thickness destruction of dermal and epidermal components.

First-degree burns involve only superficial epidermal cells and do not injure the dermal structures. They may be recognized by their dry, erythematous appearance, which is painful to the touch. The classic example of this kind of burn is a sunburn.

Second-degree burns may be either superficial or deep. The former, barring infection, may be expected to heal within 1 to 2 weeks. They may be diagnosed by the presence of skin blistering, representing separation of necrotic epithelium from underlying dermis at the level of the basement membrane. In addition, they are also painful and erythematous but appear moist. Deep second-degree burns may be difficult to distinguish from full-thickness burns, on occasion turning white and woody soon after injury. They may require up to 6 weeks to heal and are often accompanied by the unfortunate sequelae of deeper injury, including contractures, hypertrophic scarring, and increased susceptibility to infection. As alternative methods of obtaining wound coverage become available, however, differentiating these wounds, with at least some intact dermis left from their full-thickness counterparts may be important for good long-term results.

Third-degree burns affect all layers of the skin. They are typically described as insensate and can appear black, white, or dark red, secondary to fixed hemoglobin in the dermis. They are firm or woody in texture as a result of the skin having lost its suppleness through collagen denaturation. Hair follicles and sweat glands are frequently damaged or destroyed.

Many texts and reviews are available that address the complicated subject of burns in more detail.[6,33,54] Some texts classify a further type of burn injury involving deeper structures such as bone, muscle, and tendon. These injuries are typical of high-voltage burns, caustics such as hydrofluoric acid, or situations where impaired sensation prevents removal of the offending burn agent. These complex injuries must be treated on an individual basis and are not discussed further in this chapter.

Pressure ulcers

Pressure ulcers include decubitus ulcers, derived from Latin, meaning to lie down. It is true that 96% of all pressure sores occur in the lower half of the body in bedridden patients. These wounds are secondary to prolonged external pressure on the skin, producing elevated capillary pressure in the face of repetitive microtraumas, which is reflected in the fact that these ulcers only develop over areas of bony prominence such as the sacrum or calcaneus (Fig. 14-1). Direct mechanical trauma may play a critical role in the pathogenesis of pressure ulcers. If capillary pressures are elevated for prolonged periods, ischemia develops as in venous

Classification and Management of Pressure Sores

STAGE	DESCRIPTION
I	Inflammation overlying a bony prominence without ulceration
II	Superficial ulceration extending into the dermis
III	Deeper ulceration, commonly in an inverted cone shape extending into subcutaneous tissue and/or muscle
IV	Complex ulceration with widespread extension into other ulcers, along bursae, into joints, body cavities, or bone

From Shea JD: Pressure sores: classification and management, Clin Orth 112:89-100, 1975.

hypertension. The situation is more injurious, however, because the pressure is exerted both by the external environment and the bony prominence.

Shear is also an important factor. When the head of a bed is elevated 30 degrees, the epidermis of the coccygeal region is subjected to greater mechanical stress, which may lead to ulceration at lower direct pressures.[52] This may be the result of attenuated blood flow through perforating fasciocutaneous or musculocutaneous vessels, which are tethered by the deep fascia.

Systemic conditions should also not be overlooked as part of the etiology. Neurological impairment has often been implicated as a complicating factor in the creation of pressure ulcers. These patients lack the protective mechanisms of pain and/or the motor skills necessary to shift weight off danger areas. Stroke victims, paralyzed patients, and elderly patients have a particularly high risk of developing pressure ulcers.

Shea[60] classifies pressure ulcers into four grades, which should be used for the initial evaluation to help guide the response to therapy.

Pressure sores are frequently complicated by the presence of a concomitant infection. The dermal circulation is more robust than the subcutaneous fat. Pressure ulcers assume an inverted cone shape, and a large infection develops underneath dry eschar. The subcutaneous abcesses can be quite large in contrast to the small area of dermal necrosis. Wound cultures should be taken to help determine the appropriate antibiotic therapy. These wounds may be heavily colonized by mixed flora, with Proteus, Pseudomonas, and Bac-

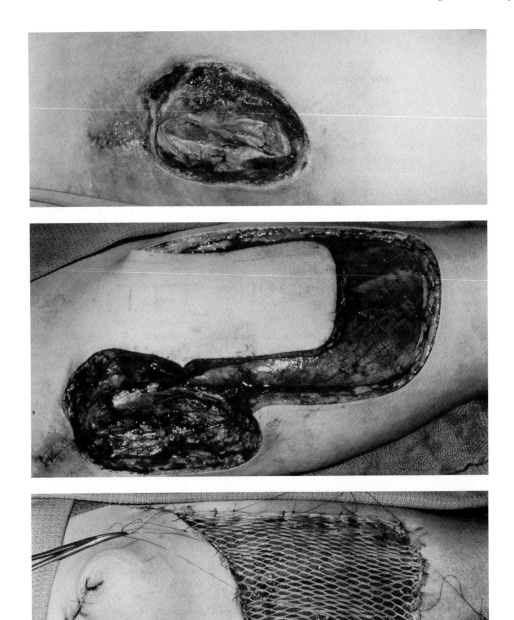

Fig. 14-1 Trochanteric pressure sore in a paraplegic patient. **A,** Shows presence of necrotic tissue. **B,** After debridement and elevation of a tensor fascia lata flap. **C,** The flap is sutured in place, and the donor site is covered with a meshed skin graft.

ETIOLOGIES DIAGNOSIS TREATMENTS

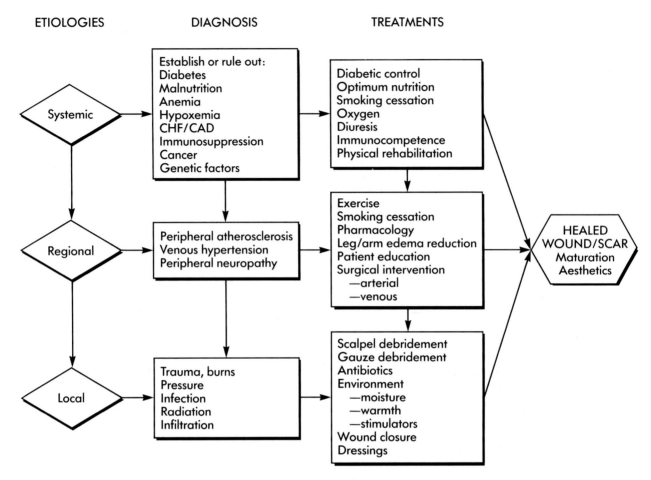

Fig. 14-2 This schema includes most etiological, diagnostic, and therapeutic considerations.

teroides species present in addition to *Staphyloccus aureus.*[60] A computed tomography (CT) scan may be helpful in delineating the extent of abcess formation.[12] However, there is no substitue for direct clinical inspection, palpation, and adequate surgical debridement. Physical examination is frequently more helpful than x-rays or even bone scans in defining bony involvement.

Infiltration injuries

Most infusion injuries are temporarily painful, causing minor inconvenience for the patient and perhaps a thrombosed vein. In the past, larger extravasation injuries have been treated expectantly or at worst with a split-thickness skin graft. Recently, however, the advent of chemotherapy using potent toxins has necessitated a specialized approach to these kinds of wounds. All agents associated with blistering, ulceration, and necrosis should be handled with special care.

The so-called vesicant agents deserve special note. These include Adriamycin and daunorubicin, as well as the Vinca alkaloids such as vinblastine and vincristine sulfate, vindesine, and some alkylating agents like mitomycin and dicarbazine.[37] Should extravasation of these substances occur, especially in the face of significant pain or skin blistering, cold packs, elevation, and early notification of the surgical team should be effected. Treatment is initiated once the degree of necrosis is determined, including excision of the ulcer and wound closure with a skin graft or local flap tissue.

Irradiated skin

The biological effects of ionizing radiation may be either direct, meaning the cell has absorbed enough energy to disrupt its intact functioning or indirect, by the secondary ionization of intracellular water, resulting in the formation of toxic-free radicals. Skin that has been damaged by irradiation exhibits dermal thinning, telangiectasias, burnlike induration, and pigmentation changes. After the acute damage, skin exhibits chronic fibrosis with markedly diminished vascularity and tends to ulcerate easily. Radiation wounds are usually quite painful and show little capacity for reepithelialization or contraction. The pathophysiology behind poor wound healing has been attributed to microvascular occlusion and subsequent tissue ischemia.[63] Damage to cellular deoxyribonucleic acid (DNA) preventing replication of keratinocytes and fibroblasts may also play a role, especially since some electron microscopy studies have failed to demonstrate obliterative microvascular changes in irradiated skin.[58]

Modern techniques, including better shielding and reduced x-ray exposure, have limited radionecrosis injuries largely to patients who have received ionizing radiation as adjunctive therapy for cancer.[53] The increased doses being used to treat cancer result in deeper tissue damage to those areas frequently treated for malignancy, including the groin, rectum, chest wall, head, and neck. These injuries are perhaps the most difficult chronic wounds to treat. They are virtually impossible to heal, except by excising all damaged tissue and bringing in healthy, well-vascularized unradiated tissue for closure.

TREATMENT

A rational basis for treatment is achieved only by understanding the varied pathophysiology of different wounds (Fig. 14-2). The patient is assured the best chance for healing by reversing any abnormal systemic conditions such as hypoxemia, malnutrition, vitamin deficiencies, organ system failure, or hyperglycemia before addressing the wound itself. Systemic antibiotic therapy is indicated to eradicate deep tissue infections not amenable to topical antibiotics.

Regional deficits can be altered by efforts to improve local blood flow, including smoking cessation, revascularization procedures, or medications designed to maximize arterial inflow. Venous hypertension may be improved by changes in life-style such as weight loss, frequent leg elevation, and the use of compression stockings or pumps. Stanozolol (Winstrol) is an anabolic steroid that has been shown to be effective in removing pericapillary fibrin and improving the condition of patients with liposclerosis.[9,13]

Local methods to improve healing should include changing position to eliminate pressure from areas of ulceration, as well as debridement, antibiotic therapy, and surgical wound closure as will be described.

Debridement

Optimal wound healing demands the relative absence of offending substances, including necrotic tissue, toxic metabolites, and bacteria, using the following debriding tools.

Gauze debridement

Gauze debridement remains the standard conservative therapy for relatively uncomplicated or indolent wounds. A sterile gauze dressing is moistened with saline, which softens eschar and permits wound substances to enter the interstices of the gauze. The dressing is allowed to dry, binding the exudate into the gauze, which is then removed. Patients often complain of pain when the dry gauze is pulled off, and therefore many clinicans remove the gauze when it is still moist.

Sharp debridement

Sharp debridement is considered the fastest way to effect debridement and remains the gold standard against which all other methods are measured. It is advocated for heavily infected wounds of all kinds, deep partial- and full-thickness burns, and traumatic wounds.[30] Drawbacks include bleeding, pain, and the potential for merely enlarging the original nonhealing wound, especially when systemic or local conditions have not been corrected.

Chemical debridement

Various chemical (enzymatic) debriding agents have been developed over the years, but only a few have gained FDA approval. Travase, derived from *Bacillus subtilus* is a mixture of proteolytic enzymes. The results of treatment with Travase have gained mixed reviews. Associated problems include pain, a prolonged course of treatment, and overwhelming sepsis. Panafil and Granulex are papain derivatives that do not digest viable tissue. They produce copious wound exudate and require multiple applications for even small surface areas. Other preparations include collagenases (Santyl, Biozume C, fibrinolysins, and desoxyribonuclease (Elase), and in Europe, streptokinase and streptodornase (SKSD).

Other topical compounds used for debridement include hydrophilic substances meant to absorb wound exudate and fibrin, leaving a clean bed of granulation tissue. Our own experience with these substances is that so far none provide a universal substitute for mechanical debridement.

Occlusive dressings

Several authors have advocated the efficacy of occlusive dressings to obtain a clean bed for wounds not already heavily contaminated.[20] It is true that moist conditions facilitate reepithelialization and that trapped exudate may loosen and even remove necrotic material. If the wound is not clean already, there can be rapid bacterial proliferation underneath the occlusive dressing, producing a clinical infection. We have used liquid-tight vinyl chambers on laboratory animals to provide an isotonic fluid environment for experimental wounds but add antibiotics to the fluid to prevent infection.

Water irrigation

Water irrigation with a hand-held shower attachment, whirlpool, or a Waterpick device is a gentle and effective method of cleaning, decontaminating, and debriding small amounts of nonviable tissue, as well as exudate from the wound surface.

Decontamination
Debridement

Surgical debridement of nonviable tissue is still the most effective way to clean a wound.

Systemic therapy

Systemic antibiotic therapy increases the concentration in the blood to a bacteriocidal level. Broad-spectrum coverage is begun when the exact organisms and their antibiotic sensitivities are unknown. Therapy is directed toward probable offenders, such as Gram positive and Gram negative bacteria in diabetes or anaerobes in necrotizing fasciitis. This is an inefficient method to treat relatively small areas and may produce toxic systemic effects. Some authors believe current local therapeutic methods are frequently inadequate in providing enough tissue penetration to decontaminate wounds.

Systemic therapy is best reserved for cellulitic wounds or those with high levels of bacteria cultured in semiquantitative fashion. It should not be viewed as a substitute for local measures.

Local applications

The Physician's Desk Reference currently lists more than 70 preparations of creams, ointments, and gels with topical antibacterial action. Many clinicians, in fact, employ irrational polypharmacy in treating wounds. The problem is exacerbated by the fact that the mere act of swabbing a wound surface for bacteria disrupts delicate reepithelialization, and the mixed flora cultured may not represent true pathogenicity.[54]

Until a suitable "tissue culture" microenvironment can be provided as an optimal local environment, we favor a conservative approach that minimizes the chances of local infection. This precludes most ointments, emollients, and occlusive dressings in wounds that are likely to be contaminated and favors the removal of as much necrotic tissue as possible by surgical debridement, coupled with methods to maximize

tissue oxygenation. Gauze debridement using broad-spectrum antibiotic solutions is used to obtain a clean base of granulation tissue, which is then suitable for grafting.

Healing phase

A little inflammation may be required to initiate the healing process, but overall attempts should be made to limit inflammation. There appears to be a quantitative effect at work here; too much inflammation results in impaired wound healing.[2] In addition, less systemic spillover of inflammatory mediators improves overall patient status. Demling[15] demonstrated significantly diminished pulmonary function in animals with elevated prostanoid production secondary to distant infected burns.

The healing phase of wounds is divided here into two main sections, epithelialization and dermal repair/contraction, with a brief discussion of potential modulators.

Epithelialization

When a wound is created, epithelial cells undergo a process termed *dedifferentiation,* which allows a reversal of the commitment to differentiation, upward migration, and senescence.[25] Keratinocytes may then undergo mitosis and move sideways in epibolic (leapfrogging) fashion until contact inhibition of such movement is reestablished and mitoses cease.[62] This outgrowth from the wound margins is slow (not more than 1 to 2 cm per month), making it impractical to heal large wounds. The process of contraction draws the edges closer together, occasionally obviating the need for immediate grafting or flap procedures, although in most cases the bridging epithelium remains fragile for a long time because of the lack of rete pegs and organization in the underlying scar tissue.

It has been suggested that a healing wound is already maximally stimulated.[67] Although this theory is controversial (and in animals, normal wound healing *can* be augmented), it is definitely true that conditions known to inhibit reepithelialization should be avoided.

Inhibitors

In a seminal paper published in 1962, Winter presented evidence that moist conditions facilitate epithelial migration.[66] Dry conditions, or substances promoting dessication, should therefore be avoided. Exposure to hypotonic fluids is also deleterious, leading to severe epidermal vesiculation and inflammation.[34] It has also been shown that ambient temperature plays a role. When wounds were experimentally subjected to temperatures below 28° C, they demonstrated diminished tensile strength early on.[32] Local infection, defined as tissue bacterial content $\geq 10^5$ colonies/g also impedes reepithelialization, and via the elaboration of collagenases, may affect contraction as well.[2] And perhaps most important, as evidenced by the underlying pathophysiological mechanisms for many of the wounds discussed, tissue ischemia is extremely deleterious.[38]

Stimulators

Eliminating the inhibitory factors merely brings the wound-healing equation back to baseline. A tremendous amount of effort and money has been expended in the quest for positive modulators of wound healing, most aiming for a significant diminution in the time required to effect reepithelialization. Some time-honored substances, such as scarlet red, have become entrenched as adjuncts in wound healing and may affect the so-called lag phase of wound healing by stimulating epithelial mitosis, but even this has not been shown to actually speed up resurfacing.[32]

Promising results with some other substances may hold potential for the future and will be discussed further.

Dermal repair and contraction

There has been great emphasis in the literature on tensile strength as a quantitative measure of healing. However, the quality of healing, including the visibility or prominence of the scar, is more important to the patient. It is the dermal elements of healing that frequently determine this quality. Functional results also depend on dermal repair and contraction, since this is what gives scar tissue its strength and determines the degree of deformation.

Collagen is the major structural component of dermis in both nonwounded and wounded skin. The difference is not merely one of tertiary structure but also biochemical composition. At last count, 11 distinct types of collagen have been characterized.[44] Collagen is synthesized by fibroblasts, and many of the known inhibitors of dermal repair exert their effects by alterations of collagen metabolism. The reader is referred to other sources for a more detailed description.[42,44]

In skin grafting, peel strength (how strongly epidermis is bonded to underlying dermal substrate) is crucial. This is a function of the desmosomal attachment of the epithelial basement membrane to the underlying dermis. The magnitude of this interaction is multiplied by the presence of involutions in the basement membrane of the epidermis, termed *rete pegs.* Many of the criticisms aimed at cultured epithelial autografts stem from the lack of a dermal substrate, resulting in graft fragility, especially over extensor surfaces. This underscores the importance of the dermis, and it is critical to determine, for example, if any viable dermis lies at the base of a burn wound and to employ tangential debridement techniques whenever possible.

Most texts give an adequate description of the difference between contraction, a normal event in wound healing [23] and contracture, a pathologic process representing the end product of contraction across joints or a derangement of collagen deposition and remodeling.[47] The clinical impact of burn-scar contractures is well appreciated, with most requiring release and reconstruction.

Although much work has been done to elucidate the mechanism of contraction with an eye toward controlling it, our understanding is far from complete. For example, knowing that myofibroblasts have intracellular elements resembling smooth muscle contractile units led to the application of smooth muscle inhibitors, which diminished the rate of contraction. However, when the substances were removed, unabated contraction resumed.[41] Likewise, steroids applied topically or given systemically may slow the process, but do not eliminate it.

Mechanical means remain the most reliable way to modify the contraction process and prevent contractures. Some success has been reported using splints, external pressure devices, or temporary skin replacements.[22]

While the pendulum appears to have swung toward myofibroblasts and away from collagen formation and remodeling as the main culprit in contracture formation, it is likely that the problem reflects a complex interaction between many cell types and the extracellular matrix.

Modulators

Much of the current research being conducted in wound healing is directed at defining the effects of various extrinsically applied modulators of the healing process such as polypeptide growth factors, hormones, electrical charge, and components of the extracellular matrix.

A list of potential growth factor regulators is provided in Table 14-1, and the most promising are briefly outlined.

In one highly publicized study, topical applications of epidermal growth factor (EGF) sped "healing" of partial-thickness donor graft sites by a little more than 1 day.[7] This paralleled effects seen in animal models, including our own that used fluid-phase therapy of porcine partial-thickness excisional wounds.

Other studies have been published, touting the effects of platelet-derived growth factor (PDGF) for enhancing breaking strength,[46,49] as well as returning diabetic animal–wound healing to normal.[28] It has been postulated that it exerts these effects via a mitogenic and chemoattractant capacity.

Table 14-1

Growth Factors Influencing Wound Healing

Factor	Source	Target
TGF-β	Platelets, macrophages, lymphocytes, bone, and most tissues	All cells
PDGF	Platelets, macrophages, endothelial cells, and smooth muscle cells	fibroblasts, smooth muscle cells, and glial cells
aFGF and bFGF (acidic fibroblast growth factor,	Macrophages	Endothelial cells and cartilage
Basic fibroblast growth factor, Heparin-binding growth factors)	Fibroblasts and the brain	Chondrocytes and glial cells
EGF	Saliva and urine	Epithelial cells and fibroblasts
MDGF (monocyte-derived growth factor)	Fibroblasts	Macrophages
		Smooth muscle cells
IGF-I (insulin-like growth factor)	Plasma, liver, and fibroblasts	Fibroblasts, endothelial cells, and fetal tissues
IL-1, IL-2 (interleukins)	Macrophages (IL-1) T lymphocytes (IL-2)	Fibroblasts and synovial cells

Adapted from McGrath MH: Peptide growth factors and wound healing, Clin Plast Surg 17:421-431, 1990.

Perhaps the most intriguing of the growth factors is TGF-β, a two-chain polypeptide synthesized by all the cells. It is believed to have an effect in wound healing. It has myriad effects, both stimulatory and inhibitory, depending on what other factors or cells are present and may play a pivotal role in orchestrating the proliferative responses in wound healing.[61]

Although the real effects of these biological mediators are still largely unknown, their study has shed some light on basic cellular processes intrinsic to the study of carcinogenesis, cellular signaling, and embryonic development. We believe that while these may eventually prove fertile to the practicing plastic or general surgeon, they should not divert attention or resources away from efforts at manipulations of the local wound environment designed to reverse the actions of known inhibitors, as outlined earlier in this chapter.

Scars

All surgeons have a vested interest in obtaining the best wound healing possible. It is the plastic surgeon, however, who often deals with the cosmetic sequelae when surface scarring fails to meet expectations or needs or when, as in the case of burn contractions, functional debilitation results from scarring gone awry.

Current thinking with regard to scars has been heavily influenced by the occasional rare event of wound dehiscence and perhaps by the researcher's need to quantify wound healing phenomena. Virtually every text or chapter on wound healing includes data on tensile strength measurements (usually parallel to a

discussion of collagen deposition and remodeling). It is our belief that in discussing quality versus the quantity of healing, it is time the balance shifted away from the latter and toward the former. In fact, as is clearly the case with hypertrophic scars and keloids, it is more important to downregulate the quantity of collagen production.

Table 14-2 displays a comparison of the two types of pathologic scarring—keloids and hypertrophic scars. Although it has been demonstrated that excess collagen production and decreased degradation are responsible for the unsightly appearance of the first keloids and hypertrophic scars, a complete explanation for their formation is lacking. Ischemia,[28] excessive mechanical stimulation of wound-exposed fibroblasts,[61] and autoimmune response[36] have all been postulated as possible causes of elevated collagen production. In addition, it has been shown that subpopulations of fibroblasts may exist within keloids, which produce abnormal ratios of type III to type I collagen.[19]

Treatment of unsatisfactory scars may include mechanical, pharmacological, radiation, surgical, or combined means, and if a patient is known to form keloids, careful attention to surgical techniques may diminish the postoperative scarring problems.

Pressure dressings may induce local ischemia, thereby decreasing collagen synthesis.

Pharmacological modalities include local injection of steroids, colchicine (which may stimulate collagenases in addition to downregulating fibroblasts), penicil-

Table 14-2

Comparison of Pathological Scars

	Hypertrophic scar	Keloid
Sex	Male = female	Female ≥ male
Age	Usually ≤ 20 years	Usually 10 to 30 years
Race	No clear predilection	Black ≥ white
Inheritance	Some familial tendency	Significant familial tendency
Natural history	Maximizes months after injury and then lessens	Maximizes quickly and rarely subsides
Location	Across flexor surfaces	Mostly face, earlobes, and anterior chest
Etiology	Tension and timing of closure	Autoimmunity and ischemia
Treatment	Steroids and colchicine	Pressure and surgical revision

From Rohrich RJ: The Biology of wound healing, SRPS 5:1-36, 1988.

lamine, and tetrahydroquinone given systemically.[10] Other agents have been tried, but none are particularly successful.[35]

Surgical scar revision is occasionally necessary, and the reader is directed to any standard text for specific techniques. It does appear to us, however, that combinations of the previously discussed modalities will prove to be far more useful than any single agent therapy.

SUMMARY

We have attempted to give a brief overview of some practical aspects of wound healing. Therapeutic intervention should be directed by first determining the correct diagnosis to ensure the best possible outcome. Identifying the level (systemic, regional, or local) of the problem is necessary for the proper diagnosis. It is only after correctable deficits have been rectified from all higher levels that attention is directed at the local environment of the problematic wound. Manipulations of that environment should first be directed to bringing the baseline to an optimum before employing potential positive modulators.

REFERENCES

1. Adzick NS et al: Comparison of fetal, newborn, and adult wound healing by histological, enzyme-histochemical, and hydroxyproline determination, J Pediatr Surg 20:315-319, 1985.
2. Alexander JW: The role of infection in the burn patient. In Boswick JAJ (ed): The art and science of burn care, Rockville, Md, 1987, Aspen Publishers Inc.
3. Bagdade J, Root R, and Bulger RJ: Impaired leucocyte function in patients with poorly controled diabetes, Diabetes 23(1):9-15, 1973.
4. Bagdade JD, Stewart M, and Walters E: Impaired granulocyte adherence: a reversible defect in host defense in patients with poorly controled diabetes, Diabetes 27(6):677-681, 1978.
5. Benson SC and LuValle PA: Inhibition of lysyl oxidase and proline hydroxylase activity in glucocorticoid treated rats, Biochem Biophys Res Commun 99(2):557-562, 1981.
6. Boswick, J.A.J. The Art and Science of Burn Care. Rockville, Md, Aspen, 1987.
7. Brown GL et al: Enhancement of wound healing by topical treatment with epidermal growth factor, NE J Med 321(2):76-79, 1989.
8. Browse NL and Burnand KG: The cause of venous ulceration, Lancet 2(8292):243-245, 1982.
9. Burnand KG et al: Venous lipodermatosclerosis: treatment by fibrinolytic enhancement and elastic compression, Br Med J 280(6206):7-11, 1980.
10. Cohen IK et al: Immunoglobulin, complement, and histocompatibility antigen studies in keloid patients, Plast Reconstr Surg 63(5):689-695, 1979.
11. Cruse PJE: A five-year prospective study of 23,649 surgical wounds, Arch Surg 107:206-210, 1973.
12. Daltrey DC, Rhodes B, and Chattwood JG: Investigation into the microbiological flora of healing and non-healing decubitus ulcers, J Clin Path 34(7):701-705, 1981.
13. Davidson JF et al: Fibrinolytic enhancement by stanozolol: a double blind trial, Br J Haematol 22:543-559, 1972.
14. Davidson MB: Diabetes mellitus—diagnosis and treatment, New York, 1986, John Wiley and Sons.
15. Demling RH et al: Endotoxin-induced prostanoid production by the burn wound can cause distant lung dysfunction, Surgery 99(4):421-430, 1986.
16. Duncan HJ and Faris IB: Skin vascular resistance and skin perfusion pressure as predictors of healing of ischemic lesion of the lower limb: influences of diabetes mellitus, hypertension, and age, Surgery 99(4):432-438, 1986.
17. Dziatkowiak H, Kowalska M, and Denys A: Phagocytic and bactericidal activity of granulocytes in diabetic children, Diabetes 31(12):1041-1043, 1982.
18. Ehrlich HP and Hunt TK: Effect of cortisone and vitamin A on wound healing, Ann Surg 167(3):324-328, 1968.
19. Ehrlich HP and Needle AL: Wound healing in tight skin mice: delayed closure of excised wounds, Plast Reconstr Surg 72(2):190-198, 1983.
20. Falanga V and Eaglestein WH: Management of venous ulcers, Am Fam Physician 33(2):274-281, 1986.
21. Firooznia H et al: Computerized tomography of pressure sores, pelvic abcesses, and osteomyelitis in patients with spinal cord injury, Arch Phys Med Rehab 63(11):545-548, 1982.
22. Frank DH, Brahme J, and Van de Berg JS: Decrease in rate of wound contraction with the temporary skin substitute Biobrane, Ann Plast Surg 12(6):519-524, 1984.
23. Gabbiani G et al: Granulation tissue as a contractile organ: a study of structure and function, J Exp Med 135(4):719-734, 1971.

24. Galpin JE, Chow AW, and Bayer AS: Sepsis associated with decubitus ulcers, Am J Med 61:346-350, 1976.

25. Gillman T and Penn J: Studies on the repair of cutaneous wounds, Med Proc 2 (suppl 3):121, 1956.

26. Goodson WH and Hunt TK: Studies of wound healing in experimental diabetes mellitus, J Surg Res 22(3):221-227, 1977.

27. Goodson WH and Hunt TK: Wound healing in experimental diabetes mellitus: importance of early insulin therapy, Surg Forum 29:95-98, 1978.

28. Grotendorst GR and Pencev D: Stimulation of granulation tissue formation by platelet-derived growth factor in normal and diabetic rats, J Clin Invest 76:2323-2329, 1985.

29. Grove GL: Physiologic changes in older skin, Dermatol Clin 4(3):425-432, 1986.

30. Haury B et al: Debridement: an essential component of traumatic wound care, Am J Surg 135(2):238-242, 1978.

31. Hunt TK: Wound healing and wound infection: theory and surgical practice, New York:, 1980, Appleton-Century-Crofts.

32. Hunt TK and Zederfeldt B: Nutritional and environmental aspects in wound healing. In Dunphy JE and Van Winkle WJ (ed): Repair and regeneration: the scientific basis for surgical practice, New York, 1969, McGraw Hill.

33. Hurt A and Eriksson E: Management of the burn wound, Clin Plast Surg 13(1):57-67, 1986.

34. Jolly M and Swan AG: The effects on rat skin of prolonged exposure to water, Br J Dermatol 103:387-395, 1980.

35. Kelly EW and Pinkus H: Oral treatment of keloids, Arch Dermatol 78:348, 1958.

36. Kischer CW, Theis C, and Chvapil M: Perivascular myofibroblasts and microvascular occlusion in hypertrophic scars and keloids, Hum Pathol 13(9):819-824, 1982.

37. Larson DL: Alterations in wound healing secondary to infusion injury, Clin Plast Surg 17(3):509-517, 1990.

38. LaVan FB and Hunt TK: Oxygen and wound healing, Clin Plast Surg 17(3):463-472, 1990.

39. Leichter SB: Diabetes patient education in hospital settings, Diabetes Educ 12(3):277-80, 1986.

40. Levenson SM, Birkhill FR, and Waterman DF: The healing of soft tissue wounds: the effects of nutrition, anemia, and age, Surgery 28:905-935, 1950.

41. Madden JW, Morton D, and Peacock EE: Contraction of experimental wounds. I. Inhibiting wound contraction by using a topical smooth muscle antagonist, Surgery 76(1):8-15, 1974.

42. Madden JW and Peacock EE: Studies on the biology of collagen during wound healing. III. Dynamic metabolism of scar collagen and remodeling of dermal wounds, Ann Surg 174(3):511-20, 1971.

43. McMurry JF: Wound healing with diabetes mellitus, Surg Clin North Am 64(4):769-778, 1984.

44. Miller EJ and Gay S: The collagens: an overview and update. In Cunningham LW (ed): Methods in enzymology: structural and contractile proteins, Orlando; 1987, Academic Press Inc.

45. Moosa HH et al: Oxygen diffusion in chronic venous ulceration, J Invest. Dermatol 84(4):A358, 1985.

46. Mustoe TA et al: Accelerated healing of incisional wounds in rats induced by transforming growth factor-β, Science 237:1333-1335, 1987.

47. Peacock EE: Wound repair, Philadelphia; 1984, WB Saunders Co.

48. Peterson JM, Barbul A, and Breslin JR: Significance of T-lymphocytes in wound healing, Surgery 102:300-305, 1987.

49. Pierce GF et al: Platelet-derived growth factor (PDGF) stimulation of wound healing, J Exp Med 167:974-987, 1988.

50. Pollack SV: Wound healing: a review. III. Nutritional factors affecting wound healing, J Dermatol Surg Oncol 5:615-619, 1979.

51. Puckett CL and Silver D: Principles and management of leg ulcers. In Georgiade NG et al (eds): Essentials of plastic, maxillofacial, and reconstructive surgery, Baltimore, 1987, Williams and Wilkins.

52. Reichel SM: Shearing forces as a factor in decubitus ulcers in paraplegics, JAMA 166:762, 1958.

53. Reinisch JF and Puckett CL: Management of radiation wounds, Surg Clin North Am 64(4):795-802, 1984.

54. Robson MC: Management of the burn wound. In Najarian J and Delaney JP (eds): Trauma and critical care surgery, Chicago, 1987, Year Book Medical Publishers.

55. Robson MC, Stenberg BD, and Heggers JP: Wound healing alterations caused by infection, Clin Plast Surg 17(3):485-492, 1990.

56. Rohrich RJ: The biology of wound healing, SRPS 5(1):1-36, 1988.

57. Roth GS, Danon D, and Kowitch MK: Promotion of wound repair in old mice by local injection of macrophages, PNAS 86:2018, 1989.

58. Rudolph R, Arganese T, and Woodward M: The ultrastructure and etiolgy of chronic radiotherapy damage in human skin, Ann Plast Surg 9(4):282-292, 1982.

59. Salomon JC, Diegelmann RF, and Cohen IK: Effects of dressings on donor site epithelialization, Surg Forum 25:516-517, 1974.

60. Shea JD: Pressure sores: classification and management. Clin Orth 112:89-100, 1975.

61. Sporn MB and Roberts AB: Peptide growth factors and inflammation, tissue repair, and cancer, J Clin Invest 78:329-332, 1986.

62. Stenn KS: Epibolin, a protein in human plasma that supports epithelial cell movement, Proc Natl Acad Sci USA 78(11):6907-6911, 1981.

63. Telok HA: Histopathological study of radiation injuries of the skin, Surg Gyn Obstet 90:335-348, 1950.

64. Uitto J and Prockop DJ: Hydroxylation of peptide-bound proline and lysine before and after chain completion of the polypeptide chains of procollagen, Arch Biochem Biophys 164:210-217, 1974.

65. Weigel PH et al: The role of hyaluronic acid in inflammation and wound healing, Int J Tiss Reac 10(6):355-365, 1988.

66. Winter GD: Formation of the scab and the rate of epithelization of superficial wounds in the skin of the young domestic pig, Nature 193:293-294, 1962.

67. Seiler WO and Stähelin HB: Treatment through five therapeutic principles, Geriatrics 40(9):30-43, 1985.

Index